S0-EGE-466

A Self-Instructional Guide:

DIAGNOSIS AND TREATMENT OF ODONTOGENIC INFECTIONS

by

Thomas H. Hohl, DDS
Robert J. Whitacre, MS, DDS
James R. Hooley, DDS
Betsy L. Williams, PhD

A Self-Instructional Guide:

DIAGNOSIS AND TREATMENT OF ODONTOGENIC INFECTIONS

(ISBN #0-89939-090-0)

by

THOMAS H. HOHL, DDS
Associate Professor
Department of Oral and Maxillofacial
  Surgery
School of Dentistry
University of Washington
Seattle, Washington

ROBERT J. WHITACRE, MS, DDS
Educational Consultant
Department of Oral and
  Maxillofacial Surgery
School of Dentistry
University of Washington
Seattle, Washington

JAMES R. HOOLEY, DDS
Dean and Professor of Oral and
  Maxillofacial Surgery
School of Dentistry
University of California, Los Angeles
Los Angeles, California

BETSY L. WILLIAMS, PhD
Research Associate Professor
Department of Periodontics
School of Dentistry
University of Washington
Seattle, Washington

Illustrated by
Thomas H. Hohl, DDS

This book is one of a series of self-instructional textbooks designed to teach concepts of oral surgery and related disciplines to dental students, dental practitioners and dental auxiliaries. The series title of **A Self-Instructional Guide to Oral Surgery in General Dentistry** was formerly used to describe this series; however, many individuals outside of the specialty of oral surgery have expressed a desire to expand the titles of these books to facilitate transmission of this material in their areas. This series includes the following self-instructional book titles:

1. **Instruments Used for Oral Surgery**
2. **The Removal of Teeth**
3. **Medications Used in Oral Surgery**
4. **Surgical Complications**
5. **Dental Asepsis**
6. **Assessment of and Surgery for Impacted Third Molars**
7. **Pre-Prosthetic Surgery**
8. **Principles of Biopsy**
9. **Diagnosis and Treatment of Odontogenic Infections**

published by

Stoma Press, Inc.

13231 42nd Avenue NE
Seattle, WA 98125
(206) 365-2665

Typeset By
CASTEEL TYPESETTING
18316 1st NE
Seattle, WA 98155
(206) 363-9054

Printed By
ATOMIC PRESS
1421 N 34th
Seattle, WA
(206) 632-0550

PREFACE

This book was written to review the **basic** concepts involved in the primary management of patients with oral and/or maxillofacial infections. It was not intended to be the definitive text on this subject.

During the development of this book we have reviewed several case histories of oral and/or maxillofacial infections which resulted in hospitalization and/or death of patients. In some cases, the patient's presenting condition was already so serious that even the best of medical care could not reverse the infectious process. In other cases, however, patients presented to their dentist with mild to moderately serious infections which subsequently developed into very serious or even fatal conditions while under the practitioner's care. In these cases, ineffective management could be traced back to initial **inadequacies in data collection, inaccurate or incomplete diagnosis, inappropriate or inadequate treatment methods**, and/or **inadequate follow up**. The **most significant** shortcoming was the **inability to recognize** the progressing severity of the infections at an early stage and refer the patients to a dental specialist and/or hospital.

Our goal in writing this book is to help you and your patients avoid the disastrous consequences which can result from dental infections. Errors in the management of oral and/or maxillofacial infections can be minimized by the use of a systematic evaluation process to elucidate the multitude of factors involved in the complex pathobiology of the infectious process. We have developed the **checklist for diagnosing and managing oral and/or maxillofacial swellings** to assist you in the systematic management of patients with oral and/or maxillofacial infections. You should, of course, remember that no textbook, no matter how thorough, can ever replace clinical experience in the management of oral infections.

In this book, considerable time and effort has been spent in correlating basic science concepts with clinical principles and in creating a feedback system for you to monitor your learning. In each Unit (chapter) we have included a section termed "**overview and objectives**" which states the essential knowledge you can expect to gain from **reading the contents** and **completing the study exercises.** We have included a **"Post-Test"** for each unit which is intended to show you what you have learned.

The **study exercises are extremely important** and you should take the time to **write the answers** in the blanks or spaces provided. You may be tempted to mentally answer the questions or skip them entirely to save time. You will **retain more of the information** you have read with much **less effort** if you take the time to write out the answers as you proceed. Considerable research in self-instructional design and learning has shown the importance of answering such study questions.

You may notice that the **study exercises** are designed for different levels of learning.

- The **first level** of study exercises are of the "fill in the blank" type. The blanks usually include "key" words or phrases taken from the content preceding the study exercise.

- The **second level** of study exercises are problem-solving tasks. Generally these take a small piece of a larger concept and allow you to focus your attention on mastery of the piece. The small pieces are then assimilated into larger concepts which can be integrated with ease.

- The **third level** of study exercises are simulations of more extensive clinical problems similar to those you will face when treating patients. Having completed the previous study exercises, you should be able to adequately cope with these. These are the most important study exercises because they more closely resemble the real world of dentistry.

Even though we have had considerable input from many experts during the writing of this book, we by no means imply that this book presents the "only way" to manage odontogenic infections. In specific clinical situations, deviations from methods described in this book may be employed by experts who have had extensive experience in treating patients with infections of the oral and maxillofacial areas.

EDITORIAL CONSULTANTS

The successful management of odontogenic infections draws upon knowledge from many areas within the fields of dentistry and basic sciences. During the eight-year development of this book, we have received considerable assistance from scholars in many academic fields. Central to our efforts was the encouragement, contributions and constructive criticism provided by the oral and maxillofacial surgeons participating in the development of the entire book series. Valuable input was also provided by experts in related fields. While the contents of this book may not totally reflect the opinions of each editorial consultant, we have attempted to integrate each of their comments (a difficult task in such a diffuse subject) into the overall project. We believe the final content in this book will be of great assistance in teaching the fundamentals of infection management to those practicing or seeking a career in general dentistry.

ORAL AND MAXILLOFACIAL SURGERY

Delmar D. Albers, DDS, MSEd, Chairman, Dept. of Oral & Maxillofacial Surgery, School of Dentistry, Marquette University, Milwaukee, Wisconsin.

Richard S. Alley, DDS, MSD, Dept. of Oral and Maxillofacial Surgery, University of Texas Health Science Center at San Antonio, Dental School, San Antonio, Texas

B.K. Arora, BDS, DMD, MS (oral surgery), FRCD, FICD, Chairman, Dept. of Oral & Maxillofacial Surgery, Faculty of Dentistry, University of Alberta, Edmonton, Alberta, Canada.

Donald F. Booth, DMD, Chairman, Dept. of Oral & Maxillofacial Surgery, Boston University, Goldman School of Graduate Dentistry, Boston, Mass.

Sidney L. Bronstein, DDS, MScD, Chairman, Division of Oral Surgery, School of Dentistry, University of Colorado, Denver, Colorado.

Bernard C. Byrd, DDS, MS, Chairman, Dept. of Oral Surgery, School of Dentistry, Loma Linda University, Loma Linda, California.

John B. Curran, BDS, FFD, RCSI, FRCD(C), Section of Oral & Maxillofacial Surgery, Dept. of Stomatology, Faculty of Dentistry, University of Manitoba, Winnipeg, Manitoba, Canada.

Duane T. DeVore, DDS, JD, PhD, Dept. of Oral & Maxillofacial Surgery, School of Dentistry, University of Maryland, Baltimore, Maryland.

Henry M. Duke, DDS, Dept. of Oral & Maxillofacial Surgery, College of Dental Medicine, Medical University of South Carolina, Charleston, So. Carolina.

Stephen E. Feinberg, DDS, MS, PhD, Dept. of Oral and Maxillofacial Surgery, College of Dentistry, University of Iowa, Iowa City, Iowa.

Leon P. Fiedler, DDS, Chairman, Dept. of Oral & Maxillofacial Surgery, School of Dentistry, University of Louisville, Louisville, Kentucky.

Raymond J. Fonseca, DMD, Chairman, Dept. of Oral & Maxillofacial Surgery, School of Dentistry, University of Michigan, Ann Arbor, Michigan.

Paul E. Gates, DDS, Dept. of Oral & Maxillofacial Surgery and Anesthesia, School of Dentistry, Fairleigh Dickinson University, Hackensack, New Jersey.

John D. Gehrig, DDS, MSD, Dept. of Oral & Maxillofacial Surgery, School of Dentistry, University of Washington, Seattle, Washington.

Anthony P. Giammusso, DMD, Dept. of Oral & Maxillofacial Surgery, College of Dental Medicine, Medical University of South Carolina, Charleston, South Carolina.

James A. Giglio, DDS, Division of Oral & Maxillofacial Surgery, School of Dentistry, Medical College of Virginia, Virginia Commonwealth University, Richmond, Virginia.

Newton C. Gordon, DDS, MS, Division of Oral & Maxillofacial Surgery, School of Dentistry, University of California at San Francisco, San Francisco, California.

Robert W. Graves, DDS, Chairman, Dept. of Oral and Maxillofacial Surgery, School of Dentistry, University of West Virginia, Morgantown, West Virginia.

Kenneth W. Hughes, DDS, Dept. of Oral & Maxillofacial Surgery, College of Dentistry, University of Illinois, Chicago, Illinois.

R. Pat Hylton, Jr., DDS, Dept. of Oral & Maxillofacial Surgery, College of Dentistry, University of Florida, Gainesville, Florida.

Thomas W. Jones, DDS, Dept. of Oral & Maxillofacial Surgery, School of Dentistry, University of Alabama, Birmingham, Alabama.

Edwin D. Joy, Jr., DDS, Chairman, Dept. of Oral Surgery, Medical College of Georgia, Augusta, Georgia.

Thomas B. Kilgore, DMD, Dept. of Oral & Maxillofacial Surgery, Boston University, Goldman School of Graduate Dentistry, Boston, Mass.

Dennis T. Lanigan, DMD, MD, Dept. of Diagnostic and Surgical Sciences, Division of Oral & Maxillofacial Surgery, College of Dentistry, University of Saskatchewan, Saskatoon, Saskatchewan, Canada.

Jeffrey L. Laskin, DDS, MS, Dept. of Oral & Maxillofacial Surgery, College of Dentistry, University of Florida, Gainesville, Florida.

Martin S. Lebowitz, DDS, MS, Chairman, Dept. of Oral & Maxillofacial Surgery, College of Dentistry, University of Florida, Gainesville, Florida.

Steven J. Levy, DDS, Dept. of Oral & Maxillofacial Surgery, Emory University School of Dentistry, Atlanta, Georgia.

Cecil Rhodes Lupton, DDS, Dept. of Oral & Maxillofacial Surgery, School of Dentistry, University of North Carolina, Chapel Hill, North Carolina.

Richard D. Mallow, DDS, MS, Dept. of Oral Surgery, School of Dentistry, University of Detroit, Detroit, Michigan.

Philip D. Marano, DDS, Director, Dept. of Oral & Maxillofacial Surgery, School of Dentistry, Oral Roberts University, Tulsa, Oklahoma.

Victor J. Matukas, DDS, MD, Chairman, Dept. of Oral & Maxillofacial Surgery, School of Dentistry, University of Alabama, Birmingham, Alabama.

Roger A. Meyer, Chairman, Dept. of Oral & Maxillofacial Surgery, Emory University School of Dentistry, Atlanta, Georgia.

Robert A. Middleton, DDS, Chairman, Dept. of Oral Surgery, School of Dentistry, University of the Pacific, San Francisco, California.

Eric P. Millar, DDS, FRCD, FICD, Associate Director, Division of Oral & Maxillofacial Surgery, Faculty of Dentistry, McGill University, Montreal, PQ, Canada.

Howard S. Misner, DDS, Dept. of Oral & Maxillofacial Surgery, College of Dentistry, University of Tennessee, Memphis, Tennessee.

Gerald R. Ott, DDS, Director of Undergraduate Surgery, College of Dentistry, University of Nebraska Medical Center, Lincoln, Nebraska.

ORAL AND MAXILLOFACIAL SURGERY (Continued)

John A. Paterson, DDS, FACD, Chairman, Dept. of Oral & Maxillofacial Surgery and Anesthesia, School of Dentistry, Fairleigh Dickinson University, Hackensack, New Jersey.

Gordon W. Pedersen, DDS, MSD, Dept. of Oral Surgery, School of Dentistry, Case-Western Reserve University, Cleveland, Ohio.

James H. Quinn, DDS, Dept. of Oral & Maxillofacial Surgery, School of Dentistry, Louisiana State University, New Orleans, Louisiana.

Monty Reitzik, BDS, FDSRCS, MB, ChB, Dept. of Oral & Maxillofacial Surgery, Faculty of Dentistry, The University of British Columbia, Vancouver, British Columbia, Canada.

Alan S. Ross, DDS, Chairman, Dept. of Diagnostic and Surgical Sciences, Division of Oral & Maxillofacial Surgery, College of Dentistry, University of Saskatchewan, Saskatoon, Saskatchewan, Canada.

Doran E. Ryan, DDS, MS, Div. of Oral & Maxillofacial Surgery, Dept. of Surgery, Medical College of Wisconsin, Milwaukee, Wisconsin.

Lawrence Salman, DDS, MPA, Chairman, Dept. of Oral Surgery, College of Dentistry, New York University, New York, New York.

Allen L. Sisk, DDS, Dept. of Oral Surgery, Medical College of Georgia, Augusta, Georgia.

Ernest W. Small, DDS, MS, Dept. of Oral & Maxillofacial Surgery, School of Dentistry, University of North Carolina, Chapel Hill, North Carolina.

Richard A. Smith, DDS, Division of Oral & Maxillofacial Surgery, School of Dentistry, University of California at San Francisco, San Francisco, California.

Albert F. Staples, DMD, PhD, Chairman, Dept. of Oral Surgery, College of Dentistry, University of Oklahoma, Oklahoma City, Oklahoma.

Martin Steiner, DDS, Dept. of Oral & Maxillofacial Surgery, School of Dentistry, University of Louisville, Louisville, Kentucky.

A.E. Swanson, DDS, MS, FRCD(C), Head, Dept. of Oral & Maxillofacial Surgery, Faculty of Dentistry, The University of British Columbia, Vancouver, British Columbia, Canada.

Lucian Szmyd, DMD, MS, Dept. of Oral Surgery, School of Dentistry, University of the Pacific, San Francisco, California.

ORAL MEDICINE

James A. Cottone, DMD, MS, Dept. of Dental Diagnostic Science, University of Texas at San Antonio, Dental School, San Antonio, Texas.

Edmond L. Truelove, DDS, MSD, Chairman, Dept. of Oral Medicine, School of Dentistry, University of Washington, Seattle, Washington.

Donald J. Soltero, DDS, MSD, Dept. of Oral Medicine, School of Dentistry, University of Washington, Seattle, Washington.

ORAL PATHOLOGY

Thomas H. Morton, Jr., DDS, MSD, Dept. of Oral Medicine and Dept. of Oral Biology, Division of Oral Pathology, School of Dentistry, University of Washington, Seattle, Washington.

DENTAL RADIOLOGY

Thomas E. Emmering, DDS, FICD, Chairman, Dept. of Dental Radiology, School of Dentistry, Loyola University, Maywood, Illinois.

ENDODONTICS

Robert J. Oswald, DDS, Chairman, Dept. of Endodontics, School of Dentistry, University of Washington, Seattle, Washington.

ORAL MICROBIOLOGY

James J. Crawford, PhD, Dept. of Endodontics, School of Dentistry, University of North Carolina, Chapel Hill, North Carolina.

John A. Molinari, PhD, Chairman, Dept. of Microbiology and Biochemistry, School of Dentistry, University of Detroit, Detroit, Michigan.

Page S. Morahan, PhD, Chairman, Dept. of Microbiology, Medical College of Pennsylvania, Philadelphia, Pennsylvania.

RESTORATIVE DENTISTRY

Robert C. Canfield, DDS, Acting Chairman, Dept. of Restorative Dentistry, School of Dentistry, University of Washington, Seattle, Washington.

DENTAL EDUCATION

Richard S. Mackenzie, DDS, MS, PhD, Chairman, Dept. of Dental Education, College of Dentistry, University of Florida, Gainesville, Florida.

FAMILY MEDICINE

Jeff Altman, MD, Diplomat, American Board of Family Practice; Director, Primary Care Unit, Student Health Center, University of Washington; Clinical Instructor, Department of Family Medicine, School of Medicine, University of Washington, Seattle, Washington

SPECIAL ACKNOWLEDGMENTS

Special acknowledgments are extended to the following persons for their unselfish contribution of clinical photographs, teaching materials, and/or diligent efforts which all made this text possible:

B.K. Arora, BDS, DMD, MS, FRCD, FICS
James J. Crawford, PhD
Donald H. Devlin, DDS
Dennis T. Lanigan, DMD, MD
Robert A. Middleton, DDS
Thomas H. Morton, Jr., DDS, MSD

James H. Quinn, DDS
Monty Reitzik, BDS, FDSRCS, MB
Susan K. Robins, DDS
Ernest W. Small, DDS, MS
Richard A. Smith, DDS

TABLE OF CONTENTS

AN UNFORTUNATE SCENARIO

The following case history illustrates the potential consequence of poorly managed dental infections. The information presented reflects a combination of data obtained from two very similar infections, both of which had a fatal outcome. The chronology is presented to emphasize the short period of time between "toothache" and death.

Background Information:

This 36-year-old patient has had "a sore right back tooth" since Sunday. When he telephoned his regular dentist on Sunday, he was instructed to see the dental emergency clinic as soon as possible because he (the dentist) was to be out of his office this coming week. The pain became worse on Monday and the patient called the dental emergency clinic and was given an appointment for Tuesday morning.

July 14, 9:00 a.m. (Tuesday)
Patient was seen in the emergency dental clinic.

Chief Complaint:
Toothache over the right side of his lower jaw and neck.

History of Present Problem:
Toothache began Sunday and his neck began to hurt Monday. In addition, the patient said he could not open his mouth and has had trouble eating and swallowing for the last two days. He has lost sleep in the last two days and is tired. He said he had no previous injury or surgery in this area but has had "bad" teeth and gums for years.

Past Medical Factors:
No history of any factors that would contribute to this problem.

Clinical Examination:
Vital Signs: Temp. 100.4°F; BP 135/90; Pulse 82; Resp. Rate 18.
Extraoral Exam: Patient has slight submandibular swelling on the right, with tender right submandibular lymph nodes. Patient appeared tired and somewhat non-responsive.
Intraoral Exam: Patient could not open his mouth to perform intraoral exam because of trismus and facial pain. A swelling of the mandibular right buccal vestibule was noted in the area of the mandibular right premolar. This tooth and other teeth in this area appeared to have moderately advanced caries. His tongue appeared larger than would be expected; however, detailed examination could not be performed.

Radiographic Examination:
No radiographs were obtained because patient could not open his mouth (no panoramic radiograph was attempted even though the equipment was available).

Diagnosis:
A diagnosis of abscessed unspecified mandibular right posterior tooth was recorded.

Treatment:
Patient was instructed to take an antibiotic (oral penicillin, 250 mg q6h), to "take it easy," and to return to the clinic the following Monday for follow-up care once the infection had "settled down."

July 17, 3:00 p.m. (Friday)
The patient returned to the emergency clinic with the help of his wife who apologized for returning earlier than instructed. She said her husband's condition had become worse. He could not swallow, and had not eaten or drunk water since Wednesday. The patient was lethargic and was only able to mumble.

Chief Complaint:
Much worse than before, increased pain, can't swallow or eat.

History of Present Problem:
Increased pain and swelling since Tuesday.

Past Medical Factors:
Same as above, except now he had the recent history of oral penicillin-V (250 mg q6h) prescription. However, the patient was unable to take the antibiotic because of problems with swallowing.

Clinical Examination:
   Vital Signs: Temp: 103.0°F; B.P. 135/90; Pulse Rate 84; Resp. Rate 20.
   Serious General Signs: Respiratory difficulties, trismus, dysphagia, dehydration, and inadequate nutrition.
   Extraoral Exam: Edematous swelling of right submandibular space with extension into submental space and contralateral submandibular space. Fluctuance was not detected. Jugulo-omohyoid and superficial and inferior deep cervical lymph nodes were bilaterally enlarged and tender.

Diagnosis:
Ludwig's angina secondary to an unspecified dental infection of the mandibular right posterior area.

Management:
Patient was immediately transported to the nearby hospital dental clinic and an oral and maxillofacial surgeon met the patient there.

July 17, 4:00 p.m. (Friday)
The patient was seen in the hospital dental clinic. The following significant signs and symptoms were noted at that time:

1. Vital signs: Temp. 103.4°F; Pulse 96; Resp. 20; BP 140/95.
2. Bilateral indurated swellings of the submental and submandibular regions.
3. Tongue elevated and protruding slightly.
4. Dysphagia and drooling.
5. Increased respiratory effort noted with accessory muscles being used for breathing.
6. Head postured in a "sniffling" position (chin forward and up).
7. Brawny swelling of neck down to clavicles.
8. Marked trismus (unable to open his mouth).
9. Speech was soft, muffled and unintelligible.

The following clinical photo and a panoramic radiograph were obtained:

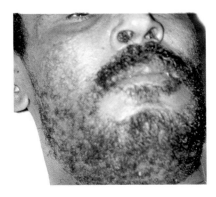 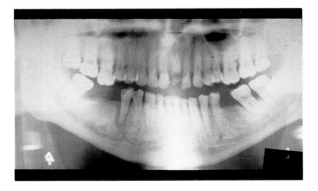

The following additional radiographs were obtained to assess the degree of cervical involvement:

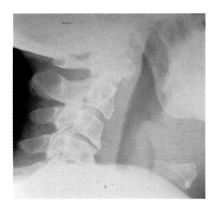

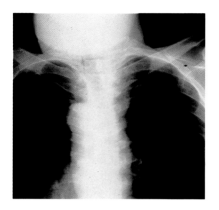

Lateral cervical view shows (1) fluid accumulation in neck below the angle of the mandible and (2) swelling of the epiglottis, base of the tongue, and pharyngeal wall with partial restriction of the airway.

P-A chest radiograph shows increased radioopacity in the cervical region consistent with the accumulation of increased fluids and/or pus.

July 17, 6:00 p.m. (Friday)
Treatment at the time of hospital admission:
1. I.V. antibiotics and fluids — 2 million units of I.V. penicillin-G every four hours.
2. Bed rest.
3. I.V. analgesics
4. Vital signs every four hours.
5. Scheduled for the operating room the next morning for incision and drainage.

July 17, 6:00 p.m. (Friday)
Following hospital admission, the patient was placed in his hospital bed in a supine position with his head elevated approximately 30°. I.V. Penicillin-G (2,000,000 units) was begun STAT, and continued at 2,000,000 units qid. Patient scheduled in operating room for next morning to perform incision and drainage and/or space decompression.

July 17, 10:00 p.m. (Friday)
The patient appeared to be more comfortable and the I.V. was running well, but he had no decrease in respiratory effort or neck swelling.

July 18, 2:00 a.m. (Saturday)
No changes were noted in vital signs, respiratory effort or neck swelling.

July 18, 6:00 a.m. (Saturday)
No changes were noted in vital signs, respiratory effort or neck swelling.

July 18, 9:00 a.m. (Saturday)
Ward rounds on the patient prior to transporting the patient to the operating room found the patient in a right lateral position without pulse or respiration. Immediate C.P.R., intubation and life support measures failed.

July 18, 10:00 a.m. (Saturday)
Patient pronounced dead.

July 24, 4:00 p.m. (Friday)
Autopsy Report:
1. Gram negative septicemia — bacteroides sp.
2. Massive neck cellulitis and tissue necrosis of the suprahyoid and infrahyoid muscles.
3. Laryngeal edema with decreased tracheal opening.

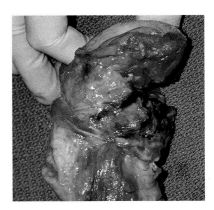

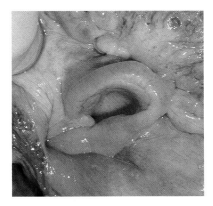

This photograph of a gross specimen from autopsy shows the base of the tongue at the top, hyoid bone near the center. Brown areas in the tissue represent necrosis of the supra- and infrahyoid muscles.

This photograph of a gross specimen from the autopsy shows the base of the tongue near the top right and edematous swelling of the epiglottis.

Cause of Death — Cardiac arrhythmia secondary to respiratory obstruction. Gram negative neck infection and septicemia originating from the mandibular right second premolar.

OVERVIEW OF THIS BOOK

The previous case history describes a tragic outcome for what intially presented as a moderately serious oral infection. While this example may seem extreme, it is by no means an isolated example of fatal outcomes resulting from the mismanagement of oral and/or maxillofacial infections. More frequently, tactical errors in the early management of mild to moderate oral infections allow these infections to become more serious, and thus require the involvement of specialists (e.g., oral and maxillofacial surgeon) and/or hospitalization for control of problems.

This book focuses on the principles of **primary** patient assessment and should help you **distinguish** between dental infections which can usually be managed by general dentists from those requiring care by specialists and/or hospitalization.

The management of oral and/or maxillofacial infections is complicated by many factors. These factors can generally be grouped into three general areas:

- The patient's general health
- The anatomical location of the problem
- The characteristics of the microorganism(s) responsible for the infection.

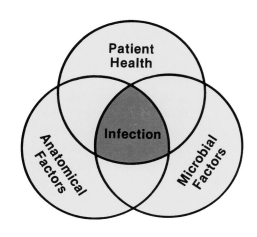

The diagram to the right illustrates the overlapping influence that **each** of these major factors can have on the other factors. When presented with a patient who has an infection of the oral and/or maxillofacial area, you should carefully collect relevant data associated with the infection in order to evaluate the contribution of each of these three general areas to the overall clinical picture. This information is essential to forming an accurate diagnosis, planning appropriate treatment or making a timely decision to refer the patient.

This book is divided into the following sections and the following topics within each section:

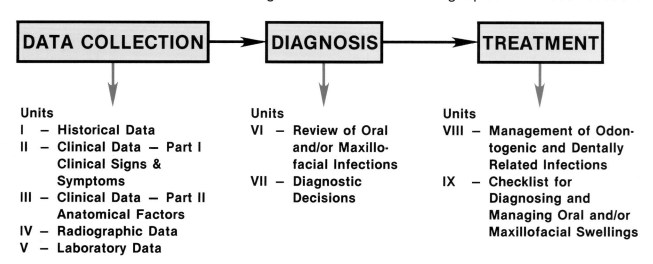

DATA COLLECTION → **DIAGNOSIS** → **TREATMENT**

Units
I – Historical Data
II – Clinical Data – Part I
    Clinical Signs &
    Symptoms
III – Clinical Data – Part II
    Anatomical Factors
IV – Radiographic Data
V – Laboratory Data

Units
VI – Review of Oral
    and/or Maxillo-
    facial Infections
VII – Diagnostic
    Decisions

Units
VIII – Management of Odon-
    togenic and Dentally
    Related Infections
IX – Checklist for
    Diagnosing and
    Managing Oral and/or
    Maxillofacial Swellings

The following flow diagram summarizes the management of oral and/or maxillofacial infections and emphasizes referral decision points and the need for monitoring treatment results.

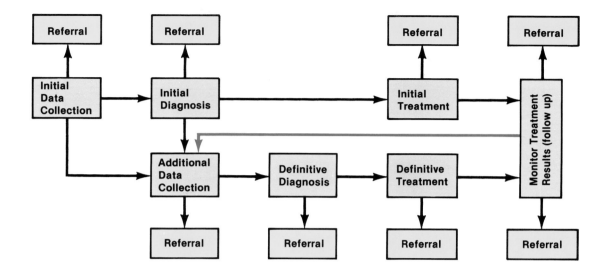

DATA COLLECTION

Each of the five units in this section presents a **checklist for summarizing a patient's signs and symptoms** and discusses the **significance** of each item on the checklist. In addition, each checklist is designed to **detect significant problems requiring referral** to a specialist or hospital.

DIAGNOSIS

Unit VI **reviews the causes of oral and/or maxillofacial swellings** (both non-microbial and microbial), and then reviews odontogenic and many dentally related non-odontogenic infections.

Unit VII presents a flow chart to aid in **diagnostic decisions** as well as provides practice in the diagnostic decision-making process.

TREATMENT

Unit VIII first describes the process of defining **management objectives** based upon the available data, then **presents various treatment options** that could be used to accomplish these objectives. Finally, this unit discusses a **system for monitoring** the results of treatment.

Unit IX **assembles all of the checklists** from each of the previous units into the Checklist for Diagnosing and Managing Oral and/or Maxillofacial Swellings, then demonstrates how the complete checklist can be useful in dental practice.

Overall Goal

The overall goal of this book is to assist you, the practitioners of general dentistry, in your management of patients with oral and/or maxillofacial infections. Our goal is to help you and your patients avoid the scenario of the introductory case. While this process may seem long and involved, it only scratches the surface of this complex topic. You should seek additional references on this subject to remain current in the management of these problems.

DATA COLLECTION

The first section of this book focuses on the **data collection process** for a patient presenting to your office with an oral and/or maxillofacial swelling. Unless appropriate data are obtained, you will not be able to formulate an accurate diagnosis, institute appropriate treatment, or make timely referrals.

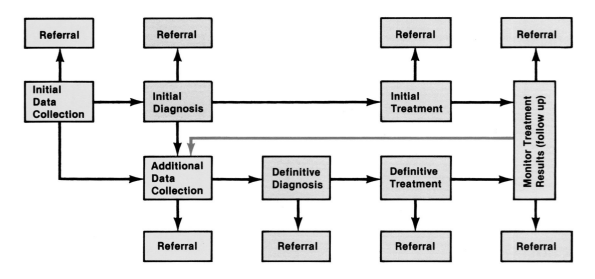

Unit I — Historical Data — This unit discusses a system for obtaining a patient's Chief Complaint, History of Present Problem, Review of Compromising Medical Factors, General Predisposing Factors and Local Predisposing Factors. Guidelines for referral are also presented.

Unit II — Clinical Data I — Signs and Symptoms — This unit first focuses on serious clinical signs requiring immediate referral to a specialist and/or hospital facility. Next it discusses evaluation of your patient's **vital signs,** signs of inflammation, and then reviews the local **predisposing** signs to infection.

Unit III — Clinical Data II — Anatomical Data — This unit presents a summary of head and neck anatomy including lymph nodes and fascial spaces. A review of the signs and symptoms associated with infections of anatomical areas is also provided.

Unit IV — Radiographic Data — This unit discusses basic dental radiographic views and reviews **additional** radiographic views which can be used to demonstrate the extent of involvement of a problem.

Unit V — Laboratory Data — This unit reviews laboratory tests that can be used to establish the presence or absence of microorganisms and to better understand the effects of microorganisms on your patients. It also discusses which laboratory data are needed, how the specimen should be collected, and how the data should be interpreted.

NOTE: Through the process of data collection, errors in diagnostic and treatment decisions can be minimized.

UNIT I
HISTORICAL DATA

OVERVIEW AND OBJECTIVES

The first step in diagnosing and treating oral and/or maxillofacial swellings is the collection of **Historical Data.** Historical data includes information you can obtain by questioning your patients about their symptoms and background history. This information includes the **chief complaint** (main problem), **history of the present problem** and **past medical history.** The purpose of this unit is to first acquaint you with the **historical data checklist** and to then describe the significance of each factor on this checklist. Following completion of this unit you will:

1. Describe the value of the **chief complaint** in terms of criteria for:
   a. Immediate hospital referral.
   b. Referral to a specialist.
   c. Continuation of the data collection process.
2. Describe how you should proceed with collection of the **history of present problem** and name nine (9) factors that should always be considered when collecting your patient's description of a problem.
3. Given a summary of data recorded from the patient interview recorded on the historical data checklist, identify information **not** obtained during the interview which could be significant to the diagnosis and management of a patient's swelling.
4. Describe how a **patient's past medical history** can influence the management of an oral and/or maxillofacial infection.
5. Given the list of medical conditions as described on page 22, describe the effect each condition can have upon host defense mechanisms.
6. Describe how each of the following categories of **medications** can affect host defense mechanisms and the common infections that may develop when a patient is taking these medications:
   a. Immunosuppressant drugs.
   b. Cytotoxic chemotherapy.
   c. Steroids.
7. Describe why it is important for you to identify any **recent history of antibiotic therapy.**
8. Describe two (2) ways in which **previous antibiotic therapy** can affect normal host flora.
9. State why identification of **allergies** can be important in management of oral and/or maxillofacial swellings.
10. Describe how **previous radiation therapy** can influence host resistance and your management of oral and/or maxillofacial swellings.
11. Describe how each of the following factors can be important in management of odontogenic infections:
a. Age	**d. Drug abuse**
b. Poor nutrition	**e. Patient's psychological condition**
c. Chronic use of alcohol	**f. Family & social environment**
12. Given a clinical simulation or description of a patient's historical data, correctly complete the **historical data checklist** and describe your course of action.

UNIT I
HISTORICAL DATA

Introduction
Chief Complaint
History of Present Problem
Past Medical History
Specific Medical Factors Pre-
disposing to Infections
Disease Processes Can Reduce
Host Defense Mechanisms
Medications Can Reduce Host
Defense Mechanisms
Allergies

Recent Antibiotic Therapy
Radiation Therapy
General Factors Predisposing to Infection
Age
Nutritional Status
Alcohol Consumption
Drug Abuse
Psychological Condition
Family and Social Environment
Medical Risk Assessment

INTRODUCTION

The purpose of this unit is to review the historical information that is needed to make valid diagnostic and treatment decisions for patients with oral and/or maxillofacial swellings.

NOTE: Historical data is information that is derived from questioning the patient. This information is a record of the patient's symptoms.

The **historical data** that should be obtained from your patient prior to the clinical examination is summarized on the following checklist.

HISTORICAL DATA

Patient Name _____ (Ref. #_____) Date of Data Collection _____
CHIEF COMPLAINT (present problem)_____
HISTORY OF PRESENT PROBLEM

☐ Onset of Illness _____
☐ Duration of Illness_____
☐ Episodic Nature _____
☐ Patient Symptoms
    a) Pain _____
    b) Swelling _____
    c) Dysfunction_____
    d) Other _____
    _____
    _____
☐ Previous Treatment _____
    _____

☐ Factors Improving Condition_____
    _____
☐ Factors Exacerbating Condition _____
    _____
☐ Local Trauma
    a) Injury_____
    b) Post surgical _____
☐ Associated Oral Disease
    a) Caries _____
    b) Periodontal disease_____
    c) Nonvital teeth_____
    d) Other _____

PAST MEDICAL FACTORS THAT WOULD COMPROMISE HOST DEFENSES

Specific Medical Factors

Yes No
☐ ☐ Disease process(es) _____ Effect _____
☐ ☐ Medication(s) _____ Effect _____
☐ ☐ Allergies _____
☐ ☐ Recent antibiotic therapy. Drug _____ Dosage _____ How long ago _____
☐ ☐ Radiation therapy_____

General Factors Predisposing to Infections

☐ ☐ Age ____ years .... ☐ Age related factors present_____
☐ ☐ Nutritional status ... ☐ Adequate ☐ Inadequate: ☐ Protein & Caloric ☐ Fluids ☐ Vitamins & minerals
☐ ☐ Alcohol consumption ☐ Non-user ☐ Low withdrawal potential ☐ High withdrawal potential
☐ ☐ Drug abuse .... Drug(s) _____ Dosage _____ Duration _____ ☐ Low Risk ☐ High Risk
☐ ☐ Psychological status . ☐ Favorable ☐ Unfavorable: Why? _____
☐ ☐ Family & social status ☐ Favorable ☐ Unfavorable: Why? _____

We will discuss each item on this checklist emphasizing the importance of each of these symptoms or historical factors. This information can be of great help in identifying the overall degree of seriousness of a problem and will be influential in defining treatment objectives and selecting treatment methods.

CHIEF COMPLAINT

The chief complaint (main problem) is an essential part of the historical data. It is obtained by asking the patient to describe his/her main problem. Occasionally a patient may be too sick to talk to you or to come into your office. Often, a relative or friend will telephone you and describe the patient's condition. **You should record this historian's name as well as their description of the patient's problem and arrange to see the patient immediately in your office or make an appropriate referral. Do not delay.** The chief complaint may sometimes reveal serious, life-threatening symptoms.

> EXAMPLE: **"I have had increasing swelling of my neck and I have some difficulty in breathing."**

NOTE: **This chief complaint is a signal for you to IMMEDIATELY REFER your patient to a specialist or physician in the emergency room of a hospital. Further data collection and diagnosis is not necessary at this time.**

Guidelines for Referral

Generally speaking, if you determine from the chief complaint that your patient's life is not immediately threatened, you should continue with the history of the present problem. Review past medical history and the clinical examination before deciding whether a referral is appropriate. This approach will enable you to make an informed referral.

The following guidelines should be used to decide whether your patient should be referred at this stage of the examination:

Immediate referral to a specialist or physician in a hospital emergency room — Should be made if patient is in an immediate life-threatening condition. Patient statements can often describe serious conditions, such as:

- Respiratory impairment
- Difficulty in swallowing
- Impairment of vision and/or eye movements
- Change in voice quality
- Severe lethargy
- Decreased level of consciousness

NOTE: **Not all physicians are experienced in management of serious maxillofacial infections. When referring a patient to a hospital you should contact a dental or medical specialist who is qualified to manage these problems. All references in this book to immediate hospital referral imply referral to a specialist experienced in management of serious oral and maxillofacial infections.**

Referral to a specialist should be made if patient is not in immediate danger, but the infection is beyond your level of training and skills. This may include such conditions as:

- Severe infectious spreading beyond the oral cavity into critical fascial spaces
- Systemic involvement
- Rapidly progressing infections
- Long-term chronic infections
- Severe trismus
- Moderate to severe dehydration
- Any treatment which may require administration under hospital conditions (e.g. I.V., antibiotics, blood cultures, or other advanced management techniques.)

HISTORY OF PRESENT PROBLEM

The next information you need to collect is the **history of the present problem**. This information is an elaboration of the patients' chief complaint or main problem. Much information can be elicited from your patients **if you give them the opportunity to describe their symptoms.**

When obtaining the **History of Present Problem** you should systematically seek data relating to the factors summarized on the following portion of the checklist.

HISTORY OF PRESENT PROBLEM

☐ Onset of Illness _____

☐ Duration of Illness_____

☐ Episodic Nature _____

☐ Patient Symptoms

    a) Pain _____

    b) Swelling _____

    c) Dysfunction_____

    d) Other _____

    _____

    _____

☐ Previous Treatment _____

    _____

☐ Factors Improving Condition_____

_____

☐ Factors Exacerbating Condition _____

_____

☐ Local Trauma

    a) Injury_____

    b) Post surgical _____

☐ Associated Oral Disease

    a) Caries _____

    b) Periodontal disease _____

    c) Nonvital teeth_____

    d) Other _____

A detailed discussion of patient interviewing techniques is beyond the scope of this book; however, these techniques are an essential ingredient in the diagnostic process. During the history-taking process, you should ask your patient for the above information using **open-ended or guided** questions. You should **avoid using prompted questions** which could evoke misleading responses or prevent your patient from describing all of his/her symptoms.

- **Example of guided question:** "Are you having discomfort at this time? Show me where it hurts."

- **Example of prompted question:** "It looks to me as though you are having pain over your left cheek and that the pain is radiating to your left ear. Is this correct?"

NOTE: You should ask your patients general questions dealing with their problem. Give your patients the opportunity to describe their symptoms. You should avoid using prompted questions which could evoke misleading answers, and thus misdirect your data collection, diagnosis, and treatment.

STUDY EXERCISES

1. *When collecting data about the* **History of Present Problem** *you should:*

    Yes   No

    _____ _✓_   *a. Ask questions that will lead your patient to describe specific details by answering "yes" or "no" to specific questions.*

    _✓_ _____   *b. Ask general open-ended questions and allow your patient to describe factors related to the problem.*

2. *Which of the following* **chief complaints** *contain information indicating* **immediate** *referral to either specialist or specialist in a hospital (***RH = Refer to hospital now; R = Refer to specialist now; P = Proceed with data collection, patient not in danger at this time***):*

    _RH_ **a. Chief Complaint:** *"Doctor, I've got this large swollen area around where you pulled my wisdom tooth and it's getting hard for me to swallow and even breathe."*

    _RH_ **b. Chief Complaint:** *"Doctor, after you started the root canal on my upper eyetooth, a swelling began over my cheek and my eye is now swollen shut."*

    _R_ **c. Chief Complaint:** *"I noticed a lump develop under my jaw after I ate dinner last night. Later it went down but came back when I ate breakfast this morning."*

For each of the following cases, **check** the categories of information obtained during collection of the **History of Present Problem.** Identify those areas in which no information was obtained.

Case #1
Chief Complaint:
"This swelling in my neck right here below and anterior to the angle of mandible has developed and gotten worse since my wisdom tooth was taken out six days ago."

History of Present Problem:
The patient's neck problem began 2 days following mandibular 3rd molar impaction surgery. Prior to surgery he had a moderate pericoronitis. Penicillin (500 mg) every 6 hours was given for 5 days to control this problem before surgery, and was continued post-surgically. Present symptoms include lateral neck swelling extending to the clavicle (which is abnormal for post-surgical swelling.) Pain is also severe and constant. Patient has problems swallowing. The swelling has continued to increase in size and extension and appears unaffected by heat or cold packs. No other factors could be identified that improved or exacerbated this condition.

CHIEF COMPLAINT (present problem) _____
HISTORY OF PRESENT PROBLEM

- ☐ Onset of Illness *2 days after surgery*
- ☐ Duration of Illness *4 days*
- ☐ Episodic Nature *severe constant*
- ☐ Patient Symptoms
  - a) Pain *severe constant*
  - b) Swelling *lateral neck to clavicle*
  - c) Dysfunction *prob. swallowing*
  - d) Other _____

  _____
- ☐ Previous Treatment *Pen 500mg every 6 hrs*

- ☐ Factors Improving Condition *ø*
  _____
- ☐ Factors Exacerbating Condition *ø*
  _____
- ☐ Local Trauma
  - a) Injury _____
  - b) Post surgical *mand. 3rd molar*
- ☐ Associated Oral Disease
  - a) Caries *ø*
  - b) Periodontal disease _____
  - c) Nonvital teeth _____
  - d) Other _____

Case #2
Chief Complaint:
"I have this painful swelling under my tongue."

History of Present Problem:
The swelling in the anterior floor of the mouth has gradually increased over the past several weeks and seems to slowly enlarge. Patient had root canal therapy for both mandibular central incisors 6 months ago without complications. He has had some problems with periodontal disease and has had composite restorations in the mandibular anterior area placed within the last month. Patient reports no accidental trauma to the area and no recent surgery.

CHIEF COMPLAINT (present problem) _____
HISTORY OF PRESENT PROBLEM

- ☐ Onset of Illness *several weeks ago*
- ☐ Duration of Illness *slowly enlarge*
- ☐ Episodic Nature *slowly enlarge*
- ☐ Patient Symptoms
  - a) Pain *yes*
  - b) Swelling *ant - floor mouth*
  - c) Dysfunction _____
  - d) Other _____

  _____
- ☐ Previous Treatment *mand. cent. inc. 6 months root canal, perio surgery, compos*

- ☐ Factors Improving Condition _____
  _____
- ☐ Factors Exacerbating Condition _____
  _____
- ☐ Local Trauma *negative*
  - a) Injury _____
  - b) Post surgical _____
- ☐ Associated Oral Disease
  - a) Caries *composite*
  - b) Periodontal disease *yes*
  - c) Nonvital teeth _____
  - d) Other _____

STUDY EXERCISE ANSWERS

1. a. **No.** Leading questions can lead to distorted data.
   b. **Yes.** This type of question will give more accurate data.
2. a. **RH** — Refer to a specialist in hospital now! Patient's life in danger.
   b. **R** — Serious problem requiring immediate effective treatment.
   c. **P** — Proceed with data collection. Patient not in acute danger.

Case #1

HISTORY OF PRESENT PROBLEM

☒ Onset of Illness _2 days after mand. 3rd molars were Ext._
☒ Duration of Illness _4 days_
☒ Episodic Nature _Continuous worsening_
☒ Patient Symptoms
    a) Pain _Severe & constant_
    b) Swelling _Lateral neck to clavicle_
    c) Dysfunction_____
    d) Other _____

☒ Previous Treatment _Penicillin q 6h for past 11 days_

☒ Factors Improving Condition _none_

☒ Factors Exacerbating Condition _none_

☒ Local Trauma
    a) Injury_____
    b) Post surgical _Impacted 3rd Molar Extraction_
☒ Associated Oral Disease
    a) Caries_____
    b) Periodontal disease _____
    c) Nonvital teeth_____
    d) Other _Previous Pericoronitis around partially impacted mandib. 3rd molar_

The **History of the Present Problem** obtained in this case included all significant information that should have been obtained during your initial interview with the patient. This information alone provides you with enough data to preliminarily conclude that the patient has a serious problem and **immediate referral to a hospital is necessary.**

Case #2

HISTORY OF PRESENT PROBLEM

◔ Onset of Illness _____
☒ Duration of Illness _several weeks_
◔ Episodic Nature _____
☐ Patient Symptoms
    a) Pain _yes_
    b) Swelling _Under tongue - anterior floor of mouth_
    c) Dysfunction_dysphagia_
    ⓓ Other _____

☒ Previous Treatment _Root canal Therapy mand central incisors 6 mo previously, Composite Rest. mand Ant. area in last month._

◔ Factors Improving Condition_____

◔ Factors Exacerbating Condition _____

☒ Local Trauma
    a) Injury _none_
    b) Post surgical _none_
☒ Associated Oral Disease
    a) Caries _____
    b) Periodontal disease _Some problems_
    c) Nonvital teeth _Root canals mand cent. Inc._
    d) Other _____ _6 mo ago_

The **History of the Present Problem** obtained in this case was insufficient and could mislead you in your diagnosis. The historical data collected **could** indicate a sublingual abscess associated with a failing root canal, pulpal necrosis resulting from placement of the composite restorations, or possibly a periodontal abscess. No information was obtained on **factors improving or exacerbating** the problem. If these questions had been asked, the patient would have said, "Previous dental treatment has not seemed to help and the swelling and pain increases whenever I eat." With this information you would not be inclined to prematurely conclude the problem to be the result of an infection process and your initial treatment would not be directed toward management of an abscess. With this information you would continue the data collection process and definitely obtain an occlusal radiograph of the anterior floor of the mouth. With this data you would have found a stone in the salivary duct near the orifice and could have provided immediate treatment of the problem or referred the patient to a specialist.

PAST MEDICAL HISTORY

The next step in collecting historical information involves a review of your patient's **past medical history.** This information adds to the data base from which you can assess your patient's overall health status. The following factors from the **past medical history** may have particular importance in the diagnosis and management of oral and/or maxillofacial swellings.

PAST MEDICAL FACTORS THAT WOULD COMPROMISE HOST DEFENSES

Specific Medical Factors

Yes No
- ☐ ☐ Disease process(es) _____ Effect _____
- ☐ ☐ Medication(s) _____ Effect _____
- ☐ ☐ Allergies _____
- ☐ ☐ Recent antibiotic therapy. Drug _____ Dosage _____ How long ago _____
- ☐ ☐ Radiation therapy _____

General Factors Predisposing to Infections
- ☐ ☐ Age ____ years .... ☐ Age related factors present _____
- ☐ ☐ Nutritional status ... ☐ Adequate ☐ Inadequate: ☐ Protein & Caloric ☐ Fluids ☐ Vitamins & minerals
- ☐ ☐ Alcohol consumption ☐ Non-user ☐ Low withdrawal potential ☐ High withdrawal potential
- ☐ ☐ Drug abuse .... Drug(s) _____ Dosage _____ Duration _____ ☐ Low Risk ☐ High Risk
- ☐ ☐ Psychological status . ☐ Favorable ☐ Unfavorable: Why? _____
- ☐ ☐ Family & social status ☐ Favorable ☐ Unfavorable: Why? _____

SPECIFIC MEDICAL FACTORS PREDISPOSING TO INFECTIONS

☐ ☐ **Disease Processes Can Reduce Host Defense Mechanisms**

Many disease processes can compromise the health of your patients and decrease their ability to combat infections. **Table I-1** (page 22) shows examples of several common disease processes and how they can alter the body's response to infection. These disease processes must be identified early in the management of any infection since a relatively simple infection in a healthy patient can become much more serious in a patient with reduced host defense mechanisms.

You will notice that several of these diseases directly affect key factors involved in host defense mechanisms resulting in:
- depressed inflammatory response
- decreased phagocytic activity
- decreased pulmonary clearance
- compromised circulation

The presence of these disease processes can
- increase the likelihood of systemic involvement
- prolong resolution time

thereby significantly increasing the risk from an otherwise uncomplicated infection. You should refer to internal medicine references for a more detailed discussion of these disease processes.

NOTE: Because of the increased patient risk associated with these disease processes, a general dentist would be well advised to consult with specialists or refer patients with these problems to a specialist for the management of an otherwise minor infection.

COMPROMISING MEDICAL CONDITIONS

CONDITION	PATHOPHYSIOLOGY	INCREASED POTENTIAL FOR INFECTIONS
Malnutrition	Impaired phagocytosis and phagocyte killing	Pneumonia, skin, gastro-intestinal, septicemia
Alcoholism	Suppressed glottic reflex, reduced phagocytic chemotaxis detoxification and impaired detoxification (impaired liver)	Pneumonia
Diabetes	Reduced chemotaxis and phagocytosis	Pneumonia, skin, soft tissue, gastrointestinal, septicemia
Heart failure, chronic lung disease	Decreased pulmonary clearance, respiration impaired	Pneumonia, tuberculosis
Heart murmur, rheumatic fever, prosthetic heart valves	Cardiac valve surface damaged	Endocarditis
Prosthetic joints	Unnatural surfaces, poor circulation around prosthesis	Localized abscesses
Influenza	Damaged respiratory epithelium	Pneumonia
Hodgkin's disease	Decreased cell-mediated immunity	Pneumonia
Cystic fibrosis	Decreased mucocilliary clearance and pulmonary phagocytosis	Pneumonia
Renal failure	Impaired chemotaxis and cell-mediated immunity	Pneumonia, wounds, urinary, septicemia, enterocolitis
Lymphoproliferative disorders (leukemia, lymphosarcoma, multiple myeloma, macroglobulinemia)	Reduced antibody synthesis	Pneumonia, skin, urinary tract, septicemia, etc.
Hereditary or acquired diseases affecting leukocytes (bone marrow transplant patients, Down's syndrome, hypogammaglobulinemia, leukemia, chronic granulomatous disease, Job's syndrome, lazy leukocyte syndrome)	Impaired chemotaxis and phagocytosis or phagocyte killing	Pneumonia, skin, soft tissue, septicemia, osteo-myelitis, etc.

Table I-1. Medical conditions that can lead to compromises in the body's resistance to infection.

STUDY EXERCISES

For each of the following medical conditions, describe the pathophysiological effect each condition has upon the patient's body defense mechanism.

Disease or Condition   **Defense Mechanism Affected**
1. Alcoholism   *glottic reflex, phagocytic chemotaxis detoxification*
2. Diabetes   *chemotaxis & phagocytosis*
3. Heart failure   *pulmonary clearance, respiration*
4. Leukemia   *antibody synthesis*

☐ ☐ **Medications Can Reduce Host Defense Mechanisms**

In addition to the disease processes that affect host defense mechanisms, numerous drugs also have effects upon the inflammatory process, phagocytic activity, and other processes involved in host defense mechanisms. Three common drug groups and their effect upon host defense mechanisms are summarized below. Also shown are systemic infections which are more likely to occur in persons taking these medications.

It is essential for you to **review all medications** a patient is taking or **has taken within the last six months** and evaluate the effects these medications could have on host defense mechanisms **before** initiating treatment. All medications **should be recorded** on the checklist.

MEDICATIONS	DEFENSE MECHANISM AFFECTED	INCREASED POTENTIAL FOR INFECTIONS
• Immunosuppressants • Cytotoxic chemotherapy • Steroids	• Decrease in circulating phagocytes • Reduced antibody synthesis	• Pneumonia, stomatitis, skin, soft tissue infections, septicemia, etc.

☐ ☐ **Allergies**

Needless to say, any history of previous allergies should be recorded. Of specific importance to the management of infections are allergies to antibiotics or pain medications.

NOTE: Any allergies must be recorded on the checklist.

☐ ☐ **Recent Antibiotic Therapy**

Identification of antibiotics your patient may have been taking prior to the onset of an infection is of particular importance. Prior administration of antibiotics can select for microorganisms which could be resistant to your antibiotic of first choice in the management of an infection. A previous history of penicillin or tetracycline therapy is of particular importance due to the wide use of these antibiotics.

NOTE: You should check this box on the checklist and identify the specific antibiotic(s). You should also record the dosage(s) of antibiotic(s) used if this information is available.

PREVIOUS ANTIBIOTIC THERAPY	DEFENSE MECHANISM AFFECTED	INCREASED POTENTIAL FOR INFECTIONS
Can lead to:	• Alteration of normal flora • Selection of resistant flora	• Pneumonia, stomatitis, urinary, vaginal infections

☐ ☐ **Radiation Therapy**

Patients who have received radiation therapy may have reduced host defense systems; thus, an otherwise minor infection is a much more serious problem for these patients. Previous irradiation of the head and neck area can **predispose these patients to osteoradionecrosis** if surgery is performed during management of infections. Whole-body irradiation can retard lymphocyte and leucocyte production. Systemic effects of irradiation include reduced antibody production and reduced leucocyte activity, thus, the risks for systemic infection is increased for these patients.

PREVIOUS RADIATION THERAPY	DEFENSE MECHANISM AFFECTED
Can cause:	• Decreased vascularity, especially of bone tissue • Decreased resistance of oral tissues • Decreased phagocytic activity • Decreased antibody synthesis • Decreased salivary flow

NOTE: Any patient having a history of radiation therapy must be managed by a dentist trained to treat post-radiation problems.

GENERAL FACTORS PRE-DISPOSING TO INFECTION

General pre-disposing factors are those systemic or lifestyle factors that can decrease host resistance to infection or make pain management more difficult. These factors include:

General Factors to Predisposing Infections

☐	☐	Age ___ years	☐ Age related factors present _____
☐	☐	Nutritional status	☐ Adequate	☐ Inadequate:	☐ Protein & Caloric	☐ Fluids	☐ Vitamins & minerals
☐	☐	Alcohol consumption	☐ Non-user	☐ Low withdrawal potential	☐ High withdrawal potential
☐	☐	Drug abuse	Drug(s) _____	Dosage _____	Duration _____	☐ Low Risk	☐ High Risk
☐	☐	Psychological status .	☐ Favorable	☐ Unfavorable: Why? _____
☐	☐	Family & social status	☐ Favorable	☐ Unfavorable: Why? _____

A summary of your analysis of these factors should be recorded on the checklist above.

☐ ☐ Age

Age is especially important if your patient is **very young,** such as in the first few months of life. During this stage, newborns do not have fully active antibody production and rely on maternal antibodies. During this time newborns are particularly sensitive to Gram negative infections. In addition, they will dehydrate rapidly, so early treatment is important.

NOTE: If you should be consulted by the parents of a newborn for what they may believe to be a dental problem, and you have not had experience in pediatric stomatology, you should refer the patient to a specialist.

Age can also have an effect on body defenses in elderly patients. As one becomes older, there may be a decrease in T-cell function which can reduce body defenses, and the probability is high that one or more medical problems have developed that could reduce body defense mechanisms (e.g., diabetes, congestive heart failure, cirrhosis of the liver). In addition, elderly patients may have poor nutrition due to financial limitations or their living conditions.

NOTE: It is particularly important for you to carefully review the medical history of older patients and to seek appropriate secondary data at the earliest opportunity. Elderly patients with seriously reduced body defenses who have oral infections should be referred to a specialist immediately.

☐ ☐ Nutritional Status

Nutritional status is a factor that contributes to your patient's:
- resistance to infection
- ability to control existing infection
- rate of recovery from infection.

Nutritional status can be less than adequate for a variety of reasons. Most causes are linked to such socio-economic factors as: living alone and not eating regular meals, insufficient finances requiring substitution of carbohydrates for protein, and prolonged fad diets. Debilitating diseases such as drug or alcohol addiction or other medical problems can also reduce nutritional status. Inadequate nutritional status is of concern not only when gross deficits are present such as in prolonged starvation or extreme fluid deprivation, but also when inadequacies in protein, vitamins or minerals have persisted for a long time (i.e., the alcoholic gets ample calories but they are all carboydrates). **When other factors of host defenses are compromised, poor nutritional status only makes things worse.** As will be discussed later, you can rapidly improve most patients' nutritional status through dietary counseling and dietary supplements, or your patients may require hospitalization in order to improve nutritional deficiencies.

☐ ☐ **Alcohol Consumption**

It is extremely important for you to identify patients who consume alcohol frequently. Alcohol can interact with narcotic analgesics (including propoxyphene) and lead to respiratory depression or arrest. Alcoholic patients can develop alcoholic withdrawal symptoms (delirium tremors = DTs) if taken off alcohol during the management of an infection.

Chronic alcohol consumption can also greatly reduce the body's defense mechanisms. This is often due to a decrease in nutritional status and an increase in local predisposing factors such as poor oral hygiene, caries, and uncontrolled periodontal disease, and other family, social, and psychological factors as well. Excessive chronic ingestion of alcohol can result in demonstrable alterations in the body's cellular immune systems. The mobilization and transport of neutrophils to infected sites as well as complement function can be abnormal in chronic alcoholic patients.

NOTE: A patient with a serious alcohol problem and also a moderate to serious infection should be referred to a specialist for management. The specialist may elect to place the patient in the hospital in order to control alcoholic withdrawal.

☐ ☐ **Drug Abuse**

Drug abusers as a group are more prone to develop oral and/or maxillofacial infections than non-users. These patients are more prone to self-induced infections through the use of unsterile needles. Some abusers will inject narcotics into the soft tissue of their mouth and thus initiate an oral infection. These patients frequently neglect caries and endodontic problems and use these problems to obtain narcotics. Infections in drug abusers **can progress more rapidly due to the following potential compromises in host defense mechanisms:**
  - **nutritional deficiencies** due to poor eating habits prior to the onset of an infection.
  - **decreased liver function** due to the effects of the drugs. This disorder may decrease the addict's ability to detoxify drugs and increases the potential for various blood disorders.

Management of infections in drug abusers can also be more difficult because of the:
  - increased potential for drug withdrawal symptoms during treatment
  - higher tolerances for narcotic analgesics
  - problems in managing the psychological aspects. Often these patients will not tell the truth during interviews, nor will they follow your instructions.

You need to evaluate the potential impact of the above factors upon the management of infections in drug abusers. You should attempt to **identify what drugs are being taken, how much is used,** and **how long drugs have been taken**, and then estimate the potential risk for drug-related complications. This information should be recorded on the checklist.

NOTE: If the potential for drug-related problems is high, you should refer the patient to a specialist or hospital dental service. Low risk drug abusers should be closely followed during treatment.

☐ ☐ **Psychological Condition**

Your patient's psychological status will often affect his/her recovery capabilities. Patients who are or become depressed with either the infection or the progress of treatment are less likely to follow your instructions. Assessment of initial psychological status will enable you to take extra measures to encourage your patient and consider a treatment approach that would minimize further depression.

☐ ☐ **Family and Social Environment**

Evaluation of your patient's family and/or social lifestyle is an important factor to consider in the assessment and ultimate management of any oral and/or maxillofacial infection. Your patient's present living environment may contribute to a decrease in host resistance through poor nutrition and increased emotional stress.

An unfavorable living environment **can decrease your patient's ability to:**
- follow your treatment recommendations
- improve nutritional status
- obtain and administer antibiotics and/or analgesics on prescribed schedules
- obtain necessary rest
- perform other self-administered treatment

Does patient live alone?

Elderly patients living alone may not have the time, energy or economic resources to obtain proper nutrition, rest and medication during the recovery period. Persons living alone may have major problems in carrying out your instructions. A more supportive environment may be preferred, i.e., nursing home, live-in houseperson, staying with relatives.

Can patients decrease their work or family responsibilities?

Evaluation of patient's ability to "take it easy" and obtain necessary rest at home is important. Frequently, a patient will have heavy responsibilities at home and his or her spouse may not be able to assume these duties. If your patient is a single parent, child care responsibilities will make it difficult for your patient to rest. Self-employed persons often do not have "sick leave" from their business duties or responsibilities.

If family and social environment is not ideal you must evaluate the options for improvement, including:
- Can a responsible person provide direct care for your patient at home? Family, friend, public health nurse, or other.
- Can your patient move in with someone who can care for him or her?
- Should patient be placed in a hospital to closely regulate living environment?

MEDICAL RISK ASSESSMENT

Assessment of your patient's overall medical health is an essential step prior to diagnosis and treatment of oral and maxillofacial swellings. However, a detailed discussion of specific systemic medical problems and drugs used to manage these problems is beyond the scope of this chapter.

You may need to consult with your patient's physician or with another dentist who has received additional training in the management of medically compromised patients if you have **any** uncertainty regarding the risk and management of any medical problem. Careful evaluation of drugs your patient may be taking can be helpful in identifying medical problems or potential drug interaction problems.

Following a thorough review of the patient's medical history you can make a decision as to the significance of the findings and then categorize your patient into one of the following general groups. These categories will be explained in more detail in Unit VII, Diagnostic Decisions.

The following interpretations should be made in this category:
- **Serious medical risk or problem.** Treatment should only be performed by a person trained to manage serious medical problems.
- **Moderate medical risk.** Patient's condition could be managed by a general practitioner in conjunction with appropriate consultations or prior laboratory tests.
- **Minor medical risk.** Some potential problems may exist; however, you should be able to adequately manage these problems in the setting of an office equipped for general dentistry.
- **Low risk.** Your patient does not have any foreseeable medical risk.

STUDY EXERCISES

*From the data presented in each of the following cases, **extract any information from the past medical history that could indicate compromises in the patient's body (host) defenses** against infections. You should refer to the checklist on page 21.*

Case #1.

A 17-year-old female presents to your office for a swelling in the base of the upper lip and pain from a cariously involved central incisor. She is 5'6" tall and weighs 85 pounds, and appears pale. You note several blue marks on her forearm. She lists a downtown hotel as her address and lists no nearest relative on her patient registration form. There is decreased muscle mass and lethargy.

Compromising Factors	Effect(s) of Compromise on Host Defense Mechanisms
malnutrition	↓ phagocytosis
drug abuse	↓ liver function
no home	depression

Case #2.

In evaluating a 42-year-old female patient who is complaining of an infected and painful front tooth, you find the following medical history: insulin dependent diabetic, allergy to sulfa drugs, just completed irradiation treatment for breast tumor, and is now undergoing cytotoxic chemotherapy and taking immuno-suppressant drugs.

Compromising Factors	Effect(s) of Compromise on Host Defense Mechanisms
diabetic	↓ phagocytosis
allergy	cannot give sulfa drugs
radiation tx	↓ phagocyte activity
chemotherapy	↓ p
immuno drugs	↓ phagocytosis

Discussion of Cases:

Case #1:

A 17-year-old female is living alone and her weight far below normal for her height. Decreased muscle mass and lack of energy may point to several medically compromising conditions. Malnutrition, malignant disease or person's alcohol or drug addiction should be considered. You should collect additional data including consultation with her physician.

Case #2:

Compromising factors include insulin dependent diabetes, radiation therapy, chemotherapy, and immunosuppressant medication. This patient should be treated by a specialist.

POST-TEST — UNIT I

Now that you have worked through Unit I, you should take the following self-test to see how much of the information you have been able to retain and use in clinical problem-solving situations.

*Please **read the following instructions and complete the following post-test for Unit I.***

- *Answer each of the following questions.*
- *Check your answers with the correct responses on page 30.*
- *If all questions are answered correctly, proceed to Unit II, page 32.*
- *If you did not answer all questions correctly, read and study the content of Unit I again.*

QUESTIONS

1. *Given the following patients' **chief complaints**, identify the appropriate course of action:*

	Immediate Hospital Referral	Refer to Specialist	Proceed with Examination
*(a) **Chief Complaint:** "I have a toothache and this little swelling on the roof of my mouth."*			X
*(b) **Chief Complaint:** "My right eye is swollen shut and is red. This problem developed last night after you began the root canal on my upper tooth."*		X	
*(c) **Chief Complaint:** "Both sides of my son's neck are sore and swollen. He can't swallow very well, and he hasn't been able to eat or drink for the past 5 days. He has a high fever, looks pale, and cannot get out of bed without help."*	X		

2. *Which of the following statements describes the correct method you should use to obtain a patient's **History of Present Problem**?*
   __X__ (a) Ask questions which elicit unprompted patient responses.
   _____ (b) Ask closed-ended questions which your patient can answer by yes or no.

3. *Given the following description of a patient's **History of Present Problem**, complete the following checklist as a summary of this data.*

   History of Present Problem: *The patient first noted a toothache in the lower left first molar region 5 days prior to his appointment with you after he was struck in the face during a fight. Swelling has steadily increased until the present time. He presents with a large left facial swelling, reports trismus (inter-incisor opening is 2 cm) and severe pain. The pain increases when he is lying down. Two days ago he took two penicillin tablets which a friend gave him. He tried four aspirin for pain relief and got none. He was able to relieve the pain by taking four Percodan tablets each day which he got from a friend. The patient last saw a dentist five years ago, at which time he was advised that six teeth were "decayed" and he should see a specialist for treatment of "gum disease."*

HISTORY OF PRESENT PROBLEM

- ☐ Onset of Illness _5 dys_
- ☐ Duration of Illness _____
- ☐ Episodic Nature _____
- ☐ Patient Symptoms
  - a) Pain _lying down_
  - b) Swelling _increased_
  - c) Dysfunction _____
  - d) Other _____
  - _____
- ☐ Previous Treatment _____
- _____

- ☐ Factors Improving Condition _____
  - _percodan_
- ☐ Factors Exacerbating Condition _____
  - _lying down_
- ☐ Local Trauma
  - a) Injury _fight_
  - b) Post Surgical _____
- ☐ Associated Oral Disease
  - a) Caries _____
  - b) Periodontal disease _____
  - c) Nonvital teeth _____
  - d) Other _____

4. *Given the following description of a patient's medical history, complete the checklist for* **past medical factors which would compromise host defenses** *and describe your probable course of action.*

   An 18-year-old male presents to your office with a large external swelling in the right submandibular region. **Medical History:** *As a child he developed rheumatic heart disease and had severe asthma and severe acne. He is allergic to penicillin. He currently is taking tetracycline (250 mg/day) and corticosteroids (10 mg/day) for control of his acne.*

PAST MEDICAL FACTORS THAT WOULD COMPROMISE HOST DEFENSES

Specific Medical Factors

Yes No
- ☐ ☐ Disease Process(es) _rheumatic heart_____   Effect _____
- ☐ ☐ Medication(s) _____   Effect _____
- ☐ ☐ Allergies _acne_____
- ☐ ☐ Recent antibiotic therapy. Drug _tetr.____ Dosage _250mg/dy___ How long ago _____
- ☐ ☐ Radiation therapy _____

5. *Given the following partial description of a patient's medical history, complete the checklist for* **general factors predisposing to infections** *and describe your probable course of action based on this information.*

   A 67-year-old male with a 20-year history of chronic alcoholism (750 ml [1 fifth] of whiskey per day) presents to the "Skid Road Medical Center" at which you are a volunteer dentist. This patient complains of a "toothache" which has caused his left eye to close shut. He lives alone in one room in a hotel with no telephone and has no immediate family or friends who can provide care. He claims to have not eaten any solid food during the previous 4 days. He also claims that "two flying horses flew through my window this morning and carried me here."

General Factors Predisposing to Infections
- ☒ ☐ Age _67_ years ..... ☐ Age related factors present _____
- ☒ ☐ Nutritional status .... ☐ Adequate ☒ Inadequate: ☐ Protein & Caloric ☐ Fluids ☐ Vitamins & minerals
- ☒ ☐ Alcohol consumption ☐ Non-user ☐ Low withdrawal potential ☒ High withdrawal potential
- ☐ ☐ Drug abuse .... Drug(s) _____ Dosage _____ Duration _____ ☐ Low Risk ☐ High Risk
- ☒ ☐ Psychological status . ☐ Favorable ☒ Unfavorable: Why? _____
- ☒ ☐ Family & social status ☐ Favorable ☒ Unfavorable: Why? _____

Post-Test Answers

1. *(a) Proceed with examination*
   (b) Refer to specialist (oral and maxillofacial surgeon)
   (c) Refer to hospital immediately

2. *(a) is correct. Do not prompt patient with closed-ended questions.*

3. *All factors on the checklist were covered with this History of Present Problem except Episodic Nature.*

HISTORY OF PRESENT PROBLEM

☒ Onset of Illness *5 days prior to appt.*

☒ Duration of Illness *5 days*

☐ Episodic Nature _____

☒ Patient Symptoms
　a) Pain _____
　ⓑ Swelling *left facial*
　ⓒ Dysfunction *trismus*
　d) Other _____
　　_____
　　_____

☒ Previous Treatment *2 tabs penicillin 2 days ago, 4 Percodan tabs*

☒ Factors Improving Condition *Percodan*
_____

☒ Factors Exacerbating Condition *lying down*
_____

☒ Local Trauma
　ⓐ Injury *fist to face - 5 days ago*
　b) Post surgical _____

☒ Associated Oral Disease
　ⓐ Caries *"6 decayed teeth" - 5 yrs. ago*
　ⓑ Periodontal disease *reports "gum disease"*
　c) Nonvital teeth _____
　d) Other _____

Discussion: This is a typical history for a patient you will see. It points out the amount of historical information that can be derived from a patient in a short period of time.

4.

PAST MEDICAL FACTORS THAT WOULD COMPROMISE HOST DEFENSES

Specific Medical Factors

Yes　No

☒　☐　Disease process(es) *RHD, asthma*　　Effect *requires premedication, ↑stress risk*

☒　☐　Medication(s) *corticosteroids, tetracycline*　Effect *immunosuppresion, altered flora*

☒　☐　Allergies *penicillin*

☒　☐　Recent antibiotic therapy. Drug *tetracycline*　　Dosage *250 mg/day*　　How long ago _____

☐　☒　Radiation therapy _____

Course of Action: Collect more data. See Unit II for clinical data collection.

*Discussion: This patient's medical history places him in the moderate to serious medical risk category. His **history of rheumatic heart disease** necessitates antibiotic premedication (with erythromycin due to his **allergy to penicillin**). His tetracycline treatment to control acne may have altered normal oral flora and established a tetracycline resistant flora. Corticosteroid therapy often results in suppressed adrenocortex activity and decreased immunological competence. Prior to treatment you should question his physician about the need for altering the steroid dosage. The patient's asthma also increases his risk status. Stress may precipitate an acute attack. All three factors above require closer monitoring of the patient during treatment. Either his asthma or corticosteroid therapy could result in emergency problems for the patient — either respiratory obstruction or shock — and you must be prepared to treat these problems if you do not elect to refer the patient to a specialist for treatment.*

5.

General Factors Predisposing to Infections

☒　☐　Age *67* years . . . . ☐ Age related factors present _____

☒　☐　Nutritional status . . . ☐ Adequate　☒ Inadequate: ☐ Protein & Caloric　☐ Fluids　☐ Vitamins & minerals

☒　☐　Alcohol consumption　☐ Non-user　☐ Low withdrawal potential　☒ High withdrawal potential

☐　☐　Drug abuse . . . . Drug(s) _____　Dosage _____　Duration _____　☐ Low Risk　☒ High Risk

☒　☐　Psychological status . ☐ Favorable　☒ Unfavorable: Why? _____

☒　☐　Family & social status　☐ Favorable　☒ Unfavorable: Why? _____

Course of Action: *Based upon this data, patient is a serious medical risk, especially considering that the problem involves his eye. Referral to a specialist and hospitalization is essential at this time.*

Discussion: *This patient has several predisposing factors which contribute to the seriousness of his problem. His age (67) coupled with chronic alcoholism should make you extremely suspicious that this infection may develop serious complications due to the patient's debilitated state of health. Also, his psychological status or possible delirium tremors (D.T.s) must be considered.*

UNIT II — CLINICAL DATA
CLINICAL SIGNS & SYMPTOMS

OVERVIEW AND OBJECTIVES

As a result of a detailed clinical examination, you will be able to collect essential information as to the clinical signs of the disease process. This information will allow you to assess the seriousness of the disease process affecting your patient.

This unit deals with an evaluation of your patient's general signs, vital signs, head and neck examination, signs of inflammation, and any local signs of factors predisposing to infections. Subsequent units will deal with the anatomic location of the problem, radiographic data, and laboratory data. Following completion of this unit you will:

1. Name five (5) serious general signs that are indicative of a **serious life-threatening problem** requiring immediate action.
2. Describe the typical signs of a patient who appears **toxic.**
3. Describe your course of action if your patient shows signs of **respiratory difficulty.**
4. Given a description of a patient's signs, identify any signs which may indicate a **central nervous system** involvement and describe your course of action if CNS involvement is suspected.
5. Given a description of a patient's signs, identify any signs which may indicate a **dehydration** problem and describe your course of action when a serious problem is discovered.
6. Describe four (4) major reasons why a patient with a serious odontogenic infection may become dehydrated.
7. Given a description of a patient's signs, identify any signs which may be associated with a long-term **inadequate diet.**
8. Name five (5) patient population groups which frequently exhibit signs of inadequate diet.
9. Describe why a patient undergoing an active weight-loss program who develops an infection should be carefully examined.
10. Given a description of a patient's **vital signs,** identify data indicative of an infection and also identify and describe any vital signs data which indicates the need for immediate hospital referral.
11. Given data from a clinical examination for signs of inflammation, complete the checklist to summarize the results.
12. Given a description of a patient's clinical signs, identify any **local factors which would predispose to infection.**

UNIT II
CLINICAL DATA
CLINICAL SIGNS & SYMPTOMS

Introduction
Serious General Signs
  Toxic Appearance
  Respiratory Difficulty
  CNS Changes
  Dehydration
  Inadequate Diet

Vital Signs
  Body Temperature
  Blood Pressure
  Pulse Rate
  Respiration
Signs of Inflammation
  Swelling
  Pain and Tenderness

Increased Temperature
Redness
Loss of Function
Local Predisposing Signs
  Recent Local Trauma
  Associated Oral
    Disease
  Altered Vascularity

The collection of **clinical data** includes collection of **specific patient signs and symptoms** and of **specific anatomical factors.** Because of the broad scope of material contained in this section we have divided **clinical data** into two units.

        Unit II — Clinical Signs & Symptoms
        Unit III — Anatomical Factors

INTRODUCTION

The collection of **clinical data** involves the collection of information by **inspection, palpation, percussion** or **auscultation.** This data is termed the **clinical signs** as opposed to data obtained by questioning your patient, which is termed the **patient's symptoms.** In this unit we will discuss the categories summarized on the checklist below. This checklist represents the major factors you should evaluate during your clinical examination of a patient with an oral and/or maxillofacial swelling.

CLINICAL DATA

SERIOUS GENERAL SIGNS   Degree of Severity & Course of Action

Yes No
☐ ☐ **Toxic Appearance** ..... _____
☐ ☐ **Respiratory Difficulty** .. _____
☐ ☐ **CNS Changes** .... _____
☐ ☐ **Dehydration** .... _____
☐ ☐ **Inadequate Diet** .... _____

VITAL SIGNS

Temp _____°F _____°C B.P. ___/___/___ mm Hg Describe Abnormality(ies)_____
Pulse Rate _____ beats/min Resp. Rate _____ cycles/min _____

SIGNS OF INFLAMMATION

Yes No
☐ ☐ **Swelling** (see details in Anatomic Areas involved)   Additional characteristics
      ☐ Intraoral size _____ ☐ Generalized ☐ Non-fluctuant _____
      ☐ Extraoral size _____ ☐ Localized ☐ Fluctuant _____
☐ ☐ **Increased Temperature of Involved Area** _____
☐ ☐ **Pain & Tenderness** .... ☐ Generalized ☐ Localized Where? _____
☐ ☐ **Redness** .... ☐ Intraoral ☐ Extraoral
                         ☐ Red ☐ Reddish purple ☐ Purple _____
☐ ☐ **Loss of Function**
      ☐ Trismus .... ☐ Slight ☐ Moderate ☐ Severe _____
      ☐ Dysphagia .... ☐ Slight ☐ Moderate ☐ Severe _____
      ☐ Respiratory Difficulty . ☐ Slight ☐ Moderate ☐ Severe _____

LOCAL PREDISPOSING SIGNS

☐ ☐ Recent Local Trauma .... ☐ Accidental injury ☐ Surgical trauma ☐ Other _____
☐ ☐ Associated Oral Diseases ☐ Caries ☐ Periodontal disease ☐ Non-vital teeth_____
☐ ☐ Altered vascularity .... ☐ Reduced vascularity ☐ Increased vascularity ☐ Radiation therapy

SERIOUS GENERAL SIGNS

The **first step** in your clinical examination should be an examination for signs of serious general problems, thus allowing you to quickly evaluate how sick your patient is. This evaluation can be of great help in deciding whether or not to refer your patient to a specialist or hospital at this time. These signs include:

SERIOUS GENERAL SIGNS   Degree of Severity & Course of Action

Yes No
☐ ☐ Toxic Appearance ..... _____
☐ ☐ Respiratory Difficulty .. _____
☐ ☐ CNS Changes .... _____
☐ ☐ Dehydration........... _____
☐ ☐ Inadequate Diet .... _____

☐ ☐ **Toxic Appearance**

A patient with a significant odontogenic infection may have a toxic appearance which means the systemic effects of the infectious process can be observed in the general appearance of the patient. The following signs might contribute to the toxic appearance.

- **Paleness**
- **Rapid respirations**
- **Rapid, thready pulse**
- **Fever**
- **Appears ill**
- **Shivering** — chills
- **Lethargic** — no energy
- **Diaphoretic** — cold clammy sweat

Figure II-1B shows a clinical example of a patient with a severe toxic appearance. Systemic toxicity developed as a result of a submandibular space infection as shown in **Figure II-1A**. In **Figure II-1C** toxicity has been controlled. This patient appears very ill in **B**. You can also notice the striking differences in patient appearance between **B** and **C** once systemic toxicity has been controlled.

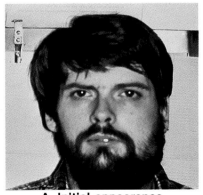   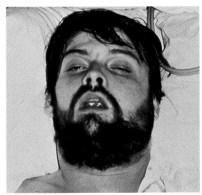   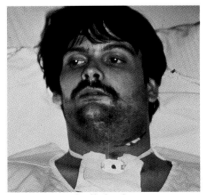

A. Initial appearance   B. Severe toxic appearance   C. Improved clinical appearance

Figure II-1. The appearance of systemic toxicity. A. Patient with serious submandibular space and lateral pharyngeal space infection. B. Same patient with systemic toxic shock. C. Resolution of toxic shock following drainage and antibiotic therapy.

While there are varying degrees of a toxic appearance, no definite rules can be stated to separate the degrees of toxicity. You will be better able to determine the significance of a toxic appearance as you gain clinical experience in the management of toxic patients.

NOTE: If your patient "looks really sick," then he/she probably is and immediate referral is indicated.

☐ ☐ Respiratory Difficulty

Upper respiratory difficulty may progress slowly or rapidly from partial to complete obstruction of the airway. In early stages a patient may experience mild difficulty in breathing, which may increase until the patient postures his head forward (a sniffing position) and uses the accessory muscles in the neck and thorax to maintain adequate respiratory exchange. In later stages **respiratory stridor** (a high pitched noisy respiratory sound like the blowing of the wind) usually occurs just prior to complete upper airway obstruction. Paradoxical breathing or "rocking chair" breathing also accompanies upper airway difficulty. **Immediate coniotomy** followed by intubation or **immediate coniotomy** followed by tracheotomy under hospital operating room conditions may be required for patients with serious respiratory difficulties.

NOTE: Any respiratory difficulty must be viewed as a serious sign and IMMEDIATE HOSPITAL REFERRAL IS NECESSARY.

☐ ☐ C.N.S. Changes

Any significant change in the central nervous system during a suspected infection is **great cause for concern and requires immediate hospitalization** of the patient. The following signs represent significant C.N.S. signs. You will notice that most of the C.N.S. changes are eye signs. The eyes develop embryonically as a direct extension of the brain, thus it is not surprising to find that changes in the central nervous system are frequently reflected as alterations in eye function.

- **Decreased level of consciousness** — Lethargy; somnolence; semi-comatose; comatose; death
- **Meningeal irritation** — Intense headache, stiff neck, vomiting
- **Edema of eyelids**
- **Abnormal eye signs** — These signs usually occur late and indicate serious CNS involvement.
  Dilated pupils
  Exophthalmos — Protrusion of the eyeballs
  Pulsating exophthalmos
  Ophthalmoplegia — Paralysis of one or more of the motor nerves of the eye
  Papilledema — Edema of the optic disc
  Abducens nerve paralysis — Causes lateral rectus paralysis with inability to laterally rotate the eye
  Edematous subconjunctiva — Fluid collection in the conjunctival tissues of the eyes
  Retinal hemorrhages — Hemorrhages in the retina of the eye
  Photophobia — Abnormal sensitivity of the eyes to light
  Lacrimation — Tearing of the eyes
  Alteration of eye reflexes

NOTE: Many of the above C.N.S. changes require diagnostic techniques that are not usually taught in dental school programs and require advanced hospital-based training. If you suspect any of these signs are involved, you should quickly refer your patient to someone qualified to make these judgments.

☐ ☐ Dehydration

The decrease in fluid and/or resultant altered electrolyte balance in a patient is **a serious problem which requires rapid treatment.** The following signs may be present in a patient with excessive loss of water and/or sodium.

- **Postural hypotension**
- **Thirst**
- **Dryness of mucous membranes**
- **Fever**
- **Loss of skin turgor**

- **Soft eyeballs**
- **Shrunken drawn face**
- **Weakness**
- **Oliguria** — Decreased urine output
- **Serum electrolyte changes**

A patient with a serious oral and/or maxillofacial infection may become dehydrated as a consequence of the following signs and symptoms:

- **Lethargy**
- **Pain on swallowing**
- **Severe weakness**
- **Generalized inability to maintain his own needs**

If any of these signs are present, your patient may need to be hospitalized for intravenous administration of fluids and restoration of electrolyte balance.

☐ ☐ Inadequate Diet

If inadequate food intake is a short-term problem, usually no physical signs may be discovered and the only evidence of inadequate diet will come from the patient's own description as discussed in Unit I. You should, however, review this factor during your clinical examination. Short periods of inadequate food intake may not have serious consequences. However, the ketoacidosis from fasting may combine with the toxic acidosis from an infectious process to impair the patient's electrolyte balance. **This could be a significant factor for any patient who develops an oral and/or maxillofacial infection while undergoing an active weight-loss program.**

SIGNS OF LONG-TERM STARVATION

- **Continued weight loss**
- **Muscle wasting**
- **Signs of multiple vitamin deficiency**
- **Edema of ankles and feet**
- **Hair may be dry, sparse, brittle**
- **Lethargy**
- **Swollen abdomen**

CONDITIONS PREDISPOSING TO LONG-TERM STARVATION

- **Chronic alcoholism**
- **Drug addiction**
- **Elderly patients receiving inadequate care**
- **Very low income**
- **Transients**
- **Anorexia nervosa**

In many parts of the world, severe malnutrition is a major problem and must always be considered in the management of infections.

Once you have evaluated **serious general signs** you should record this information on the following checklist. You may also wish to comment on the significance of any serious general sign on the overall management of your patient.

SERIOUS GENERAL SIGNS   Degree of Severity & Course of Action

Yes No
☐ ☐ Toxic Appearance ..... _____
☐ ☐ Respiratory Difficulty .. _____
☐ ☐ CNS Changes .... _____
☐ ☐ Dehydration .... _____
☐ ☐ Inadequate Diet .... _____

STUDY EXERCISES

1. *The first step in your clinical examination is to examine your patient for any* ____ __general__ *problems. This should involve evaluation for:* 1) ~~toxic appearance~~ 2) ~~resp. difficulty~~ 3) ~~CNS~~ 4) ~~dehydration~~ 5) ~~inadequate diet~~

2. *If your patient "looks sick" then he/she probably* __is__ *. This appearance can be a serious general sign and requires* __immediate attention__ *.*

3. *If a patient with a mandibular swelling appears to have forced breathing and must lean forward to breathe, then these signs could be serious general signs of* __resp__ __difficulty__ *.*

4. *If a patient has dry mucous membrane, loss of skin turgor, is weak and has postural hypotension, then he/she may be suffering from serious* _dehydration_ .

5. *If an elderly, low-income, alcoholic patient shows signs of muscle wasting, weight loss, swelling of ankles and feet, he/she may be suffering from long-term* _starvation_ _____ .

6. *If a patient presents to you with signs of edema of eyeballs, severe lethargy, inability to rotate his eyeballs, he may be suffering from* _central_ _nervous_ _system_ *changes.*

7. *For conditions 2-6 above, what is the appropriate course of management as soon as you detect these problems?* _hospitalization_ _____

Complete the clinical data checklist *for the following cases and indicate the appropriate course of action:*

Case #1 — *Historical data indicates that a healthy 26-year-old male has symptoms associated with infraorbital swelling. During your clinical examination for serious general signs you find the patient: looks pale, has a high fever with chills (shivering) and then cold sweats. Patient is also thirsty and his mucous membranes are dry.*

SERIOUS GENERAL SIGNS   Degree of Severity & Course of Action

Yes No
☒ ☐ **Toxic Appearance** . . . . .   _____
☐ ☒ **Respiratory Difficulty** . .   _____
☐ ☒ **CNS Changes** . . . .   _____
☒ ☐ **Dehydration** . . . .   _____
☐ ☒ **Inadequate Diet** . . . .   _____

Case #2 — *Historical data indicates this 39-year-old male has symptoms associated with a mandibular swelling extending into the neck area on both sides. When evaluating* **serious general signs** *you find this patient has slight difficulty in breathing and swallowing; however, the patient says this has happened before when he had an infection around a partially erupted wisdom tooth.*

SERIOUS GENERAL SIGNS   Degree of Severity & Course of Action

Yes No
☐ ☒ **Toxic Appearance** . . . . .   _____
☒ ☐ **Respiratory Difficulty** . .   _____
☐ ☒ **CNS Changes** . . . .   _____
☐ ☒ **Dehydration** . . . .   _____
☐ ☒ **Inadequate Diet** . . . .   _____

Discussion of Cases

Case #1. *In this case, signs of* **systemic toxicity** *and* **dehydration** *are present. The combination of high fever with chills, pale appearance, and dry mucous membranes indicates serious systemic* **toxicity** *and* **dehydration. Hospital referral should be made immediately.**

Case #2. *In this case, signs of* **respiratory obstruction** *are present in combination with bilateral neck swelling. The patient may not be aware of the seriousness of these findings; thus you must impress upon him the seriousness of his problem.* **Immediate hospital referral is imperative.**

VITAL SIGNS

Measurement of your patient's vital signs is essential for determining the patient's physiological response to a pathological process. **The greater the effect of the infection on a patient's vital signs the more serious is the infection.** Vital signs which should be evaluated include:

- ☐ **Body temperature**
- ☐ **Blood pressure**
- ☐ **Pulse rate**
- ☐ **Respiration**

☐ **Body Temperature**

An elevation in body temperature is a highly predictable sign of acute infections. However, chronic or very minor infections may not cause an elevation in body temperature. Moderate to severe infections always produce an elevated temperature. A temperature increase above 99.5°F (37.5°C) usually indicates infection. If a patient's temperature is above 38.5°C you should consider taking a blood culture during this period of pyrexia. This degree of temperature elevation often indicates septicemia. Extremely high temperatures (greater than 41°C) in adults may lead to irreversible hyperthermia and thus require immediate hospitalization.

The term **fever** (pyrexia) describes a body temperature above the range of normal. The term **hyperthermia** is reserved for body temperatures equal to or greater than 41°C (105.8°F). Above this temperature the body's heat-regulating mechanisms are ineffective and the body temperature will continue to rise unless controlled by artificial means. The term **hypothermia** describes a body temperature that is below the range of normal. **Table II-1** summarizes the terminology used to describe body temperature.

TERMS	DEGREES CELSIUS	DEGREES FAHRENHEIT
Hyperthermic	Above 41.	Above 105.8
Pyrexic	37.6 to 41.	99.6 to 105.8
Normal Range	35.5 to 37.5	96. to 99.5
Hypothermic	Below 35.5	Below 96.

Table II-1. Terminology used to describe body temperature.

NOTE: **When measuring a patient's vital signs you should NOT be tempted to diagnose the patient's problem with vital signs data alone. You must consider all other data before diagnosing the problem.**

☐ **Blood Pressure**

In general, a patient's blood pressure may show minor to no change during localized infections. However, **a patient in septic shock or with septicemia may show a significant decrease in blood pressure** due to:

- • **Shock**
- • **Decreased blood volume**
- • **Vasodilatation**
- • **Decreased blood pressure may also be associated with severe dehydration, especially when postural hypotension is present.**

In this book, we will use the three-number blood pressure record system currently recommended by the American Heart Association. The **first number** is the systolic pressure. The **second number** is the pressure at which the heart sounds begin to diminish (phase 4 diastolic). The **third number** is the pressure at which the last sound is heard (phase 5 diastolic).

☐ **Pulse Rate**

The **pulse rate usually rises** as part of the normal physiologic response to infection and shock. In a toxic patient or a patient in septic shock, the pulse may be both **rapid** and **weak** (thready). Increased heart rate follows a rise in body temperature. When a fever is not accompanied by increased heart rate, the temperature increase may be artificial (e.g., patient just exercised or drank hot liquids).

☐ Respiration

Evaluation of respiration involves analysis of the following characteristics:

- **Rate**
- **Rhythm**
- **Depth**

NOTE: If any difficulty in breathing is observed in a patient with an infection involving the head and neck, the patient should be hospitalized IMMEDIATELY.

In general, the rate of respiration increases during a mild to moderate infection. The depth and rhythm will usually be normal.

NOTE: In a toxic patient respiration may become rapid and shallow. There may even be disturbances in the normal rhythm.

Table II-2 summarizes changes in adult vital signs which accompany oral and/or maxillofacial infections. You will note that **significant changes can occur** and **immediate** hospital referral is necessary. While you will rarely see patients with serious problems in your dental office, their problems may rapidly progress to this degree after leaving your office.

SIGN	NORMAL RANGE	MILD TO MODERATE INFECTION	OF EXTREME SIGNIFICANCE
TEMPERATURE	35.5-37.5°C 96.-99.5°F	> 37.5°C > 99.5°F	**> 41°C, > 105.8°F Hyperthermia — Acute medical emergency**
BLOOD PRESSURE	Systolic 120 to 140 mm Hg Diastolic 60 to 90 mm Hg	Usually little to no change	**Significant decrease may indicate systemic shock. Hospitalize immediately.**
PULSE RATE	60-80 beats/min.	90-100 beats/min. Increases but strong	**> 100 beats/min. Increased & weak pulse signifies toxic or septic shock — HOSPITALIZE IMMEDIATELY**
RESPIRATION Airway	Clear	Clear	**OBSTRUCTION — Hospitalize immediately — May need coniotomy or tracheotomy NOW!**
Rate	12-18 cycles/min.	18-20 cycles/min. Slight increase	**> 22 cycles/min. If rate increases with shallow depth and even irregular rhythm, a toxic condition may be present. Refer to hospital immediately.**
Rhythm	Regular	No change	
Depth	Normal	No change	

Table II-2. Summary of changes in adult vital signs occurring in a patient with an odontogenic infection. Numerical values listed are intended as general guidelines and are not necessarily absolute.

You should record your patient's vital signs on the checklist in the space provided and comment on the significance of any abnormal values in the space provided.

VITAL SIGNS

Temp _____°F _____°C   B.P. ___ / ___ / ___ mm Hg   Describe Abnormality(ies) _____

Pulse Rate _____ beats/min   Resp. Rate _____ cycles/min   _____

STUDY EXERCISES

Vital signs that should be routinely measured when evaluating a patient with an oral and/or maxillofacial swelling are:

a. *bp*

b. *resp*

c. *temp*

d. *pulse*

A highly predictable sign of moderate to serious acute infections is elevation of body *temp* *. Mild to moderate infections (may/may not)* *may not* *cause an increase in temperature. Patients with* **body temperatures** *above* *41* *°C or* *105.8* *°F are considered hyperthermic and thus should be referred to a* *hospital* *immediately.*

A patient's **blood pressure** *usually shows* *minor* *to* *no* *change during localized infections. However, blood pressure may significantly* *decrease* *in patients with septic* *shock* *or* *septicemia* *.*

The **pulse rate** *usually* *increases* *as part of the physiological response to infection and shock. In toxic patients or patients with acute septicemia, the pulse rate may be both* *rapid* *and* *weak* *.*

In mild to moderate infections, **respiratory rate** *(increases/decreases/is unchanged)* *increase* *while the depth and rhythm will usually be* *remain the same* *. In toxic patients respiration may become* *rapid* *and* *shallow* *. In addition, the rhythm may become* *irregular* *.*

Indicate which set(s) of vital signs data indicate presence of a problem and which set(s) indicate conditions requiring **immediate hospital referral.**

1. Temp _____°F ___39.4___°C   B.P. ___150/85/83___ mm Hg   Describe Abnormality(ies) _____
   Pulse Rate ___90___ beats/min   Resp. Rate ___22___ cycles/min   *ok*

2. Temp _____°F ___41.8___°C   B.P. ___160/82/80___ mm Hg   Describe Abnormality(ies) _____
   Pulse Rate ___100___ beats/min   Resp. Rate ___26___ cycles/min

3. Temp ___103.5___°F _____°C   B.P. ___140/70/70___ mm Hg   Describe Abnormality(ies) _____
   Pulse Rate ___80___ beats/min   Resp. Rate ___20___ cycles/min   *ok*

SIGNS OF INFLAMMATION

Inflammation is one of the significant signs used in diagnosing infections. Classically there are five primary signs of inflammation as summarized on the following checklist.

SIGNS OF INFLAMMATION

Yes	No				Additional characteristics
☐	☐	**Swelling** (see details in Anatomic Areas involved)			
		☐ Intraoral size _____	☐ Generalized	☐ Non-fluctuant	_____
		☐ Extraoral size _____	☐ Localized	☐ Fluctuant	_____
☐	☐	**Increased Temperature of Involved Area** _____			
☐	☐	**Pain & Tenderness**	☐ Generalized	☐ Localized	Where? _____
☐	☐	**Redness**	☐ Intraoral	☐ Extraoral	_____
			☐ Red	☐ Reddish purple	☐ Purple _____
☐	☐	**Loss of Function**			
		☐ Trismus	☐ Slight	☐ Moderate	☐ Severe _____
		☐ Dysphagia	☐ Slight	☐ Moderate	☐ Severe _____
		☐ Respiratory Difficulty .	☐ Slight	☐ Moderate	☐ Severe _____

☐ ☐ **Swelling**

You should identify and record the **size,** the anatomical **location of any swelling,** and whether it is **intraoral** and/or **extraoral.** You can also determine whether the swelling is **generalized** or **localized.** You may also be able to tell if the swelling is:

• **fluctuant** — swellings filled with fluid such as blood or suppuration
• **non-fluctuant** — swellings having a wide range of descriptive characteristics such as firm, indurated, boardlike, phlegmonous, etc.

The characteristics of a swelling can be very important to the diagnosis of non-infectious processes as well as non-odontogenic and odontogenic infections.

☐ ☐ **Pain and Tenderness**

Pain is a symptom which your patients will describe. **Tenderness is a sign** in which pain is elicited by the clinician usually BY PALPATION. Palpation to determine the areas of tenderness can help you in identifying the extent of involvement.

Pain and tenderness always accompany minor as well as major infections. **There is no direct relationship between the degree of pain and the seriousness of the infection.** The magnitude and severity of pain and tenderness will depend upon multiple factors including the anatomic location, amount of sensory nerve endings in the involved area, the patient's psychological state and others.

☐ ☐ **Increased Temperature**
☐ ☐ **Redness**

Swellings associated with most **acute infections** will show an elevated temperature compared with adjacent, unaffected areas when palpated. These swellings may also appear red or reddish-purple due to increased vascularity in the area of involvement.

Swellings associated with **subacute** or **chronic infections** may not exhibit an increase in temperature. **Chronic infections** appear more reddish-purple to purple in color. The depth of a swelling will influence your ability to detect changes in temperature and color. If an infection is near the surface (mucosa or skin), these signs will be more evident than if it is located deeper in tissues. Frequently, deeper swellings are more difficult to diagnose and may require additional data to establish an accurate diagnosis.

NOTE: **Beware of any swellings that lack signs of inflammation. These swellings may be of non-infectious origin. You should record the color and temperature characteristics of any swelling, especially if the swelling does not exhibit other signs of inflammation.**

☐ ☐ **Loss of Function**

Loss of function is frequently associated with inflammation. The following signs and symptoms are frequently associated with infections of the head and neck area.

☐ **Trismus**

Trismus is a sign of decreased ability to fully open the mouth. In severe infections involving the floor of the mouth, neck and muscles of mastication, the trismus may be so severe that a patient may be unable to open his/her mouth more than a centimeter. Severe trismus can reduce the patient's ability to eat properly. More significantly, trismus can greatly impede your ability to perform an intraoral examination or obtain intraoral radiographs. **Mild** — "hurts when opening mouth." **Moderate** — "noticeable decrease in mouth opening." **Severe** — "very little opening possible."

☐ **Dysphagia**

Difficulty in swallowing may develop with moderate to severe infections in the floor of the mouth and neck. Signs of dysphagia may include **drooling** and **inability to swallow** food or fluids. **These signs are danger signs and indicate the need for immediate hospitalization. Mild** — "hurts when swallowing." **Moderate** — "hurts when swallowing, but can eat small amounts." **Severe** — "can't swallow."

☐ **Respiratory Difficulty**

Any patient who shows **any difficulty in breathing or signs of respiratory obstruction requires immediate hospitalization.**

STUDY EXERCISES

The five (5) **classic signs of inflammation** *are:*
a. _redness_   c. _swelling_   e. _↓ function_
b. _pain_   d. _incr temp_

Fluctuant swellings *are those filled with* _blood_ *or* _suppuration_ .
Non-fluctuant swellings *are swellings which are* _firm_ .

Increased temperature *of a swelling is usually associated with* _acute_
infections while _chronic_ *or* _subacute_ *infections may show
no detectable increase in temperature.*

Most **acute infections** *will appear* _red_ *to* _red purple_ *in color while* **chronic**
infections *will often appear more* _red_ - _purple_ *to* _purple_ *in color.
Observable color changes are influenced by the amount of* _depth_
overlying the problem.

The **loss of function** *factors frequently associated with head and neck infections include:*
1) _trismus_   2) _dysphagia_   3) _resp. difficulty_ .

Trismus *is the term used to describe a patient's inability to* _open_ *his/her* _mouth_ .
Trismus can reduce: **1)** *patient's ability to* _open_ *properly and* **2)** *impede your access
to perform an* _intra oral_ *examination and obtain* _intra oral_ *radiographs.*
Dysphagia *is the term used to describe a* **difficulty in swallowing.** *Typical signs
include* _drooling_ *and inability to* _swallow_ *food or liquids. These signs are*
serious signs *and necessitate immediate* _hospital_ *referral.*

Any **respiratory difficulty** *should be viewed as a serious sign requiring immediate*
hospital _referral_ .

LOCAL PREDISPOSING SIGNS

Your clinical examination should also include evaluation of any **local predisposing signs** that may contribute to or actually cause a disease process. Periodontal disease, caries or associated oral diseases should be identified. Trauma to tissues and necrotic or avascular tissues may be viewed as directly or indirectly contributing to the infectious process. This data should be recorded on the checklist in the space provided.

LOCAL PREDISPOSING SIGNS

☐ ☑	Recent Local Trauma	☐ Accidental injury	☐ Surgical trauma	☐ Other _____
☐ ☑	Associated Oral Diseases	☐ Caries	☐ Periodontal disease	☐ Non-vital teeth _____
☐ ☑	Altered vascularity	☐ Reduced vascularity	☐ Increased vascularity	☑ Radiation therapy

☐ ☐ Recent Local Trauma

Recent local trauma can cause intra- or extra-oral swellings. The two most common causes of traumatic swellings are **accidental injury** and **surgical trauma.** When there is a history of such trauma, there may also be foreign bodies present (splinters, glass fragments, retained sutures, root tips, surgical debris, etc.) which may contribute to infectious swelling.

However, both **infectious** and **non-infectious** swellings can also result from trauma associated with dental procedures, including: injection of local anesthetics, injury from dental appliances, placement of retraction cord and impression procedures, subgingival procedures, and endodontic treatment.

☐ ☐ Associated Oral Diseases

Associated oral diseases, primarily **caries** and **periodontal** disease frequently predispose a patient to odontogenic infections. In your examination procedure you should identify any teeth with extensive caries and perform vitality tests. Occasionally you will discover a non-vital tooth that appears clinically normal. Other causes of pulpal necrosis include recently placed restorations, accidental injury, traumatic occlusion and others. A complete discussion of all causes of pulpal death is beyond the scope of this book.

The presence of periodontal disease can also predispose to the development of perio-dontal abscesses. Closely related to periodontal disease is inflammation in the pericoro-nal sulcus of partially erupted mandibular third molars.

☐ ☐ **Altered Vascularity**

Localized areas of tissue with an **inadequate blood supply** can result from previous use of surgical flaps. Infections in areas of reduced blood supply can lead to tissue necrosis. Localized avascularity may also develop during the course of an infection if suppuration is confined to a relatively non-distendable area. This avascularity can lead to tissue necrosis as seen in osteomyelitis and Ludwig's angina.

Localized areas of **increased blood supply** can develop as granulation tissue from wound healing. This tissue is more prone to infection and is more difficult to manage surgically.

Radiation Therapy of the head and neck will alter the health of local tissues such that infection of soft tissue and/or bone is more likely. **You should avoid performing surgical procedures on patients with a past history of radiation therapy without first consulting a specialist in the management of medically compromised patients.**

STUDY EXERCISES

Intra- and extra-oral swellings may be a result of local ___trauma___ *rather than infection.*

Two associated oral diseases which can predispose patients to maxillofacial infections are ___caries___ *and* ___periodontal___ *disease. Pulpal necrosis and subsequent odontogenic infection can result from recently placed* ___restoration___ *, accidental or traumatic* ___injury___ *.*

Altered vascularity resulting from ___periodontal___ *therapy,* ___traumatic___ *injury, improperly designed* ___surgical___ ___flap___ *, or confined* ___suppuration___ *can increase the likelihood of oral and/or maxillofacial infections as well as delaying healing.*

Case: A 19-year-old female presented to another dentist with a large, red, tender swelling of the gingival tissue overlying an impacted lower third molar. This dentist removed the impacted third molar and in so doing severely crushed and tore the tissue overlying the third molar. The patient was displeased with the work by this previous dentist and thus presented to your office. During your clinical examination you observe a swollen, dark purple mass of tissue surrounding the extraction site and the patient complains of pain and trismus.

Complete the following checklist for local predisposing signs for this case.

LOCAL PREDISPOSING SIGNS

☐	☒	Recent Local Trauma	☐ Accidental injury	☒	Surgical trauma	☐	Other _____
☐	☐	Associated Oral Diseases	☐ Caries	☐	Periodontal disease	☐	Non-vital teeth _____
☐	☒	Altered vascularity	☒ Reduced vascularity	☐	Increased vascularity	☐	Radiation therapy

Case Analysis: The following local predisposing signs can be identified:
- *Signs of local trauma from the poor surgical technique.*
- *Altered vascularity as the purple tissue represents an area of lowered blood flow. This traumatized tissue is more susceptible to infection than healthy tissue. In addition, the patient's capacity for tissue healing is reduced. Both of these factors will influence your management of any developing infection and will delay resolution of the problem.*

POST TEST — UNIT II

- Answer each of the following questions.
- Check your answers with the correct responses on page 47.
- If all questions are answered correctly, proceed to Unit III, page 49.
- If you do not answer all questions correctly, read and study the content of this Unit.

QUESTIONS

1. *Name five (5) serious general signs that can be indicative of a serious, life-threatening problem requiring immediate action.*

   a. ↓ resp _____   d. inadequate diet _____

   b. dehydration _____   e. _____

   c. altered CNS _____

2. *From the following list of general signs, check those signs associated with a* **toxic appearance.**

✕ a. appears ill	___ g. dry mucous	___ m. respiratory stridor
✕ b. decreased	membranes	___ n. postural hypotension
consciousness	___ h. loss of skin turgor	___ o. dilated pupils
✕ c. looks pale	✕ i. lethargic	___ p. exophthalmos
___ d. paradoxical breathing	___ j. oliguria	___ q. photophobia
✕ e. rapid respiration	___ k. vomiting	✕ r. tremors
___ f. muscle wasting	✕ l. fever	___ s. edema of eyelids

3. *From the following list of general signs, check those signs associated with a* **respiratory obstruction.**

___ a. appears ill	___ g. dry mucous	✕ m. respiratory stridor
___ b. decreased	membranes	___ n. postural hypotension
consciousness	___ h. loss of skin turgor	___ o. dilated pupils
___ c. looks pale	___ i. lethargic	___ p. exophthalmos
✕ d. paradoxical breathing	___ j. oliguria	___ q. photophobia
___ e. rapid respiration	___ k. vomiting	___ r. tremors
___ f. muscle wasting	___ l. fever	___ s. edema of eyelids

4. *From the following list of general signs, check those signs associated with a* **central nervous system (CNS) involvement.**

✕ a. appears ill	___ g. dry mucous	___ m. respiratory stridor
___ b. decreased	membranes	___ n. postural hypotension
consciousness	___ h. loss of skin turgor	✕ o. dilated pupils
___ c. looks pale	✕ i. lethargic	✕ p. exophthalmos
___ d. paradoxical breathing	___ j. oliguria	✕ q. photophobia
___ e. rapid respiration	___ k. vomiting	___ r. tremors
___ f. muscle wasting	___ l. fever	✕ s. edema of eyelids

5. *From the following list of general signs, check those signs associated with a* **dehydration.**

✕ a. appears ill	✕ g. dry mucous	___ m. respiratory stridor
___ b. decreased	✕ membranes	___ n. postural hypotension
consciousness	✕ h. loss of skin turgor	___ o. dilated pupils
___ c. looks pale	___ i. lethargic	___ p. exophthalmos
___ d. paradoxical breathing	___ j. oliguria	___ q. photophobia
___ e. rapid respiration	___ k. vomiting	___ r. tremors
___ f. muscle wasting	___ l. fever	___ s. edema of eyelids

6. *From the following list of general signs, check those signs associated with a* **long term inadequate diet.**

✕ a. appears ill	___ g. dry mucous	___ m. respiratory stridor
___ b. decreased	membranes	___ n. postural hypotension
consciousness	___ h. loss of skin turgor	___ o. dilated pupils
___ c. looks pale	___ i. lethargic	___ p. exophthalmos
___ d. paradoxical breathing	___ j. oliguria	___ q. photophobia
___ e. rapid respiration	___ k. vomiting	___ r. tremors
✕ f. muscle wasting	___ l. fever	___ s. edema of eyelids

7. Describe four (4) major reasons a patient with a serious odontogenic infection may become dehydrated.

a. *pain swallow*   c. *inability to care for oneself*

b. *lethargy*   d. *weakness*

8. Name four (4) population groups which are likely to have inadequate diets .

a. *elderly*   c. *poor*

b. *transients*   d. *drug addicts*

9. For each of the following sets of vital signs data indicate which sets may indicate the presence of an infection and which sets indicate serious conditions requiring hospital referral.

Temp _____ °F __39.4__ °C   B.P. __150/85/80__ mm Hg   Describe Abnormality(ies) *pyrexic ↑ pulse*

Pulse Rate __90__ beats/min   Resp. Rate __20__ cycles/min   _____

Temp _____ °F __39.7__ °C   B.P. __140/70/65__ mm Hg   Describe Abnormality(ies) *pyrexic*

Pulse Rate __80__ beats/min   Resp. Rate __20__ cycles/min   _____

Temp _____ °F __40__ °C   B.P. __90/50/40__ mm Hg   Describe Abnormality(ies) *pyrexic ↑ pulse ↑ resp*

Pulse Rate __105__ beats/min   Resp. Rate __24__ cycles/min   *↓ bp — septic shock*

10. In the following list of clinical signs select those that are signs of **inflammation:**

_____ a. rapid, shallow breathing   _____ e. polyuria   __✗__ i. redness

__✗__ b. increased temperature   _____ f. dyspnea   __✗__ j. loss of function

_____ c. postural hypotension   __✗__ g. pain   _____ k. vomiting

__✗__ d. swelling   _____ h. exophthalmos   _____ l. scoliosis

11. A 52-year-old male presents to your office with a 4x4 cm swelling below the left angle of the mandible. His vital signs are normal. He reports no pain and it is not tender to palpation. The area feels quite firm to palpation and does not feel warmer than adjacent tissue. There is no color change of the surface tissue. He reports no trismus, breathing or swallowing difficulty. Complete the checklist below.

SIGNS OF INFLAMMATION

✗ ☐ **Swelling** (see details in Anatomic Areas involved)   Additional characteristics

     ☐ Intraoral size_____   ☐ Generalized   ☒ Non-fluctuant _____

     ☒ Extraoral size_____   ☒ Localized   ☐ Fluctuant _____

☐ ☒ **Increased Temperature of Involved Area** _____

☐ ☒ **Tenderness** . . . .   ☐ Generalized   ☐ Localized   Where? _____

☐ ☒ **Redness** . . . .   ☐ Intraoral   ☐ Extraoral

     ☐ Red   ☐ Reddish purple   ☐ Purple _____

☐ ☒ **Loss of Function**

     ☐ Trismus . . . .   ☐ Slight   ☐ Moderate   ☐ Severe _____

     ☐ Dysphagia . . . .   ☐ Slight   ☐ Moderate   ☐ Severe _____

     ☐ Respiratory Difficulty . .   ☐ Slight   ☐ Moderate   ☐ Severe _____

LOCAL PREDISPOSING SIGNS

☐ ☐ Recent Local Trauma . . . . .   ☐ Accidental injury   ☐ Surgical trauma   ☐ Other _____

☐ ☐ Associated Oral Diseases .   ☐ Caries   ☐ Periodontal disease   ☐ Non-vital teeth _____

☐ ☐ Altered vascularity . . . .   ☐ Reduced vascularity   ☐ Increased vascularity   ☐ Radiation therapy

12. *A 27-year-old male presents with a 3x3 cm fluctuant swelling under his tongue. He complains of difficulty swallowing and pain when eating. The mucosa is normal color, and there is slight tenderness to palpation. Complete the checklist below.*

SIGNS OF INFLAMMATION

Yes No

☒ ☐ **Swelling** (see details in Anatomic Areas involved)   Additional characteristics
   ☒ Intraoral   size _____   ☐ Generalized   ☐ Non-fluctuant   _____
   ☐ Extraoral   size _____   ☒ Localized   ☒ Fluctuant   _____

☐ ☐ **Increased Temperature of Involved Area** _____
☒ ☐ **Pain & Tenderness** ....   ☐ Generalized   ☒ Localized   Where? _____
☐ ☒ **Redness** ....   ☐ Intraoral   ☐ Extraoral   _____
                      ☐ Red   ☐ Reddish purple   ☐ Purple
☒ ☐ **Loss of Function**
   ☐ Trismus ....   ☐ Slight   ☐ Moderate   ☐ Severe   _____
   ☒ Dysphagia ....   ☐ Slight   ☐ Moderate   ☐ Severe   _____
   ☐ Respiratory Difficulty .   ☐ Slight   ☐ Moderate   ☐ Severe   _____

13. *Complete the following portion of the clinical signs checklist and summarize the risk potential for this patient.*

A 69-year-old female presents to your office complaining of pain in her lower left jaw. She lives alone — in her own words, "my husband passed away two months ago and none of my children will take me in." She weighs 90 pounds and reports no alcohol consumption. Her medications include Valium, aspirin q2h for arthritis, and anticoagulants. Her temperature is 38°C (101°F). Blood pressure 170/95/92, and pulse rate is 85. Respiratory rate is 18 cycles/min. She recently received 7000 rads of radiation to her left mandibular region for a malignant neoplasm. Three days ago another dentist attempted to extract the lower left first molar, but was unable to complete the extraction.

The left first molar is severely carious, and the tissue surrounding it is purple with bleeding evident. A 1x1 cm fluctuant swelling is present on the alveolus buccal to this third molar. The swollen area is red, warm and tender when palpated. The patient reports slight pain when she swallows.

VITAL SIGNS

Temp *101* °F *38* °C   B.P. *170/95/92* mm Hg   Describe Abnormality(ies) _____
Pulse Rate *85* beats/min   Resp. Rate *18* cycles/min

SIGNS OF INFLAMMATION

Yes No

☒ ☐ **Swelling** (see details in Anatomic Areas involved)   Additional characteristics
   ☒ Intraoral   size _____   ☐ Generalized   ☐ Non-fluctuant   _____
   ☐ Extraoral   size _____   ☐ Localized   ☒ Fluctuant   _____

☒ ☐ **Increased Temperature of Involved Area** _____
☒ ☐ **Pain & Tenderness** ....   ☐ Generalized   ☒ Localized   Where? _____
☒ ☒ **Redness** ....   ☒ Intraoral   ☐ Extraoral   _____
                      ☐ Red   ☒ Reddish purple   ☐ Purple
☒ ☐ **Loss of Function**
   ☐ Trismus ....   ☐ Slight   ☐ Moderate   ☐ Severe   _____
   ☒ Dysphagia ....   ☒ Slight   ☐ Moderate   ☐ Severe   _____
   ☐ Respiratory Difficulty .   ☐ Slight   ☐ Moderate   ☐ Severe   _____

LOCAL PREDISPOSING SIGNS

☒ ☐ Recent Local Trauma ....   ☐ Accidental injury   ☒ Surgical trauma   ☐ Other _____
☐ ☐ Associated Oral Diseases   ☒ Caries   ☐ Periodontal disease   ☐ Non-vital teeth _____
☐ ☐ Altered vascularity ....   ☐ Reduced   ☐ Increased   ☒ Radiation therapy
                                   vascularity   vascularity

Risk Potential: *high due to rad tx* _____
_____
_____

ANSWERS

1. a. *Respiratory obstruction*   b. *Toxic appearance*   c. *CNS changes*
   d. *Dehydration*   e. *Inadequate diet*

2. **Signs of toxic appearance** *are: a) appears ill; c) looks pale; e) rapid respiration;*
   i) lethargic; l) fever; r) shivering.

3. **Signs of respiratory obstruction** *are: d) paradoxical breathing; m) respiratory stridor.*

4. **Signs of CNS involvement** *are: b) decreased consciousness; i) lethargic; o) dilated*
   pupils; q) photophobia; s) edema of eyelids.

5. **Signs of dehydration** *are: g) dry mucous membranes; h) loss of skin turgor; i) lethargic;*
   j) oliguria; l) fever; n) postural hypotension.

6. **Signs of inadequate diet** *are: f) muscle wasting.*

7. *a) lethargy; b) pain on swallowing; c) weakness; d) generalized inability to maintain*
   their own basic needs.

8. *a) chronic alcoholics; b) drug addicts; c) elderly patients receiving inadequate care;*
   d) very low income persons; e) transients.

9. *Vital signs interpretation:*

Temp _____ °F __39.4__ °C   B.P. __150/85/80__ mm Hg   Describe Abnormality(ies) pyrexic, ↑pulse, ↑resp. rate;
Pulse Rate __90__ beats/min   Resp. Rate __20__ cycles/min   probably moderate infection

Temp _____ °F __39.7__ °C   B.P. __140/70/65__ mm Hg   Describe Abnormality(ies) pyrexic, other vital signs normal;
Pulse Rate __80__ beats/min   Resp. Rate __20__ cycles/min   possibly infection but should evaluate for other causes of temperature elevation.

Temp _____ °F __40__ °C   B.P. __90/50/40__ mm Hg   Describe Abnormality(ies) pyrexic, ↓BP, weak, elevated pulse,
Pulse Rate __105__ beats/min   Resp. Rate __24__ cycles/min   shallow, elevated rate respiration; These are serious vital signs, indicating serious infection, possibly septicemia and/or septic shock.

10. *Signs of inflammation include: b) increased temperature; d) swelling; g) pain; i) redness;*
    j) loss of function

11.

SIGNS OF INFLAMMATION

Yes No

☒ ☐ **Swelling** (see details in Anatomic Areas involved)   Additional characteristics
    ☐ Intraoral   size _____   ☐ Generalized   ☒ Non-fluctuant   _____
    ☒ Extraoral   size 4×4 cm   ☒ Localized   ☐ Fluctuant   _____
☐ ☒ **Increased Temperature of Involved Area** _____
☐ ☒ **Pain & Tenderness** ....   ☐ Generalized   ☐ Localized   Where? _____
☐ ☒ **Redness** ....   ☐ Intraoral   ☐ Extraoral   _____
              ☐ Red   ☐ Reddish purple   ☐ Purple

☐ ☒ **Loss of Function**
    ☐ Trismus ....   ☐ Slight   ☐ Moderate   ☐ Severe   _____
    ☐ Dysphagia ....   ☐ Slight   ☐ Moderate   ☐ Severe   _____
    ☐ Respiratory Difficulty .   ☐ Slight   ☐ Moderate   ☐ Severe   _____

LOCAL PREDISPOSING SIGNS

☐ ☒ Recent Local Trauma ....   ☐ Accidental injury   ☐ Surgical trauma   ☐ Other _____
☐ ☒ Associated Oral Diseases   ☐ Caries   ☐ Periodontal disease   ☐ Non-vital teeth _____
☐ ☒ Altered vascularity ....   ☐ Reduced vascularity   ☐ Increased vascularity   ☐ Radiation therapy

Analysis: *This patient shows only one sign of inflammation (swelling). Some inflammatory signs such as redness and increased temperature may be present but not evident if masked by overlying tissue. In diagnosing his problem you must consider non-inflammatory processes (such as neoplasm).*

12.

SIGNS OF INFLAMMATION

Yes No

☒ ☐ **Swelling** (see details in Anatomic Areas involved)   Additional characteristics
    ☒ Intraoral   size *3×3 cm*   ☐ Generalized   ☐ Non-fluctuant   _____
    ☐ Extraoral   size _____   ☒ Localized   ☒ Fluctuant   _____

☐ ☒ **Increased Temperature of Involved Area** _____

☒ ☐ **Pain & Tenderness** ....   ☐ Generalized   ☒ Localized   Where? *Under tongue when eating*

☐ ☒ **Redness** ....   ☐ Intraoral   ☐ Extraoral   _____
                                  ☐ Red   ☐ Reddish purple   ☐ Purple   _____

☒ ☐ **Loss of Function**
    ☐ Trismus ....   ☐ Slight   ☐ Moderate   ☐ Severe   _____
    ☒ Dysphagia ....   ☒ Slight   ☐ Moderate   ☐ Severe   *associated with eating*
    ☐ Respiratory Difficulty .   ☐ Slight   ☐ Moderate   ☐ Severe   _____

Analysis: *This case includes 3 signs of inflammation but does not present the others. Diagnosis will require more date, but your differential diagnosis must include non-inflammatory causes as well as inflammation. These signs are consistent with blockage of the mandibular salivary gland duct resulting in obstruction of flow and swelling of the gland. If you prematurely assumed this patient had an infection and simply prescribed an antibiotic, you would see no relief of his problem. **This case should be referred to a specialist.***

13.

VITAL SIGNS

Temp _____°F *38* °C   B.P. *170/ 95 /92* mm Hg   Describe Abnormality(ies) *Fever, ↑ BP, ↑ resp.*
Pulse Rate *85* beats/min   Resp. Rate *18* cycles/min   *↑ pulse rate*

SIGNS OF INFLAMMATION

Yes No

☒ ☐ **Swelling** (see details in Anatomic Areas involved)   Additional characteristics
    ☒ Intraoral   size *1×1 CM*   ☐ Generalized   ☐ Non-fluctuant   _____
    ☐ Extraoral   size _____   ☒ Localized   ☒ Fluctuant   _____

☒ ☐ **Increased Temperature of Involved Area** _____

☒ ☐ **Pain & Tenderness** ....   ☐ Generalized   ☐ Localized   Where? *Over swelling on buccal alveolus*

☒ ☐ **Redness** ....   ☒ Intraoral   ☐ Extraoral   _____
                                  ☐ Red   ☒ Reddish purple   ☐ Purple   _____

☒ ☐ **Loss of Function**
    ☐ Trismus ....   ☐ Slight   ☐ Moderate   ☐ Severe   _____
    ☒ Dysphagia ....   ☐ Slight   ☐ Moderate   ☐ Severe   _____
    ☐ Respiratory Difficulty .   ☐ Slight   ☐ Moderate   ☐ Severe   _____

LOCAL PREDISPOSING SIGNS

☒ ☐ Recent Local Trauma ....   ☐ Accidental injury   ☒ Surgical trauma   ☐ Other _____
☒ ☐ Associated Oral Diseases   ☒ Caries   ☐ Periodontal disease   ☐ Non-vital teeth _____
☒ ☐ Altered vascularity ....   ☐ Reduced vascularity   ☐ Increased vascularity   ☒ Radiation therapy

Analysis: *This patient shows many signs of inflammation as well as local predisposing signs. The prior trauma and radiation therapy increase the likelihood of infection due to vascular changes. The risk for osteoradionecrosis is significant following high dose radiation therapy. An infection in this case may spread rapidly into other areas (her dysphagia suggests this has already begun) and the decreased tissue vascularity compromises her capacity to combat the infection. These factors greatly increase her medical risks from this infection and **referral to a specialist for management is appropriate.***

UNIT III
CLINICAL DATA
PART II — ANATOMICAL FACTORS

OVERVIEW & OBJECTIVES

The purpose of this unit is for you to learn or to review the basic structures of the head and neck so as to assess the specific anatomical location of intraoral or extraoral swellings. Common fascial space infections are described, the most common odontogenic sources are illustrated and patterns of spread to other areas identified. This unit also shows you how to record this data on a checklist for summarizing anatomical data. Following completion of this unit you will:

1. Given a description of lymph node swelling or tenderness, identify the specific anatomical group of nodes involved and correctly record this information on the anatomical data checklist.

2. Correctly label the anatomical structures illustrated in all anatomical drawings of the head and neck presented in this unit.

3. Correctly identify the various fascial spaces or potential spaces or anatomical areas from the anatomical drawings of the head and neck presented in this unit.

4. Given a clinical photograph and statement of signs and symptoms, diagram the fascial space(s) involved on the anatomical data checklist and name the space(s) involved.

5. Describe the most frequent origin of odontogenic infections which have spread to the fascial spaces or anatomical areas of the head and neck.

6. Describe the usual pattern(s) for spread of infections to and between the various fascial spaces of the head and neck.

7. Using the criteria presented in this unit, classify the degree of risk (high, moderate, low) associated with infections in any of the facial spaces or anatomical areas of the head and neck.

8. Describe why the degree of risk (high, moderate, low) is assigned to each of the fascial space or anatomical area infections.

9. Given photographs or clinical description of oral or maxillofacial swellings, correctly locate the swelling on the anatomical drawings on the anatomical data checklist and check the appropriate facial space(s) or anatomical area(s) involved in the space provided on this anatomical data checklist.

Unit III
CLINICAL DATA
PART II — ANATOMICAL DATA

Head and Neck Examination
Review of Head & Neck Anatomy
Review of Lymph Nodes and Lymphatic
    Drainage
Review of Fascial Spaces & Areas
Estimating the Degree of Risk for
    Involved Anatomical Areas
Infectious Swellings of the
    Dento-alveolar Ridges
Swellings of and Below the Mandible
    Facial Vestibule of Mandible
    Space of the Body of Mandible
    Mentalis Space
    Submental Space
    Sublingual Space
    Submandibular Space
    Ludwig's Angina
    Summary of the Spread of Infections
        of and Below the Mandible
Swellings of the Cheek and Lateral
    Face
    Buccal Vestibule of Maxilla
    Buccal (Buccinator) Space

Submasseteric Space
Temporal Spaces
Parotid Space
Summary of Infectious Swellings of
    the Lateral Face & Cheek
Swellings of the Pharyngeal Area
    Pterygomandibular Space
    Parapharyngeal Spaces
        Lateral Pharyngeal Space
        Retropharyngeal Space
        Peritonsillar Space
    Summary of Infectious Swellings
        of the Pharyngeal Area
Swellings of the Midface Region
    Palatal Area
    Infraorbital Area (canine fossa)
    Periorbital Area
    Base of the Upper Lip
    Spread to Maxillary Sinuses
    Summary of Spread to Anterior
        Maxillary Areas
Recording Anatomical Data

A thorough examination of the head and neck region should be performed as part of your clinical examination of any oral and/or maxillofacial swelling and the results of your examination recorded. This unit is divided into the following sections to assist you in systematic collection of anatomical data.

- **Head and Neck Examination**
- **Review of Basic Head and Neck Anatomy**
- **Review of Lymph Nodes and Lymphatic Drainage**
- **Review of Fascial Spaces and Anatomical Areas**

HEAD AND NECK EXAMINATION

You should record any general comments resulting from examination of the head and neck in the space provided on the anatomical checklist.

HEAD AND NECK EXAMINATION
    General Comments _____
    _____

REVIEW OF BASIC HEAD AND NECK ANATOMY

The following drawings illustrate the basic anatomical structures of the head and neck as seen from various planes of view. You may find it helpful to orient yourself to these drawings before progressing into the discussion of head and neck infections. Additional drawings from other perspectives will be presented in the discussion of some fascial spaces or anatomical areas; however, in these drawings you should be able to identify the various muscles and bony structures involved from a review of these drawings.

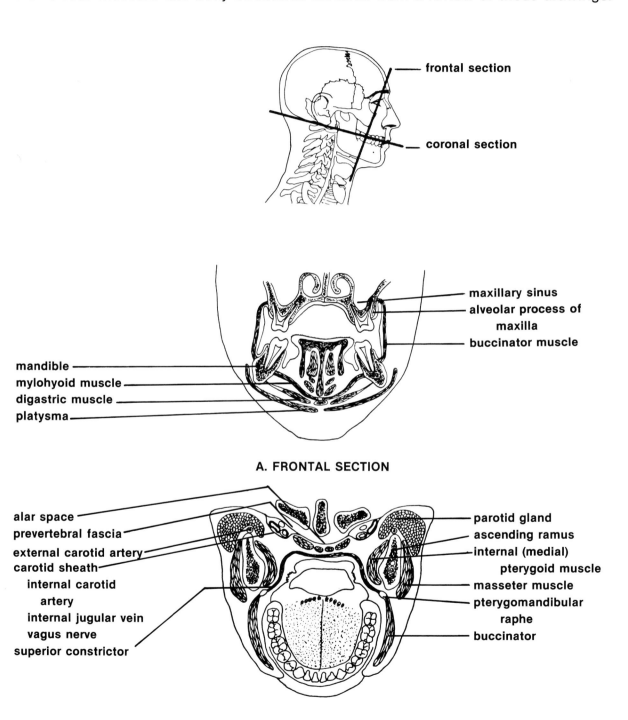

Figure III-1. Review of the basic anatomical structures of the head and neck area. A. Frontal View; section through the first molar area. B. Coronal View; section above the level of the mandibular teeth.

REVIEW OF LYMPH NODES AND LYMPHATIC DRAINAGE

As a part of your clinical examination of the head and neck you should evaluate the condition of regional lymph nodes and record this data on the anatomical data checklist. This information can be extremely important in diagnosing the cause of oral and/or maxillofacial swellings and **determining the degree of regional involvement** of both infectious or non-infectious processes. Major lymph node groups are summarized in **Figure III-2.**

LYMPH NODES & LYMPHATIC DRAINAGE

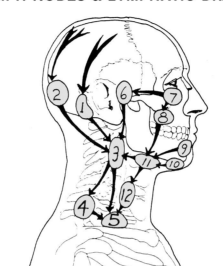

LYMPH NODE GROUPS
1. **Posterior auricular**
2. **Occipital**
3. **Superficial cervical**
4. **Posterior cervical**
5. **Inferior deep cervical**
6. **Anterior auricular**

LYMPH NODE GROUPS
7. **Infraorbital**
8. **Buccal**
9. **Mental**
10. **Submental**
11. **Submandibular**
12. **Jugulo-omohyoid**

Figure III-2. **Major lymph node groups and lymphatic drainage of the head and neck.**

Palpation of lymph nodes may establish the following signs, which should also be recorded on the checklist:
- Tenderness
- Enlargement
- Induration
- Fixation to deeper tissue

If multiple lymph nodes or groups are involved either unilaterally or bilaterally, mark each involved group and describe the specific signs by marking the appropriate location. If multiple lymph node involvement is found, describe the degree of involvement of each group in the space provided.

You should record the data on the following checklist for lymph node involvement by marking the involved area(s) on the drawings and describing the signs of involvement.

LYMPH NODE INVOLVEMENT:

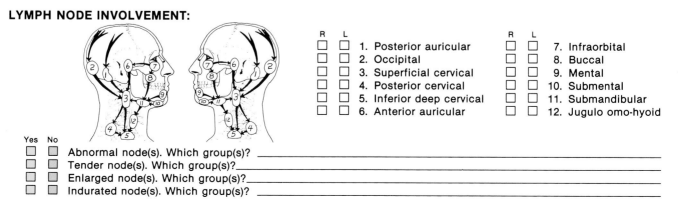

R	L		R	L	
☐	☐	1. Posterior auricular	☐	☐	7. Infraorbital
☐	☐	2. Occipital	☐	☐	8. Buccal
☐	☐	3. Superficial cervical	☐	☐	9. Mental
☐	☐	4. Posterior cervical	☐	☐	10. Submental
☐	☐	5. Inferior deep cervical	☐	☐	11. Submandibular
☐	☐	6. Anterior auricular	☐	☐	12. Jugulo omo-hyoid

Yes No
☐ ☐ Abnormal node(s). Which group(s)? _____
☐ ☐ Tender node(s). Which group(s)?_____
☐ ☐ Enlarged node(s). Which group(s)?_____
☐ ☐ Indurated node(s). Which group(s)? _____

STUDY EXERCISES

Name the areas or structures shown on the following illustrations.

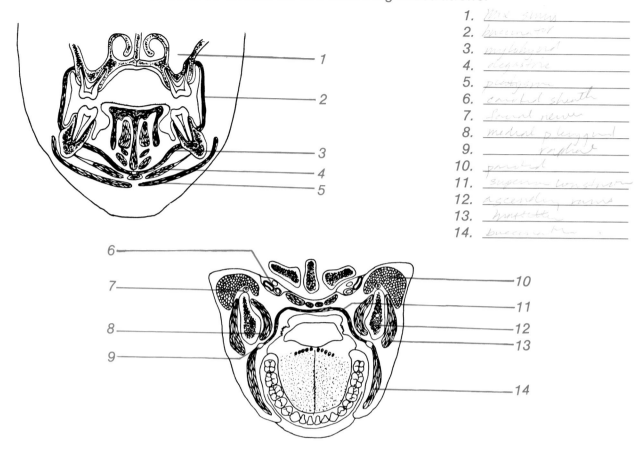

1. _mx. sinus_
2. _buccinator_
3. _mylohyoid_
4. _digastric_
5. _platysma_
6. _carotid sheath_
7. _facial nerve_
8. _medial pterygoid_
9. _raphe_
10. _parotid_
11. _superior constrictor_
12. _ascending ramus_
13. _masseter_
14. _buccinator m._

A patient presents to your office with pain and swelling around her mandibular left third molar. An infection in this tooth could involve which of the following lymph nodes?
  a) submental b) anterior auricular c) submandibular d) superficial cervical e) c and d

Match the number for each lymph node group shown on the illustration with its corresponding name.

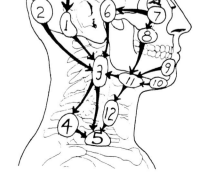

_5_ a. inferior deep cervical
_1_ b. occipital
_2_ c. posterior auricular
_4_ d. posterior cervical
_6_ e. anterior auricular
_3_ f. superficial cervical

_7_ g. mental
_8_ h. buccal
_12_ i. jugulo-omohyoid
_7_ j. infraorbital
_10_ k. submental
_11_ l. submandibular

REVIEW OF FASCIAL SPACES AND ANATOMICAL AREAS OF THE HEAD AND NECK

A clinical examination of the head and neck is necessary to determine the degree of involvement of the fascial spaces and/or anatomical areas. This information is essential to the diagnosis of oral and/or maxillofacial swellings. Whether the swelling is diagnosed as a non-infectious problem or either an odontogenic or non-odontogenic infection, precise data as to the anatomical location of the problem can greatly influence the management of the problem.

NOTE: Throughout this unit we will stress the spread of odontogenic infections to various fascial spaces. However, you should NOT PREMATURELY ASSUME THAT ALL SWELLINGS ARE THE RESULT OF INFECTIOUS PROCESSES ORIGINATING FROM TEETH OR TOOTH-RELATED STRUCTURES.

Infections originating from teeth or tooth-related structures can progress from the dento-alveolar ridges to neighboring anatomical areas, fascial spaces or maxillary sinuses. **The important factor that determines which anatomical structures or areas are affected first is the specific location at which the infective process penetrates the mandible or maxilla in relationship to areas of muscle attachment.** The area or location of swelling often has signs that can guide you to the origin of the problem and help you decide if the problem is or is not tooth related. This information will also be of assistance in identifying the overall degree of seriousness associated with anatomical factors.

In this section of this book we will discuss the location of each of the fascial spaces and anatomical areas of the head and neck, the typical signs and symptoms associated with infections involving these spaces or areas, the probable odontogenic origin of infections of these spaces or areas, and the most common routes of spread to other fascial spaces or anatomical areas. **Figure III-3** illustrates some multiple routes of spread for odontogenic infections.

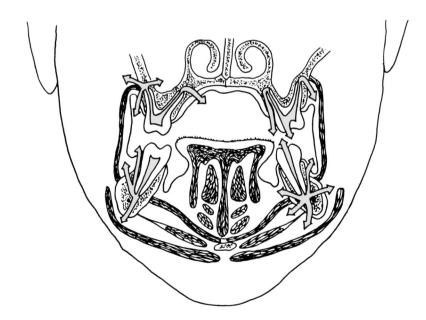

Figure III-3. Spread of odontogenic infections from tooth to surrounding structures and fascial spaces. Once spread has occurred to one fascial space, it may then spread to adjacent spaces unless adequately managed.

For the purpose of this book, we have grouped the various fascial spaces and anatomical areas of the head and neck into the following groups. This grouping is based upon the usual clinical signs associated with each space or area.

SUMMARY OF INVOLVED ANATOMICAL AREAS

Involves dento-alveolar ridges
☐ Maxillary ridge. Where? _____
☐ Mandibular ridge. Where? _____

Mandible & Below
☐ 1 Facial vestibule of mandible
☐ 2 Body of mandible
☐ 3 Mentalis space
☐ 4 Submental space
☐ 5 Sublingual space
☐ 6 Submandibular space

Cheek & Lateral Face
☐ 7 Buccal vestibule of maxilla
☐ 8 Buccal space
☐ 9 Submasseteric space
☐ 10 Deep Temporal space
☐ 10 Superficial Temporal
☐ 11 Infratemporal
☐ 12 Parotid space

Pharyngeal Spaces
☐ 13 Pterygomandibular
☐ 14 Parapharyngeal
   – Lateral pharyngeal
   – Retropharyngeal
☐ 15 Peritonsillar

☐ 16 Cervical Spaces

Mid-face Region
☐ 17 Palatal
☑ 18 Infraorbital
☐ 19 Periorbital
☑ 20 Base of upper lip
☐ 21 Maxillary sinus

You will notice that we have included some spaces which cause internal swelling with others causing external swellings. For example, sublingual space infections usually produce elevation of the tongue and no external swelling but are grouped with infection below the mandible due to the close anatomical relationship between the sublingual space and the submental and submandibular spaces and the frequent spread of infections between these spaces. The numbers next to each space will enable you to clinically identify the location of the swelling and then look up the details of each space in the text of this unit.

ESTIMATING THE DEGREE OF RISK FOR INVOLVED ANATOMICAL AREAS

Once you have identified the specific fascial space(s) or areas involved with an oral and/or maxillofacial swelling, you can quickly review the anatomic details of the area by turning to the number coded sections of this unit and then make a decision to treat or refer the problem since most oral and/or maxillofacial swellings result from infections. We have **color-coded** each anatomical location as to its potential degree of severity for most general practitioners.

☐ Problem involves **low-risk anatomical areas** and is generally treatable with intraoral measures by a general practitioner. Potential for spread to higher risk areas is low and infections in these areas will **not usually require referral to a specialist.**

☐ Problem involves **moderate-risk areas.** Infections of these areas are often treatable with intraoral measures by general practitioners; however, the potential for spread to higher risk areas is much greater. Infections involving these areas must be closely monitored. As a general practitioner, you should carefully evaluate all other patient data associated with infections of these areas and strongly consider referral to a specialist. Prompt referral should be made if initial treatment does not resolve the problem.

☐ Problem involves **high-risk areas.** Infections in these areas are or can quickly become life threatening. **Immediate referral to a specialist or hospital is indicated.**

☑ Problem involves moderate-risk areas; however, infections of these areas may **rapidly progress to cavernous sinus thrombosis** through retrograde blood flow. Infections in these areas are usually treated effectively by general practitioners, however, if not closely followed can develop into a life-threatening problem.

NOTE: In development of these categories we realize that extreme variation exists within each category and that anatomical location is only one of many variables that must be considered in evaluation of the degree of seriousness of a patient's problem. This rating system is intended to serve only as a guideline and may require modification based on the specific data for each individual patient.

STUDY EXERCISES

When considering the spread of head and neck infections, what factor initially determines which anatomical areas of the head and neck will be involved? _____
_____

INFECTIOUS SWELLINGS OF THE DENTO-ALVEOLAR RIDGES

Frequently, dental infections are confined to the dento-alveolar ridges (processes). Endodontic or periodontal abscesses can burrow through alveolar bone and periosteum and involve the soft tissue (usually mucosa) covering the alveolar ridges and form abscesses or "gum boils" on the ridges. With rupture of these abscesses, a fistula is formed which establishes drainage into the oral cavity. Generally, this pathological process does not produce significant **systemic** signs or symptoms and thus infections confined to alveolar ridges have extremely low potential for serious systemic complications.

NOTE: **Your training in endodontics and periodontics provides you with the diagnostic and treatment procedures for managing infections confined to the dento-alveolar ridges.**

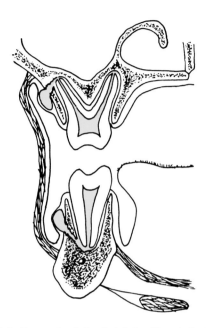

Figure III-4. Spread of dental infection into the soft tissue of the maxillary dento-alveolar ridge.

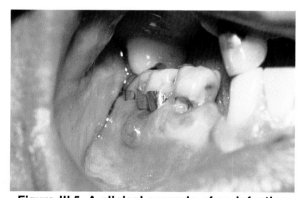

Figure III-5. A clinical example of an infection confined to the dento-alveolar ridge.

SWELLINGS OF AND BELOW THE MANDIBLE

Infectious swellings of the floor of the mouth and those adjacent to the body of the mandible include involvement of the following fascial planes and potential fascial spaces:

- ☐ 1 **facial vestibule of the mandible**
- ☐ 2 **space of the body of the mandible**
- ☐ 3 **mentalis space**
- ☐ 4 **submental space**
- ☐ 5 **sublingual space**
- ☐ 6 **submandibular space**

In addition to infections of these spaces we will discuss **Ludwig's angina** which is a life-threatening involvement of multiple fascial spaces in this area.

☐ 1 Facial Vestibule of the Mandible

The facial vestibule is the area located between the buccinator muscle and the oral mucosa and is inferiorly bounded by the insertion of the buccinator into the mandible.

Signs and Symptoms

Infections of the facial vestibule cause swellings over the buccal and labial mandibular alveolus which may obliterate portions of the mandibular buccal vestibule.

Odontogenic Origin

Swelling of the facial vestibule of the mandible most frequently originates from periodontal abscesses which are superficial to bone. If developing pus cannot drain via the sulcus, it will extend through soft tissue into the facial vestibule. Facial vestibule infections may originate from periapically involved mandibular premolars and molars or from buccal periodontal abscesses from canines, premolars, and molars. However, infection from any of the mandibular teeth which perforate the buccal cortical plate above the insertion of the buccinator muscle will also cause infection of this area.

Pattern of Spread

Infections in the mandibular facial vestibule may spread through the buccinator muscle into the **buccal space** especially if molars are involved. **Rarely do these infections spread below the mandible.**

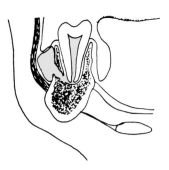

Figure III-6. Anatomical location of the mandibular facial vestibule. The facial vestibule is often divided into buccal and labial components.

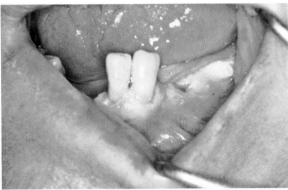

Figure III-7. An example of an infection involving the mandibular facial vestibule.

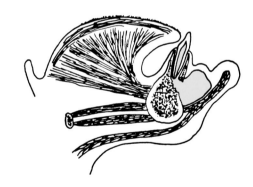

Figure III-8. Spread of dental infection to the facial vestibule of the mandible.

STUDY EXERCISES

Swelling of the facial vestibule of the mandible may be a result of infection of mandibular teeth which has perforated the _____buccal_____ _____cortical_____ plate or from a _____periodontal_____ abscess which cannot drain via the sulcus. An infection in the facial vestibule of the mandible will cause a swelling located above the insertion of the _____buccinator_____ muscle. This swelling may spread into the _____buccal_____ space.

☐ 2 Space of the Body of the Mandible

The space of the body of the mandible is the potential space between the body of the mandible and its periosteum and extends from the mandibular symphysis to the anterior border of the masseter and medial pterygoid. Dental infections generally start at the apex of the tooth, burrow through the bone to first elevate the periosteum and then penetrate the periosteum to involve adjacent spaces. If the periosteum is elevated rather than perforated, the infection will spread along this potential space. Inflammations of this could also be termed **Subperiosteal Abscesses. Post-surgical subperiosteal** infections of this space result from the introduction of microorganisms below full-thickness flaps.

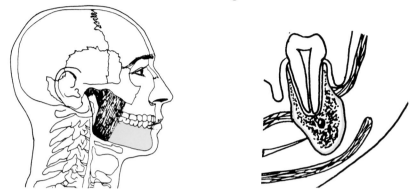

Figure III-9. The space of the body of the mandible as indicated in yellow is the potential space between the mandibular cortex and its overlying periosteum.

Signs and Symptoms

A firm painful swelling adjacent to mandibular body, lying beneath periosteum is characteristic of infections of the space of the body of the mandible. Usually no increase in redness of the oral mucosa is seen.

Odontogenic Origin

Infections of this space can originate from any of the mandibular teeth and establish an infection between bone and periosteum (periostitis). Post-surgical infections of this space can occur, especially if care is not taken to remove surgical debris from below full-thickness surgical flaps.

Pattern of Spread

Infections of the space of the body of the mandible may spread to the **sublingual, submental, buccal, mentalis, facial vestibule,** or **submandibular spaces.**

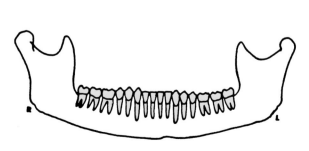

Figure III-10. Dental origin of infections involving the body of the mandible. Post-surgical infections can also develop in this potential space.

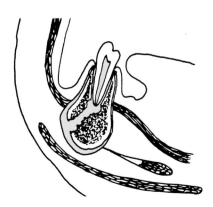

Figure III-11. Spread of infection to the space of the body of the mandible. This process can affect the lateral, medial or inferior surface of the mandible.

☐ 3 Mentalis Space

The bilateral mentalis spaces are located between the **anterior surface of the mandible on either side of the mandibular symphysis** and below the **mentalis** and **inferior labialis muscles** and superior to the **platysma** and chin prominence.

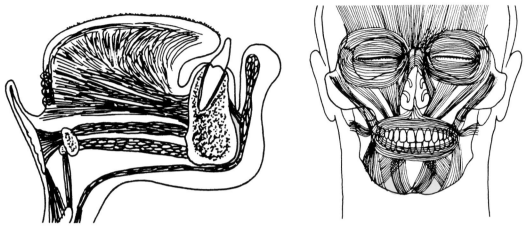

Figure III-12. Anatomical location of the mentalis space is outlined in yellow.

Signs and Symptoms

Infections involving the mentalis space may present as a slight bulging of mandibular labial vestibule. More commonly, these infections cause swelling of soft tissues of the chin prominence.

Odontogenic Origin

Mentalis space infections usually develop from the four mandibular incisors when an abscess of these teeth breaks through the labial plate at a level below the insertion of the mentalis muscle and below the vestibule.

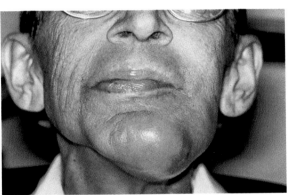

Figure III-13. An example of an infection involving the mentalis space.

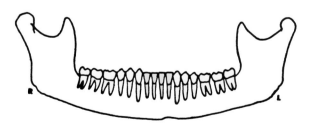

Figure III-14. The usual odontogenic source of mentalis space infections is the mandibular incisors.

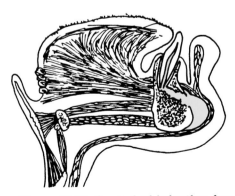

Figure III-15. Spread of infection from mandibular incisors to the mentalis space.

Pattern of Spread

Mentalis space infections can spread to the **submental space,** then may spread to one or both **submandibular** spaces.

☐ **4 Submental Space**

The submental space lies between the **mylohyoid** and **platysma** superio-inferiorly and between the diverging **anterior bellies of the digastric muscles** laterally. It communicates with the **submandibular** space posteriorly.

Principal Contents

The principal structures in the submental space are the **submental lymph nodes.**

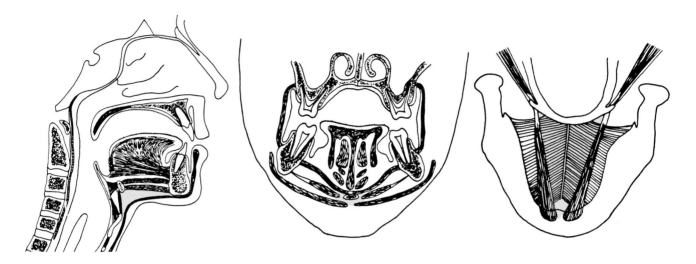

Figure III-16. Outline of submental space and its relationship to anatomic landmarks. A. Midsaggital view. B. Cross-sectional view. C. View from below the mandible. Yellow indicates extent of submental space.

Signs and Symptoms

Patients with a submental space abscess will have a swollen area beneath the chin in the **middle third of the mandible.** They may experience some difficulty in swallowing. Elevation of the tongue is usually not seen.

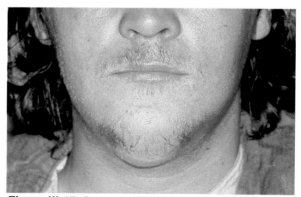

Figure III-17. An example of an odontogenic infection involving the submental space.

Odontogenic Origin

The submental space is not usually involved separately. When it is, it is usually due to an infection from a midline structure such as a mandibular central incisor, chin, lower lip or tip of tongue.

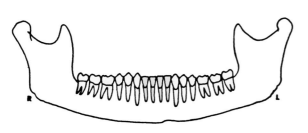

Figure III-18. Usual odontogenic origin
for submental space infection.

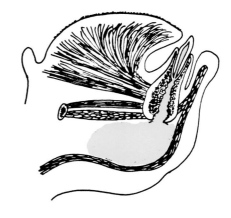

Figure III-19. Spread of odontogenic
infection to the submental space.

Patterns of Spread

Infections of the submental space can:
- spread to **submandibular space** unilaterally or bilaterally and then to the **parapharyngeal space(s)**;
- move inferiorly to involve **fascial planes of the neck;**
- move superiorly to involve the **sublingual space.**

STUDY EXERCISES

If a patient presents to you with an infection of the space of the **body of the mandible** would you expect the swelling to be firm or soft? _firm_

Which teeth can cause infection of this space?
- a. mandibular molars
- b. mandibular premolars
- c. mandibular canines
- d. mandibular incisors
- e. c & d
- f. a, b, c, & d

If not successfully treated, into what spaces might the infection spread?
- a. _buccal_
- b. _mental_
- c. _submandibular_
- d. _submental_

Infection of the **mentalis space** will cause swelling of what area? _labial vestibule_

These infections can spread to the ___submental___ space and then to one or both of the ___submandibular___ spaces.

Infections in which of the following spaces may originate from the mandibular incisors?
- a. submental
- b. mentalis
- c. body of the mandible
- d. facial vestibule of mandible

Submental space infection may spread to:
- a. _submental_
- b. _sublingual_
- c. _both parapharyngeal_
- d. _facial planes of neck_

If infection from a central incisor spreads into the **submental space,** it would cause a swelling where? _chin_ Would the tongue be elevated? (Yes/No) _No_ What other symptoms might also be associated with a submental abscess? _difficult to swallow_

□ 5 Sublingual Space

The sublingual space is a V-shaped trough which lies above (superior to) the **mylohyoid muscle** and below (inferior to) the **mucosa of the floor of the mouth.** The lingual surface of the mandible makes up the anterior and lateral boundaries. The **hyoglossus, geniohyoid, and genioglossus muscles** can divide this space into two compartments. Anterior to the tongue there is easy access to the opposite side via the floor of the mouth. The sublingual space communicates posteriorly with the bilateral submandibular spaces.

Principal Contents

The principal structures found in the sublingual space are the **sublingual salivary glands,** the **submandibular ducts,** the **lingual** and **hypoglossal nerves,** and the **tongue.**

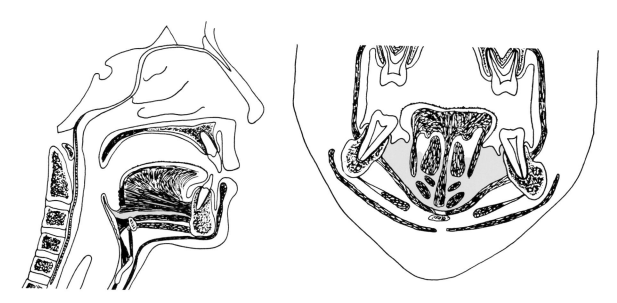

Figure III-20. Outline of the sublingual space (yellow) and its anatomic landmarks.

Signs and Symptoms

There is usually no external swelling with sublingual space infections. Patients will experience discomfort during swallowing and may have elevation of the tongue. Both unilateral and bilateral involvement occurs clinically.

Odontogenic Origin

A sublingual space abscess is usually caused by an infection of any mandibular tooth that has its apex **above the mylohyoid muscle.** These include mandibular incisors, canines, premolars and mesial roots of the first molars.

NOTE: **Any infection which discharges suppuration into the soft tissues on the lingual aspect of the mandible above the mylohyoid can cause infection of the sublingual space.**

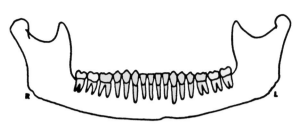

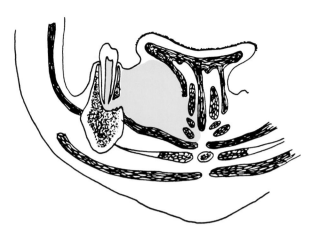

Figure III-21. Usual odontogenic origins for sublingual space infections.

Figure III-22. Spread of odontogenic infection to the sublingual space.

Routes of Spread

Infections of the sublingual space can spread:
- Posterio-inferiorly into the **submandibular space**
- Posterio-laterally into the **parapharyngeal spaces**
- Posterio-laterally into the **pterygomandibular space** (rare)

STUDY EXERCISES

The **sublingual space** lies above the ___mylohyoid___ muscle and below the ___mucosa___ of the ___floor___ of the mouth. Infection in this space can cause which of the following signs and symptoms?

a. difficulty swallowing
b. swelling below the chin
c. elevation of the tongue
d. firm swelling along lingual border of the mandible

e. trismus
f. cavernous sinus thrombosis
g. sinusitis
h. speech alteration

What determines whether an infection of a mandibular tooth will spread into the sublingual space? ___the mylohyoid space___

Infections of the sublingual space can spread into what 3 spaces? ___parapharyngeal submandibular pterygomandibular space___

☐ 6 Submandibular Space

The submandibular space lies inferior to the **mylohyoid muscle**, which separates it from the sublingual space. It is located medial to the mandibular body. The **mylohyoid** and **hypoglossus muscles** comprise its medial boundary, while the **platysma and the body of the mandible** form the lateral boundary. The **anterior and posterior belly of the digastric muscle**, with the **lower border of the mandible**, forms the submandibular triangle.

Principal Contents

The principal structures in this space are the **submandibular salivary gland (and its duct, which leads into the sublingual space)**, the **submandibular lymph nodes**, and the **facial artery and vein.**

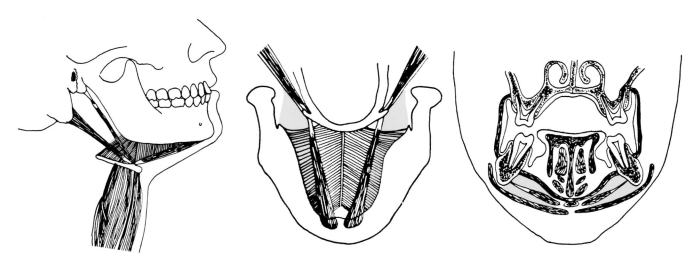

Figure III-23. Outline of the submandibular space and its relationship to anatomic landmarks. A. Lateral view. B. Mandible viewed from below. C. Cross-sectional view. Yellow area indicates extent of the submandibular space.

Signs and Symptoms

Infections of the submandibular space produce external swellings of the submandibular region. Since the pus will localize deep to the platysma muscle, the swelling will feel very hard. There is a moderate limitation to mouth opening due to interference of muscle and jaw function. These patients may appear toxic due to the large volume of suppuration which can accumulate in this space as well as the higher potential of systemic spread from this space.

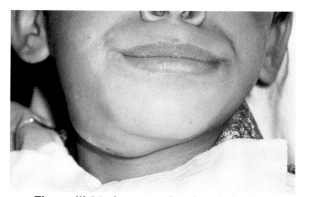

Figure III-24. An example of an infection involving the submandibular space.

Odontogenic Origin

Dental abscesses, pericoronitis of mandibular molars (primarily 3rd molars), and post-surgical infections are the most frequent causes of infections of the submandibular space. Dental abscesses which penetrate the lingual cortical plate **below** the attachment of the mylohyoid discharge into this space. Soft tissue infections in the retromolar area may spread directly into this space.

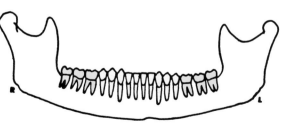

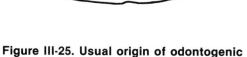

Figure III-25. Usual origin of odontogenic submandibular space infections.

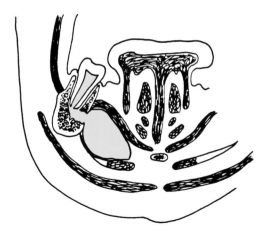

Figure III-26. Spread of infection from posterior mandibular teeth to the submandibular space.

Patterns of Spread

Infection of the submandibular space may spread:
- To the **sublingual space** by extension around the posterior border of the mylohyoid or by perforating the mylohyoid
- Medially to the opposite **submandibular space**
- Inferiorly to the **fascial planes of the neck**
- Posteriorly to the **parapharyngeal** or **pterygomandibular spaces.**
- Superioposteriorly to the **deep temporal space.**

STUDY EXERCISES

The **submandibular space** lies below the *mylohyoid* muscle. It lies *inferior* and *medial* to the posterior part of the mandible. The *mandible* and *platysma* muscles form its lateral boundary.

Infection of the submandibular space is most often caused by dental abscesses or pericoronitis of mandibular *molars* when these infections penetrate the lingual cortical plate below the insertion of the *mylohyoid* muscle.

Infection can spread from the submandibular space into the *sublingual* space, medially to the opposite *submandibular* space, inferiorly to the *neck*, posteriorly to the *parapharyngeal* or *pterygomandibular* spaces or superioposteriorly to the deep *temporal* space.

A patient with an infection of the submandibular space may present with: (choose any that apply)
a. external facial swelling
b. swelling of the tongue
c. dysphagia
d. moderate limitation of mouth opening
e. no symptoms related to limited functions

☐ Ludwig's Angina

Ludwig's angina is a clinical term used to describe a massive bilateral phlegmonous cellulitis involving mandibular fascial spaces including the sublingual, submandibular and submental spaces. In addition, the pharyngeal spaces usually become involved and may lead to respiratory difficulty. See **Figure III-27.**

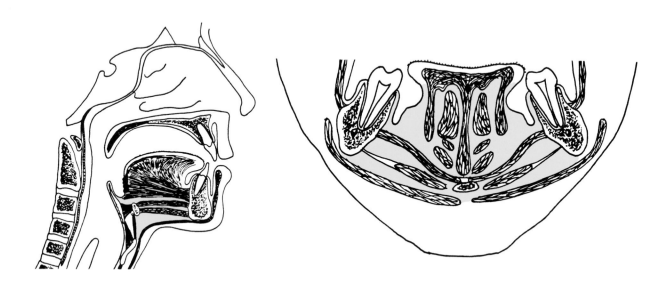

Figure III-27. Fascial spaces involved with Ludwig's angina. Yellow indicates location of infection. Notice complete involvement of spaces below the mandible.

Signs and Symptoms

This is an alarming and **life-threatening condition which can lead rapidly to respiratory obstruction and asphyxiation.** Swelling may displace the tongue upwards and backwards, thus totally blocking the pharyngeal airway. Edema of the glottis is a late complication.

The external clinical appearance is striking. There is usually an indurated massive bilateral submandibular swelling, which extends down the anterior part of the neck to the clavicles. Swallowing is difficult and drooling is evident. Breathing may be labored.

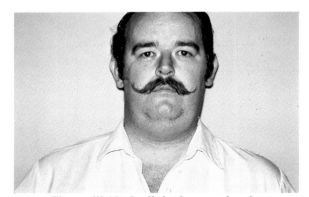

Figure III-28. A clinical example of a patient with Ludwig's angina.

Patients are frequently very ill with temperatures up to 40°C (104°F). Swallowing is difficult and breathing becomes progressively more labored. If left untreated, edema of the glottis causes a complete respiratory obstruction. Difficulty in intubation of such a patient may require an emergency coniotomy (cricothyrotomy) followed by intubation and/or tracheostomy.

Odontogenic Origin

Infections originating from any of the mandibular teeth can spread to the submental space, submandibular spaces and sublingual spaces. The spread of infection from a single space to all of these other spaces constitutes the clinical syndrome termed Ludwig's angina.

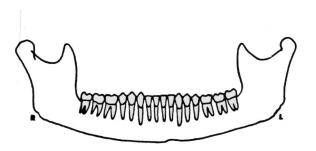

Figure III-29. Ludwig's angina may originate from odontogenic infections of any of the mandibular teeth.

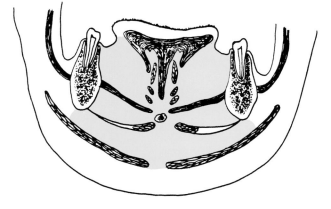

Figure III-30. Illustration of the fascial spaces involved in Ludwig's angina. Note that the parapharyngeal spaces may also be involved.

Route of Spread — Ludwig's angina may:
- spread to the **mediastinum** via **fascial planes in the neck.**
- cause **glottic edema** and rapidly lead to **respiratory obstruction.**

NOTE: Ludwig's angina is an acute medical emergency requiring IMMEDIATE HOSPITAL-IZATION and may necessitate that an emergency coniotomy (cricothyrotomy) be performed.

STUDY EXERCISES

Ludwig's angina is a term used to describe an infection which is (bilateral/unilateral) ___bilateral___ *and includes the* ___mandibular___ ___facial___ *and* ___submental___ *spaces. The* ___submandibular___ *spaces are also usually involved as well as the* ___sublingual___ *spaces. This infection can originate from which groups of mandibular teeth?*
  ☒ *incisors*   ☐ *cuspids*   ☒ *bicuspids*   ☒ *molars*

Ludwig's angina is a life-threatening condition because ___swelling___ *is very difficult resulting in poor nutrition and dehydration. Swelling in the glottis area can cause complete* ___respiratory___ ___obstruction___. *This acute medical emergency requires immediate* ___hospitalization___.

SUMMARY OF THE SPREAD OF INFECTIONS OF AND BELOW THE MANDIBLE

Dental infections can spread from the mandibular dento-alveolar ridges to the following fascial spaces or areas:

- facial vestibule of the mandible
- space of the body of the mandible
- mentalis space
- submental space
- sublingual space
- submandibular space

Infectious swellings of the floor of the mouth and below the mandible most frequently originate from periapical or periodontal infections of the mandibular teeth. The fascial space or area first involved is determined by the location at which suppuration penetrates the mandible in relationship to muscle insertions. These infections may range from localized swellings with minimal functional interferences to acute, life-threatening swellings (acute cellulitis) which may cause dysphagia and respiratory obstruction. **Any infection in this area should be considered serious and close monitoring is essential.**

From these primary spaces an infection can spread to **adjacent spaces** and extend to the **parapharyngeal space, fascial planes of the neck,** and other **fascial spaces of the head.**

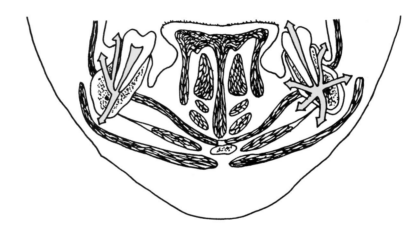

Figure III-31. Summary of swellings of the floor of the mouth and below the mandible resulting from odontogenic infections.

LOCATION OF SWELLING	OTHER UNIQUE SIGNS & SYMPTOMS	FASCIAL SPACES OR AREAS	MOST COMMONLY INVOLVED TEETH
Facial vestibule and lower cheek	None	Facial vestibule	Mandibular canines, premolars & molars
Periosteum of mandible	Firm and tender	Body of mandible	All mandibular teeth
Chin	None	Mentalis	Incisors
Midline under chin and mandible	Hard swelling, dysphagia	Submental	Incisors
Tongue and floor of the mouth	Dysphagia, elevation of tongue	Sublingual	Incisors, canines, premolars, mesial root of 1st molars
Under the body of the mandible	Dysphagia	Submandibular	Molars

Table III-1. Summary of the fascial spaces and the teeth associated with swellings of the floor of mouth and below the mandibular dento-alveolar ridges.

STUDY EXERCISES

1. The patient pictured at the right complains of pain when he swallows or opens his mouth. The swollen area feels hard. He has several severely decayed teeth. His temperature is 37.8° C (100° F) and he appears tired. What fascial space is swollen? _submandibular_

Which of his teeth might be the source of this infection? _molars_

If your initial treatment is unsuccessful and the infection spreads, what space(s) may be involved next? _____ _subling_

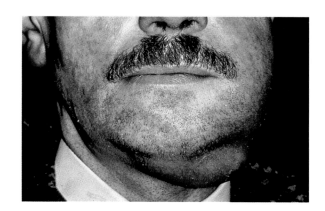

2. Label the fascial spaces (or potential spaces) indicated on the diagrams below.

Space
a. _sublingual_
b. _body_
c. _submand_
d. _submental_

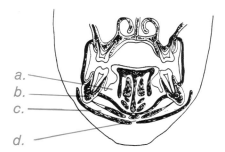

a.
b.
c.
d.

3. The patient shown here reports that a lower left incisor has been sensitive for several days when he eats. What fascial space does this infection appear to involve? _Submentalis   mentalis_

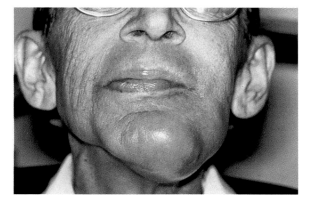

4. A patient presents to your office with severe pericoronitis involving a partially erupted mesioangular impacted mandibular right 3rd molar. You curette the area, prescribe saline rinses and an oral antibiotic. If your initial treatment fails to control the infection, into what fascial space(s) is this infection likely to spread? _____
   a. mental
   b. body of mandible
   c. submental
   d. submandibular
   e. sublingual
   f. buccal vestibule

The patient returns 2 days later complaining of soreness when swallowing (dysphagia). Which of the above spaces could now be involved? _submandibular_

5. For each fascial space listed below, match the teeth which could be the source for infections spreading into the area.

mentalis _B_____   a. all mandibular teeth
submental _B_____   b. mandibular incisors
sublingual _E_____   c. mandibular canines, premolars &
submandibular _A_____   molars
facial vestibule _C_ A_____   d. mandibular molars
body of the mandible _A_____   e. mandibular incisors, premolars,
                                    canines & mesial roots of 1st molars

6. The swelling pictured to the right is fluctuant. The patient reports no trismus or
dysphagia but has had episodic pain in
the lower second molar for the past year.
What fascial space or area is swollen?
_facial vestibule_____

_____ What space might this
infection spread into if not treated?
_buccal_____

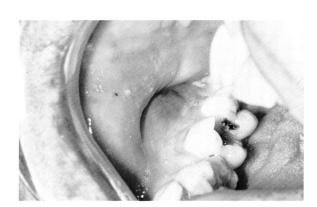

7. The patient pictured is febrile (39° C) and
tells you that he has not eaten for 3 days
because he finds it difficult to swallow.
What space appears to be involved?
_Submand_____

_____ What
should you do for this patient? _____
_hospitalize_____

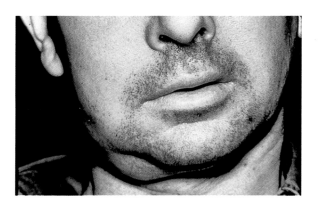

Answers

1. Submandibular. Mandibular molars. Fascial planes of the neck, parapharyngeal space, pterygomandibular space, sublingual space, deep temporal space

2. a. sublingual space   c. submandibular space
   b. body of the mandible   d. submental space

3. mentalis space

4. b, d, f; submandibular

5. Mentalis — b. mandibular incisors. Submental — b. central mandibular incisors. Sublingual — e. mandibular incisors, canines, premolars, mesial roots of first molars. Submandibular — d. mandibular molars. Buccal vestibule — c. canines premolars & molars. Body of the mandible — a. all mandibular teeth.

6. facial (buccal) vestibule; buccal space

7. submandibular

SWELLINGS OF THE LATERAL FACE AND CHEEK

Swellings of the lateral face and cheek can be a result of infection spread to the following fascial spaces:

- ☐ 7 **buccal vestibule of maxilla**
- ☐ 8 **buccal space**
- ☐ 9 **submasseteric space**
- ☐ 10 **deep temporal**
- ☐ 10 **superficial temporal**
- ☐ 11 **infratemporal space**
- ☐ 12 **parotid space**

☐ 7 Buccal Vestibule of the Maxilla

The maxillary buccal vestibule is the area of tissue medial to the buccinator muscle, inferior to the insertion of this muscle below the zygomatic process of the maxilla.

Signs & Symptoms

Infections in the maxillary buccal vestibule will present as swelling in the buccal vestibule. Externally, this will present as **distension of the posterior corner of the upper lip** or swelling of the cheek, posteriorly or anteriorly.

Odontogenic Origin

Infection originating from any of the maxillary posterior teeth can cause vestibular swelling in the maxillary arch if the abscess penetrates the maxilla below the insertion of the buccinator muscle.

Spread to Adjacent Spaces

These infections may spread:
- superiorly into the **buccal space**
- superiorly into the **infraorbital area**
- via facial vein, angular vein, and ophthalmic vein **to cavernous sinus**

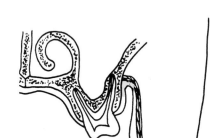

Figure III-32. Anatomical location of the maxillary buccal vestibule and how odontogenic infections spread to this area.

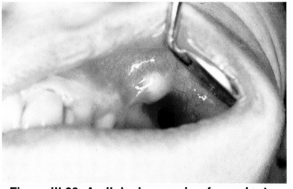

Figure III-33. A clinical example of an odontogenic infection of the maxillary buccal vestibule.

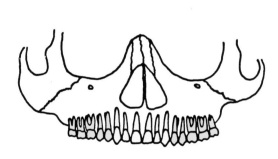

Figure III-34. Teeth most frequently associated with infections of the maxillary buccal vestibule.

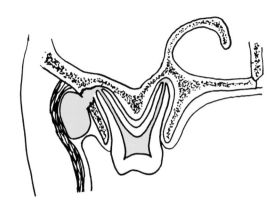

Figure III-35. Spread of odontogenic infection to the maxillary buccal vestibule.

□ 8 Buccal (Buccinator) Space

The buccal space is bounded anteromedially by the **buccinator muscle,** posteromedially by the **masseter** and anterior border of the ramus of the mandible and covered laterally by skin and subcutaneous tissue together with an extension of fascia from the parotid capsule. The superior portion of this space is often called the **buccinator space.**

Principal Contents

The buccal space contains the buccal fat pad.

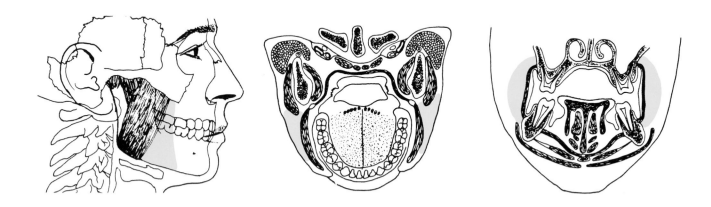

Figure III-36. Anatomical location of the buccal space.

Signs and Symptoms

Buccal space infections usually produce an external swelling of the cheek just behind the corner of the mouth, extending down to the lower border of the mandible and extending posteriorly to the anterior border of the ascending ramus. Infections of the posterior area frequently involve the submasseteric space as well. Thus, in this area, precise clinical diagnosis is difficult. Generally, buccal space infections do not cause trismus. The patient may be toxic and have an elevated temperature.

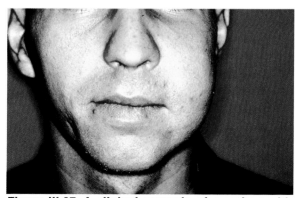

Figure III-37. A clinical example of a patient with a buccal space abscess.

Odontogenic Source

Infections of the buccal space are usually caused from infections of the maxillary or mandibular molars. The infection penetrates the outer cortex of the alveolar process superior or inferior to the attachment of the buccinator muscle or the infection may burrow through the buccinator to reach the buccal space.

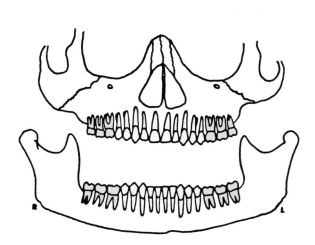

Figure III-38. Usual origin of odontogenic buccal space infections.

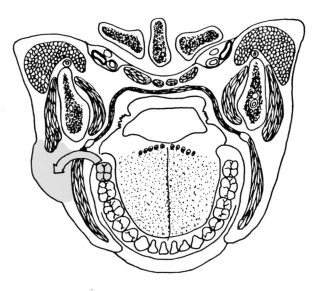

Figure III-39. Spread of odontogenic infection to the buccal space.

Route of Spread

Infections of the buccal space may spread:
- posteriorly to involve the **pterygomandibular space** or **submasseteric space**
- superiorly and medially to the **deep temporal space**
- superiorly and laterally to the **superficial temporal space**
- posteriorly to involve the **lateral pharyngeal space**

STUDY EXERCISES

Buccal space infections may originate from infections of which teeth? _*Max & mand*_ _*molars*_ Buccal vestibule infections originate from infected _*max molars*_.

The buccal space is bounded medially by the _*buccinator*_ and _*masseteric*_ muscles and laterally by the _*skin*_.

Infections can spread into the buccal vestibule of the maxilla from which maxillary teeth? _*post premolar & molar*_ From the vestibule, the infections may spread into what space(s)? _*deep & superficial temp*_ _*lat. pharyngeal, submasseter*_

□ 9 Submasseteric Space

Location

The submasseteric space is the potential space located between the masseter muscle and the lateral surface of the mandibular ramus.

From an anatomical point of view, there is no true submasseteric space. There is, however, a zone of insertion of the masseter muscle, which is less dense, thus permitting detachment of the periosteum in that region with the subsequent accumulation of pus.

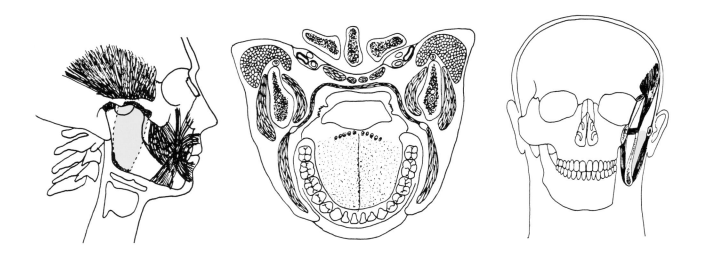

Figure III-40. Anatomical location of the potential submasseteric space.

Signs and Symptoms

The most striking signs of a submasseteric space infection are severe trismus, and a deep-seated throbbing pain. This pain occurs because pus is tightly confined by the masseter muscle and pressure cannot be relieved by expansion of tissue. Any external facial swelling is only moderate in extent and is confined to the middle region of the lateral surface of the ramus.

The patient's systemic response varies considerably. The infection may smolder for a long time setting up an osteomyelitis or it may cause a more acute response, in which case the patient is often seriously ill.

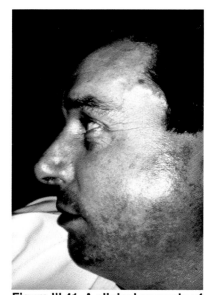

Figure III-41. A clinical example of a patient with a submasseteric space infection.

Odontogenic Origin

Infections of the submasseteric space are uncommon except for distoangularly impacted mandibular third molars since, anatomically, it is difficult for pus to burrow as far posteriorly as the lateral surface of the ramus of the mandible.

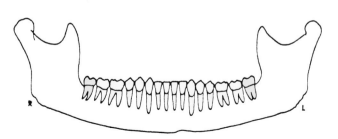

Figure III-42. Usual odontogenic origin for submasseteric space infection.

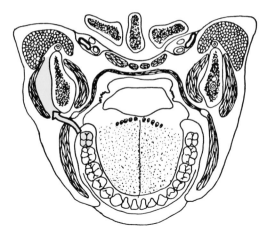

Figure III-43. Spread of odontogenic infection to the submasseteric space.

Pattern of Spread

Infections of the submasseteric space may spread:
- superiorly to involve the **superficial temporal spaces**
- anteriorly and laterally to involve the **buccal space**

□ 10 Deep and Superficial Temporal Spaces

The **superficial temporal space** is the space between the temporal fascia and the temporalis muscle with the inferior boundary being the zygomatic arch.

The **deep temporal space** is the space between the temporalis muscle and the underlying bony skull and is contiguous inferiorly with the pterygomandibular space around the lateral pterygoid. The most inferior portion of the deep temporal space is often termed the **infratemporal space.**

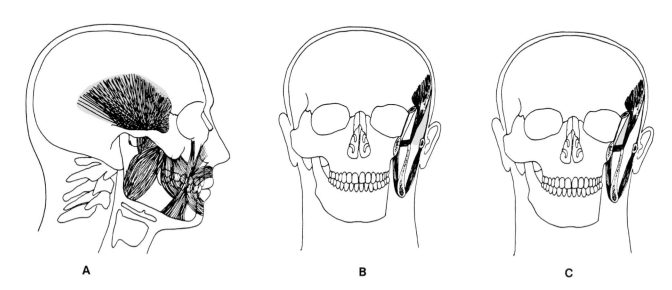

A   B   C

Figure III-44. Summary of the anatomical location of the temporal spaces. A. Lateral view.
B. Superficial temporal space. C. Deep temporal space.

Signs and Symptoms

Infections of the temporal spaces present with swelling over the temporal region above the zygomatic arch, and pain which will cause trismus.

Superficial temporal space infections usually produce external swelling, however swelling is much less than is seen in other soft tissue areas.

Deep temporal space infections are often difficult to detect because they lie below the temporalis muscle and external swelling is minimal.

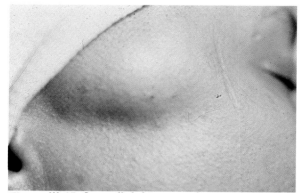

Figure III-45. Superficial temporal space infection. The swelling in this photo is located just superior to the zygomatic arch which is located between the eye and ear.

Odontogenic Origin

Most temporal space infections are **secondary** to infections spreading from the maxillary or mandibular posterior teeth via pterygomandibular or submasseteric spaces.

Pattern of Spread

Infections involving the temporal spaces may spread:

- inferiorly to the **pterygomandibular** and **submasseteric spaces**
- postero-inferiorly to the **para-pharyngeal spaces**

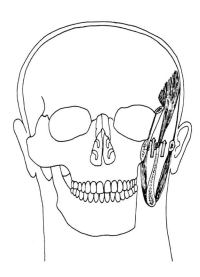

Figure III-46. Diagram of the spread of infection to the temporal spaces from the submasseteric and pterygomandibular spaces.

STUDY EXERCISES

Infections of the ___superficial___ temporal space usually produce swelling over the lateral head region (above/below) ___above___ the zygomatic arch. Infection of the ___infratemp-___ temporal space generally does not produce external facial swelling because it lies below the ___temporalis___ muscle.

Temporal space infections are usually secondary to infections spreading from posterior teeth via the ___submasseteric___ or ___pterygomandibular___ spaces.

□ 11 Infratemporal Space

The infratemporal space is the upper extremity of the pterygomandibular space. It is bounded laterally by the medial surface of the mandible and temporalis muscle and tendon. Medially its wall is made up of the medial and lateral pterygoid muscles. The inferior head of the lateral pterygoid muscle is the boundary between the pterygomandibular space and the infratemporal space.

Principal Contents

The principal contents include the maxillary artery and pterygoid plexus of veins.

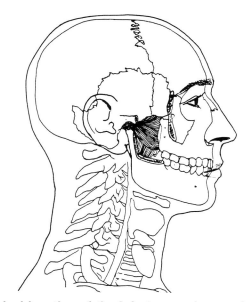

Figure III-47. The anatomical location of the infratemporal space is indicated in yellow.

Signs and Symptoms

A marked limitation of opening (severe trismus), bulging of the temporalis muscle, and very ill appearing patient in acute infections. Spread to intracranial involvement through retrograde movement via the pterygoid plexus may produce serious signs of cavernous sinus thrombosis, brain abscess, etc.

Odontogenic Source

Infections of the infratemporal space most often arise from infections involving maxillary 3rd molars or following local anesthetic injections into the infratemporal space, if a contaminated needle is used or the injection site is not properly disinfected prior to injection.

Pattern of Spread

Infections of the infratemporal space may spread:
- superiorly to involve the **deep temporal space.**
- inferiorly to involve the **pterygomandibular space.**
- intracranially via the pterygoid plexus to involve the **cavernous sinus** and produce a septic thrombosis of the cavernous sinus.

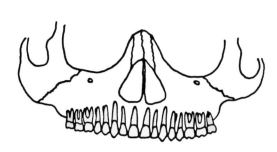

Figure III-48. Odontogenic origin for infections of the infratemporal space.

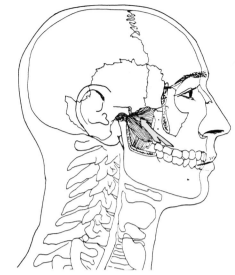

Figure III-49. Pathway for spread of odontogenic infections to the infratemporal space.

NOTE: Infections of the infratemporal space must be regarded as extremely serious because of the intracranial access via the pterygoid plexus. Any signs of meningeal irritation or any changes in C.N.S. signs must be viewed as necessitating immediate hospitalization.

An infratemporal space infection may spread to the ___deep___ ___temporal___ space ___, the ___pterygomandibular___ space or the ___Cavernous___ ___sinus___.

Why should infratemporal space infections be regarded as extremely serious? ___intracranial access___

An infection of the infratemporal space will result in severe ___trismus___, bulging of the ___temporalis___ ___muscle___, and a patient who appears very ___ill___.

An infratemporal space infection may originate from an infected maxillary ___3rd molar___ or from a ___contaminated needle___ in this space.

☐ 12 Parotid Space

The parotid space is the space occupied by the parotid salivary gland and enclosed by the fibrous capsule of the parotid gland. Parotid gland and duct and facial nerve are the principal contents of the parotid space.

Parotid space infections

Infections of the parotid space **rarely develop from odontogenic origin.** They usually develop from a retrograde flow of oral flora along the parotid duct to the gland or result from viral infections such as mumps.

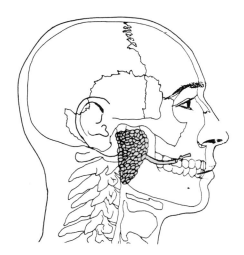
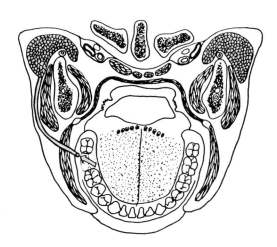

Figure III-50. Anatomical location of the parotid space.

Signs and Symptoms

Infections of the parotid space present as an extremely painful swelling in the area of the parotid gland (like mumps). Parotid space infections are located in the posterior area of the mandible. Other clinical signs of parotid space infections include: suppuration from parotid duct; inflamed parotid duct papilla; and toxic appearance.

Odontogenic Source

Infections of the parotid gland are usually **not of odontogenic origin.**

Route of Spread

Infection of the parotid may spread to:
- superficially involve the **skin with fistula**
- may move medially to involve the **parapharyngeal spaces**
- may move superiorly to the **deep temporal space**

NOTE: Infections of the parotid space should be referred to an oral and maxillofacial surgeon or other appropriate specialist.

Figure III-51. A clinical example of a parotid space infection.

SUMMARY OF INFECTIOUS SWELLINGS OF THE CHEEK & LATERAL FACE

Odontogenic infections can spread from the maxillary and/or mandibular dento-alveolar ridges directly to the **buccal vestibule, buccal space,** and **submasseteric space.**

Pterygomandibular space infections (generally produces swellings of the anterior tonsillar pillar) are not externally visible. Infections associated with this space can spread to the **deep temporal space, superficial temporal space, lateral pharyngeal space** (by spreading around the anterior border of the medial pterygoid muscle), and the **buccal space.**

Swellings of the parotid space are generally **not** of odontogenic origin but can be confused with odontogenic infections which have spread to the submasseteric space. **Figure III-52** summarizes the spread of infection to the cheek and lateral face.

INFECTIOUS SWELLINGS OF THE CHEEK & LATERAL FACE

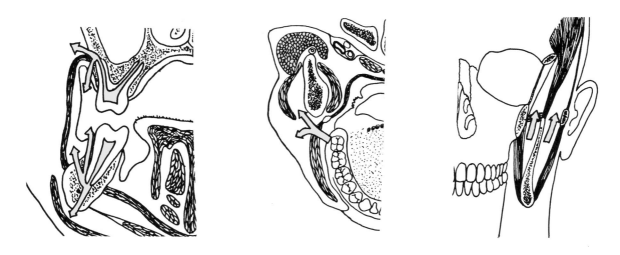

Figure III-52. Summary of the spread of infection to the cheek and lateral sides of the face.

LOCATION OF SWELLING	OTHER SIGNS & SYMPTOMS	FASCIAL SPACE INVOLVED	MOST COMMON TEETH INVOLVED
Buccal vestibule & upper cheek	Deep-seated throbbing pain	Buccal vestibule	Maxillary premolars & molars
Cheek below center of eye	Pain	Buccal space	Maxillary & mandibular molars
Swelling is generally not present. May cause slight bulge over the masseter	Pain and trismus	Submasseteric space	Mandibular 3rd molars
Between ear and lateral corner of eye above zygomatic arch	Pain	Superficial temporal space	From pterygomandibular space
Cheek anterior to the Masseter	Pain and Trismus	Infratemporal	Maxillary 3rd molars. Needle track infections
Around posterior border of the mandible	Extremely painful, suppuration from parotid duct, inflamed duct papilla, exacerbation with eating	Parotid space	Generally not of odontogenic origin

Table III-2. Summary of the fascial spaces and the odontogenic origin
associated with swellings of the cheek and lateral face.

STUDY EXERCISES

The patient pictured complained of severe pain in his lower first molar. What fascial space is involved? _Submasseteric_

If the infection is not effectively treated, what spaces may it spread into? _____

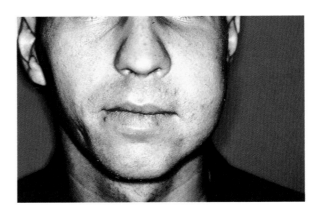

Identify each space or area numbered in the diagrams below, and indicate the most likely teeth associated with infections of the numbered spaces or areas.

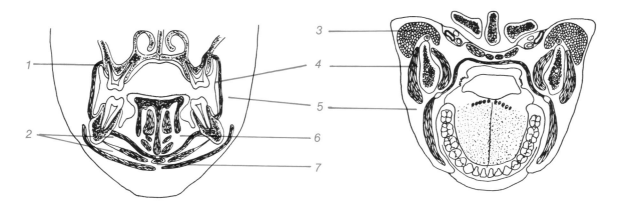

SPACE	TEETH MOST LIKELY TO CAUSE INFECTION OF THIS SPACE
1. _Buccal vestibule_	_max molar_
2. _submandibular_	_mand molars_
3. _parotid_	_duct_
4. _Submasseter_	_mand 3RD_
5. _buccal_	_max & mand 3RD_
6. _Sublingual_	_mand inc_
7. _submental_	_mand inc_

A patient presents with slight swelling over the lateral aspect of the ramus of the mandible. What three fascial spaces may be involved? a) _buccal_
b) _submasseter_ c) _parotid_. Describe additional symptoms which could help you determine which of these spaces is involved.

Space a) _no trismus_
Space b) _severe trismus_
Space c) _pus from duct, inflammed duct_

Infections in which of the following spaces may cause trismus?
  a. Buccal space
  b. Buccal vestibule of mandible
  (c.) Submasseteric space
  d. Parotid space
  e. Deep temporal
  f. Superficial temporal

What specific clinical signs and symptoms will help you identify infections of the parotid space? _pus from duct_
inflammed duct

SWELLINGS OF THE PHARYNGEAL AREAS

If your patient **does not show signs of external swelling,** and yet the signs and symptoms of infection are present (such as trismus, fever, toxicity, etc.), then examination of the pharyngeal area may reveal anterior pillar or pharyngeal area swelling. Pharyngeal swelling may ultimately develop from infections of most other fascial spaces.

Pharyngeal swelling may be due to **odontogenic infections** or it may be the result of **tonsillar inflammation** or **infections of the ear.**

The fascial spaces to be discussed in this section include:

- ☐ **Pterygomandibular space**
- ☐ **Parapharyngeal spaces**
  - **Lateral pharyngeal space**
  - **Retropharyngeal space**
- ☐ **Peritonsillar space**

NOTE: Any infection in the pharyngeal area must be considered extremely serious.

☐ 13 Pterygomandibular Space

The pterygomandibular space is located in the area between the medial surface of the ramus of the mandible and the lateral surface of the medial pterygoid muscle. This space is limited superiorly by the lateral (external) pterygoid which separates this space from the infratemporal space.

Principal Contents

The principal structures are the inferior alveolar neuro-vascular bundle and the lingual nerve and the chorda tympani.

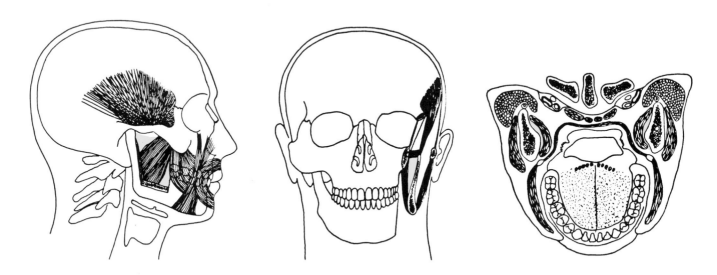

Figure III-53. Anatomical location of the pterygomandibular space.

Signs and Symptoms

As with submasseteric space infections, infections involving the pterygomandibular space produce moderate to severe trismus. There is only moderate swelling of the tonsillar pillar medially. Tenderness can be elicited over the medial aspect of the mandible; however, this symptom would be difficult to recognize in the presence of severe trismus. We would like to show you a photograph of an infection of this space; however, due to the difficulties of photographing this area we could not obtain a good example.

Odontogenic Source

Some pterygomandibular space infections result from pericoronitis associated with partially erupted mandibular third molars. Infections of this space most often develop following inferior alveolar block anesthesia if a contaminated needle is used or the injection site is not disinfected prior to the injection. Mandibular second molar infections may also spread into this space.

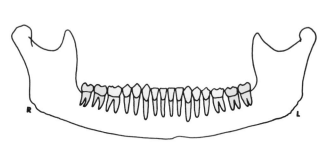

Figure III-54. Usual odontogenic source for pterygomandibular space infections.

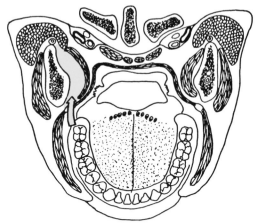

Figure III-55. Spread of odontogenic infection to pterygomandibular space.

Pattern of Spread

Infections of the pterygomandibular space may spread:
- superiorly to involve the **temporal spaces**
- antero-medially, then posteriorly to involve **parapharyngeal spaces**
- anteriorly and laterally to involve the **buccal and submasseteric spaces**
- anteriorly to the **infratemporal space**
- anteriorly and inferiorly to the **submandibular space.**

NOTE: Infections of the pterygomandibular space should be regarded as EXTREMELY SERIOUS due to the close proximity to the lateral pharyngeal, retropharyngeal spaces and fascial planes of the neck. These infections REQUIRE CLOSE SUPERVISION BY SPECIALISTS and frequently involve hospitalization of the patient.

STUDY EXERCISES

The pterygomandibular space is located between the medial surface of the ‾ramus‾ and the lateral surface of the ‾medial‾ ‾pterygoid‾ muscle.

Infections of the pterygomandibular space may be caused by pericoronitis of mandibular ‾3rd‾ molars; however, they are usually caused by ‾contaminated‾ needles when performing injections to block the ‾inf.‾ ‾alveolar‾ nerve. A third possible source is infection of mandibular ‾2nd‾ ‾molars‾.

A patient presents to your office with moderate trismus and pain over the posteriomedial aspect of the mandible that began seven days after you prepared a complete crown on a mandibular second premolar. You determine that an infection is present in the pterygomandibular space. Examination of mandibular teeth reveals no deep caries, non-vital teeth, or pericoronitis. What might be the cause of this infection? ‾injection for‾ ‾nerve block‾

Moderate to severe ‾trismus‾ is a symptom present when the pterygomandibular space is infected. This occurs because pressure builds up between the ‾mandible‾ and the ‾medial pterygoid‾ muscle (boundaries of the space).

☐ 14 Parapharyngeal Spaces

Lateral Pharyngeal Spaces
Retropharyngeal Spaces

Location

The **lateral pharyngeal space** is a potential cone-shaped space with the skull as the roof, while the apex is closely associated with the carotid sheath below. It is located between the medial pterygoid muscle laterally and the superior constrictor muscle and extends inferiorly to the hyoid bone. Below the hyoid bone this space is contiguous with the deep cervical fascia which leads to the mediastinum.

The **retropharyngeal space** is a potential space located posterior to the superior constrictor and is anterior to the carotid sheath and prevertebral fascia.

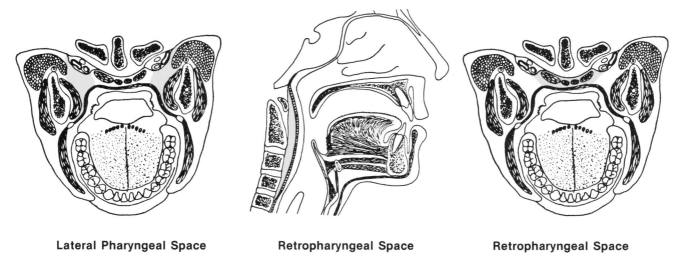

Lateral Pharyngeal Space   Retropharyngeal Space   Retropharyngeal Space

Figure III-56. The anatomical location of the lateral pharyngeal and retropharyngeal spaces.

Signs and Symptoms

There is usually a high fever and significant malaise associated with a parapharyngeal infection.

Pain on swallowing is extreme and there is some limitation of opening, but not as extreme as a pterygomandibular space abscess. The tonsil and lateral pharyngeal wall are pushed towards the opposite side of the mouth, the uvula is also deflected medially, but the soft palate is not affected. There may be slight external swelling seen with infections of the lateral pharyngeal space.

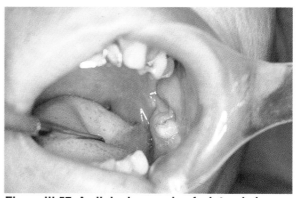

Figure III-57. A clinical example of a lateral pharyngeal space infection. Notice swelling of left pharyngeal wall medial to the ascending ramus.

Odontogenic Origin

Most parapharyngeal infections result from infections of the mandibular third molar area. Peritonsillar abscesses may also spread to the lateral pharyngeal space.

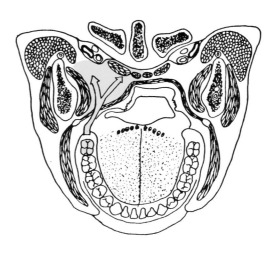

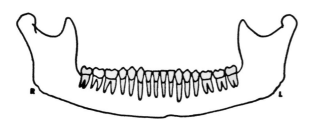

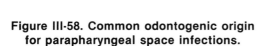

Figure III-58. Common odontogenic origin for parapharyngeal space infections.

Figure III-59. Spread of odontogenic infection to parapharyngeal spaces. Note that infection first progresses to the lateral pharyngeal space, then into the retropharyngeal space.

Pattern of Spread

Infections of the parapharyngeal spaces may spread:
- inferiorly via carotid sheath and fascial planes of the neck to the **mediastinum** and **pericardium**.
- superiorly to the **temporal spaces, base of skull, foramen ovale,** and **brain**.

NOTE: Infections of parapharyngeal spaces are EXTREMELY SERIOUS and require IMMEDIATE hospitalization. Their anatomical location and serious complications require immediate, aggressive, and expert care.

STUDY EXERCISES

What is the most likely dental source of parapharyngeal space infections? _mandibular_
___3RD___ _molars_

Check the following symptoms which could indicate a parapharyngeal space infection.
- ☐ marked trismus
- ☑ slight trismus
- ☐ severe external swelling
- ☐ extreme dysphagia
- ☐ elevation of tongue
- ☐ slight dysphagia
- ☐ severe internal swelling
- ☒ malaise & fever
- ☑ respiratory obstruction

Parapharyngeal space infections require immediate _care_ because the anatomic location requires aggressive expert care.

Parapharyngeal infections can be fatal because of several possible consequences, including:

a. Spread inferiorly via the ___carotid___ sheath to mediastinum and ___heart___ .

b. Spread superiorly to the temporal spaces, base of skull, foramen ___ovale___ and ___rotundum___ .

☐ 16 Cervical Spaces

The fascial planes of the neck are sub-divided into the **superficial** and **deep cervical fascia**. The deep cervical fascia contains six layers: 1) the **external (investing) layer** (which covers the entire neck); 2) the **middle layer** (which is below the external layer and envelops the inferior strap muscles); 3) the **visceral (pretracheal) layer** (which covers the thyroid, trachea, esophagus and is the cervical extension of the retropharyngeal space; 4) the **carotid sheath**; 5) the **alar fascia** (which is just anterior to the prevertebral fascia behind the pharynx); 6) **prevertebral** fascia which covers the vertebrae, spinal column, and associated muscles.

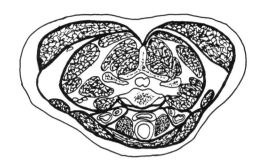

Figure III-60. Cross-section of the neck showing the numerous fascial planes (heavy black).

Signs & Symptoms

Infections involving the cervical fascia can vary in clinical appearance depending upon the specific fascia or layer involved. The following may be involved:

- **Brawny swelling of the neck**
- **Difficulty in swallowing**
- **Difficulty in breathing**
- **Obliteration of the sternal notch**
- **Signs of inflammation** can vary depending upon the depth of the involved space from the skin

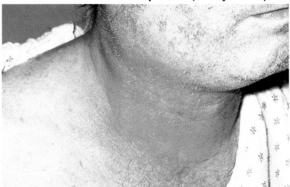

Figure III-61. In this patient an abscessed second molar resulted in the spread of infection to the parapharyngeal space and progressed to involve the fascial planes of the neck. Notice the bulging of the neck on the patient's right.

Odontogenic Sources

Dental infections involving most fascial spaces of the head can spread directly or indirectly to the fascial planes of the neck.

NOTE: The seriousness of any infection (regardless of source) involving any of the cervical fascia cannot be over-emphasized and immediate referral to a specialist or hospital is essential!

STUDY EXERCISES

You should immediately __refer__ any patient who has an infection involving the neck.

☐ 15 Peritonsillar Space Infections

Peritonsillar infections are not usually of odontogenic origin. Peritonsillar abscess will be briefly described here, since anatomically it is adjacent to the lateral pharyngeal space and may be confused with pterygomandibular and lateral pharyngeal space infections.

The peritonsillar space is located between the connective tissue bed of the faucial tonsil, between the tonsils and the superior constrictor.

The peritonsillar abscess is not considered a fascial space infection. It is an infection that develops between the superior constrictor muscle and the mucous membrane. It can be unilateral or bilateral.

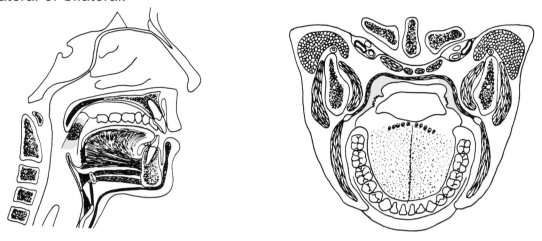

Figure III-62. Anatomical location of peritonsillar space.

Signs and Symptoms

There is acute pain on one side of the throat radiating to the ear. The patient has difficulty swallowing. Speech becomes awkward. There may be a tense swelling of the anterior pillar of the fauces and a bulge in the soft palate on the affected side, marked uvular edema. Trismus is usually absent.

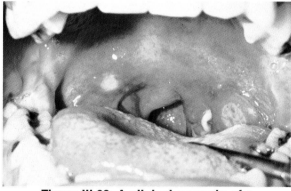

Figure III-63. A clinical example of a peritonsillar abscess.

Route of Spread

Infections of the peritonsillar space may spread to:
- the **lateral pharyngeal spaces**
- **pterygomandibular** and **deep temporal spaces**

Infections in the peritonsillar space may spread to the ___lateral___ ___pharyngeal___ *spaces or the* ___pterygomandibular___ *and* ___deep___ ___temporal___ *spaces.*

What signs and symptoms would you expect if an infection involves the peritonsillar space?

1) ___swelling___

2) ___marked uvular edema___

3) ___pain radiating from throat to ear___

4) ___speech akward___

SUMMARY OF INFECTIOUS SWELLINGS OF THE PHARYNGEAL AREA

Pharyngeal area swellings are associated with three (3) major anatomical areas or spaces. These include:
- **pterygomandibular space**
- **parapharyngeal spaces**
  - lateral pharyngeal space
  - retropharyngeal space
- **peritonsillar space or area**

Swellings associated with the peritonsillar space infection may resemble lateral pharyngeal space infections.

As shown in **Table III-3,** odontogenic infections can spread directly from maxillary and mandibular posterior teeth to the pterygomandibular space, lateral and retropharyngeal spaces or indirectly to this area from neighboring fascial spaces.

SPREAD TO PHARYNGEAL AREA FROM

- Infected tooth — maxillary or mandibular
- Buccal space
- Pterygomandibular space
- Submasseteric space
- Sublingual space
- Submandibular space
- Deep temporal space
- Palatal subperiosteal

Table III-3. Summary of spread of odontogenic infections to the fascial spaces of the pharyngeal area.

NOTE: **Virtually all infections of the fascial spaces contiguous with the oral cavity can directly or indirectly spread to the parapharyngeal area and further spread to the fascial planes of the neck and mediastinum. ANY SWELLINGS OF THE PARAPHARYNGEAL AREA SHOULD BE CONSIDERED EXTREMELY SERIOUS AND MUST BE REFERRED TO A SPECIALIST OR HOSPITAL IMMEDIATELY.**

STUDY EXERCISES

If a patient presents with swelling of the parapharyngeal area, how should you manage this problem? refer

*Infections from which teeth can spread **directly** into the parapharyngeal space?* mand max posterior teeth *Infections from which teeth frequently spread to the pterygomandibular space?* 2nd 3rd molars

Can infections of other teeth spread indirectly into these spaces from other spaces? (yes/no) yes *. If so, which spaces and which teeth?* Buccal, pterygomand, submasseteric, sublingual, submandibular, deep temporal, palatal subperiosteal

Label the spaces indicated on the following diagram:

parapharyngeal

sub-masseter

peri-tonsillar

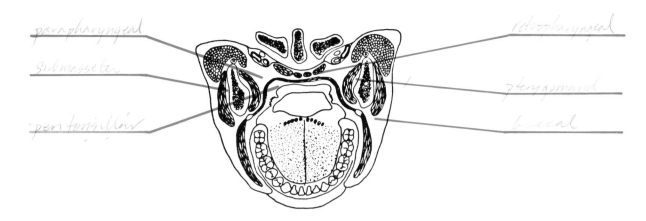

retropharyngeal

pterygomand

buccal

Name the fascial spaces associated with the following clinical signs and symptoms:

Symptoms	Space
Severe pain when swallowing, some trismus, tonsil and lateral pharyngeal wall displaced medially	parapharyngeal
Moderate to severe trismus, swelling of tonsillar pillar medially	pterygomandibular
Pain, difficulty swallowing, swelling of tonsillar pillar, uvular edema, swelling of soft palate	peri-tonsillar

SWELLINGS OF THE MIDFACE REGION

Swellings of the midface region include:
- **palatal subperiosteal area**
- **infraorbital area (canine fossa)**
- **periorbital area**
- **base of the upper lip**
- **maxillary and ethmoid sinuses**

Infections of these areas are most frequently associated with odontogenic infections of the maxillary teeth as shown in **Figure III-64** below.

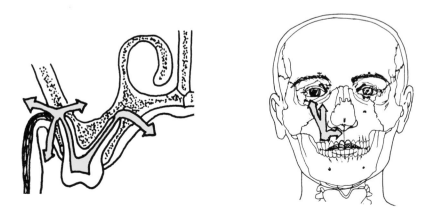

Figure III-64. Spread of odontogenic infections to the midface regions.

☐ 17 Palatal Subperiosteal Area

Anatomical Location

A subperiosteal abscess of the palate is not strictly considered a fascial space infection. Infections of maxillary teeth will frequently erode through the palatal cortical bone and delaminate the palatal mucoperiosteum from the maxilla producing palatal swelling.

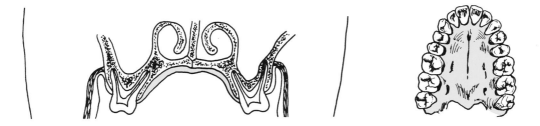

Figure III-65. Summary of the anatomical location of the palatal area.

Signs and Symptoms

The primary sign is a circumscribed fluctuant swelling usually confined to one side of the palate.

Odontogenic Origin

Frequently palatal subperiosteal abscesses develop from infections of maxillary teeth, almost always the lateral incisors or maxillary first premolars. As with all suspected infections, a differential diagnosis would include cystic lesions, salivary gland lesions and malignancies.

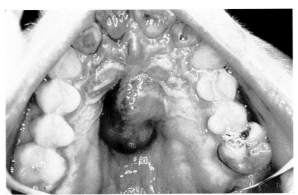

Figure III-66. Clinical example of a palatal abscess.

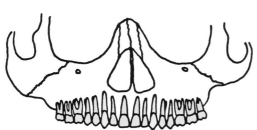

Figure III-67. Dental source for palatal area infections.

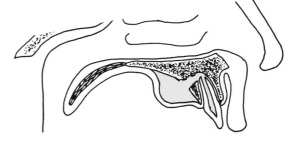

Figure III-68. Spread of infection from a maxillary lateral incisor, creating an infectious swelling of the palate.

Spread to Adjacent Areas

Infections of the palatal area seldom spread into adjacent fascial spaces.

☑ 18 Infraorbital Area (Canine Fossa)

The infraorbital area (canine fossa) is bounded superiorly by the levator muscles, anteriorly by the orbicularis oris and posteriorly by the buccinator muscle.

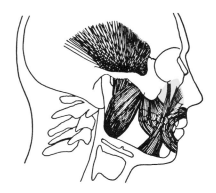 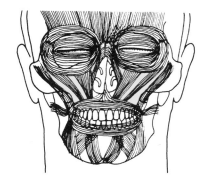

Figure III-69. Anatomical location of the infraorbital area or canine fossa.

Signs and Symptoms

Swelling may cause obliteration of the nasolabial fold and produce edema of the upper lip and lower eyelid. Intraorally, swelling of the infraorbital area (canine fossa) is seen as a bulging of the maxillary buccal vestibule anterior to the zygomatic buttress.

Odontogenic Sources

Infections of the maxillary canines and first premolars may discharge into the infraorbital area.

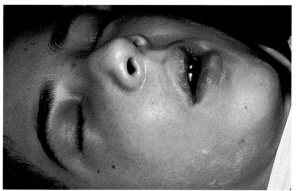

Figure III-70. A clinical example of an infection of the infraorbital area.

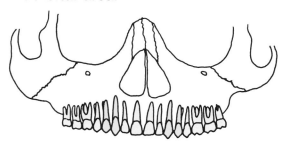

Figure III-71. Usual source of odontogenic infections of the infraorbital area.

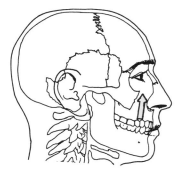

Figure III-72. Spread of odontogenic infection to the infraorbital area.

Spread to Adjacent Areas

Infections of the infraorbital area may spread:

- to the **cavernous sinus** via the facial vein, angular vein, and ophthalmic vein or by direct extension.
- posteriorly and laterally to involve the **buccal space,** then into the **deep temporal space.**
- superiorly to the **periorbital area;** however, this is rare.

Infections of the infraorbital area have significant risk for cavernous sinus involvement. Infections of this area are usually effectively treated by general practitioners; however, they can develop into life-threatening cavernous sinus infections if not closely monitored.

☐ 19 Periorbital Area

Anatomic Location

This space is located under the orbicularis oculi. Retrograde venous drainage into the ophthalmic vein can easily occur from this area.

Signs and Symptoms

Infection of the periorbital space will cause swelling of the eyelids (upper and lower), often severe enough to block vision.

Odontogenic Sources

Infections from any maxillary tooth can spread into the periorbital area; maxillary canine and first premolar infections can spread via the **infraorbital** area; maxillary molars and second premolar infections can spread via the buccal space; and maxillary incisor infections can spread via the base of the upper lip and infraorbital area.

Spread to Adjacent Areas

Infections of the periorbital space may spread to the **cavernous sinus** via the facial vein, angular vein, and ophthalmic vein and by direct posterior extension.

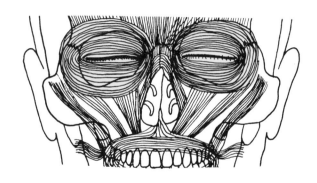

Figure III-73. Anatomic location of the periorbital areas.

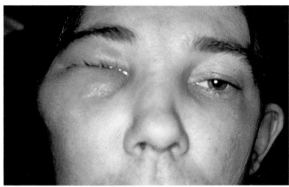

Figure III-74. A clinical example of an odontogenic infection involving the periorbital area.

NOTE: Any oral and/or maxillofacial infection which has signs and symptoms of periorbital space involvement should be regarded as extremely serious and thus referred to a specialist.

STUDY EXERCISES

For the signs and symptoms described below, state the area which is most likely infected.

Signs & Symptoms	Area
1. Circumscribed fluctuant swelling of the palate (usually unilateral)	1. *palatal subperiosteal*
2. Swelling of the upper and lower eyelid	2. *periorbital*
3. Swelling of the upper lip and lower eyelid, which often obliterates the naso-labial fold	3. *infraorbital*

☑ 20 Base of the Upper Lip

While there is no true fascial space associated with the base of the upper lip, infections of the upper incisors and canines can discharge into the various muscle layers of this area. These infections **can be very dangerous** because of their potential for spread to the **infraorbital** and **periorbital** spaces. A **cavernous sinus thrombosis** can then result from extension from the superior labial venous plexus to the angular vein and then via the ophthalmic veins to the **cavernous sinus.** Since the veins of the upper face have no valves, ascending infections are more likely in this location.

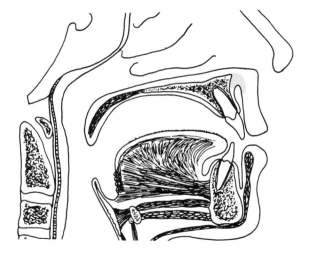

Figure III-75. Anatomical location for infections at the base of the upper lip.

Signs and Symptoms

Typical signs and symptoms include: pain, swelling involving upper lip (may be extensive), elevation of the alar base and nasal tip, obliteration of maxillary labial vestibule.

Odontogenic Source

The usual source of infections of the base of the lip are the maxillary incisors.

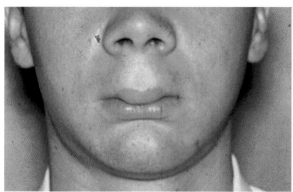

Figure III-76. Clinical example of an infection of the upper lip.

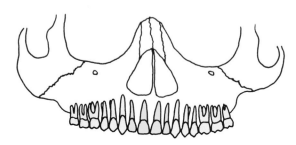

Figure III-77. Odontogenic sources for infections of the base of the lip.

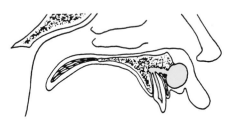

Figure III-78. Spread of odontogenic infections to the base of the upper lip.

Pattern of Spread

Infections of the base of the lip may spread:
- to involve the **infraorbital area** and then to the **periorbital space**
- **to the cavernous sinus** via facial vein, angular vein, ophthalmic vein, and direct extension

Infections involving the base of the upper lip may spread into the *infraorbital* area, the *cavernous* sinus, or the *periorbital* space via the *infraorbital* area.

What is the usual odontogenic source for infections in the base of the upper lip? *incisors*

Would you consider an infection in the base of the upper lip potentially dangerous for your patient? *yes* Why or why not? *may spread to infraorbital & periorbital area*

□ 21 Spread to Maxillary Sinuses

Signs and Symptoms

Infection of the maxillary sinus may cause headache, stuffiness, or pain. Frequently it will be difficult to distinguish maxillary sinus infections originating from maxillary teeth from those arising from other causes. Radiographs of an infected maxillary sinus will often show increased opacity. A panoramic view is helpful because bilateral comparisons can be made.

Odontogenic Sources

Odontogenic infections of the maxillary sinus **may result from any of the maxillary molars or premolars.** Maxillary sinus infections may also develop post-surgically following extraction of maxillary teeth, especially if an oro-antral communication was formed during surgery and/or a root tip has been displaced into the sinus.

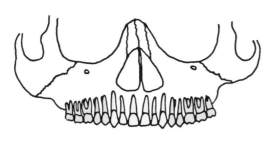

Figure III-79. Odontogenic sources for infections of the maxillary sinus

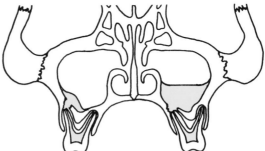

Figure III-80. Spread of infection into the maxillary sinus.

Pattern of Spread

Maxillary sinus infections can spread to the paranasal sinuses and orbits.

SUMMARY OF THE SPREAD OF INFECTION TO MAXILLARY ANTERIOR AREAS

Infection may spread from maxillary teeth into the buccal space, **base of the upper lip, infraorbital area** and/or **periorbital area.** Spread into these areas increases the seriousness of the infection because of the risk of involvement of the cavernous sinus. Infections in the infraorbital space can spread into the cavernous sinus by retrograde flow via the facial, angular and ophthalmic veins. Two other areas which may be involved following infections of maxillary teeth are the palatal area and maxillary sinus.

AREAS	ODONTOGENIC SOURCE	SPREAD TO
Infra-orbital	Maxillary canines & first premolars	Buccal space, deep temporal space, cavernous sinus, orbit
Periorbital	Any maxillary tooth	Cavernous sinus via facial, angular and ophthalmic veins
Base of upper lip	Maxillary incisors	Infraorbital area, cavernous sinus
Palatal subperiosteal	Any maxillary tooth	Maxillary sinus
Maxillary sinus	Any maxillary posterior tooth	Paranasal sinuses, orbit

Table III-4. Summary of origins and spread of infections to spaces in the anterior maxillary region.

RECORDING DATA ON THE ANATOMICAL DATA CHECKLIST

An essential component of clinical data collection is identifying and recording the involved anatomical areas. The following checklist has been developed to facilitate you in gathering anatomical data and assist you in describing the location of any swelling relative to the fascial spaces, areas, and osseous structures of the head and neck. You should mark the extent of involvement on the appropriate diagrams and check the areas involved according to the numbers.

NOTE: Clinically it may be difficult to specifically categorize discrete areas due to extensive facial swelling and edema; however, this process will help reinforce terminology easily forgotten.

ANATOMICAL LOCATION OF SWELLING

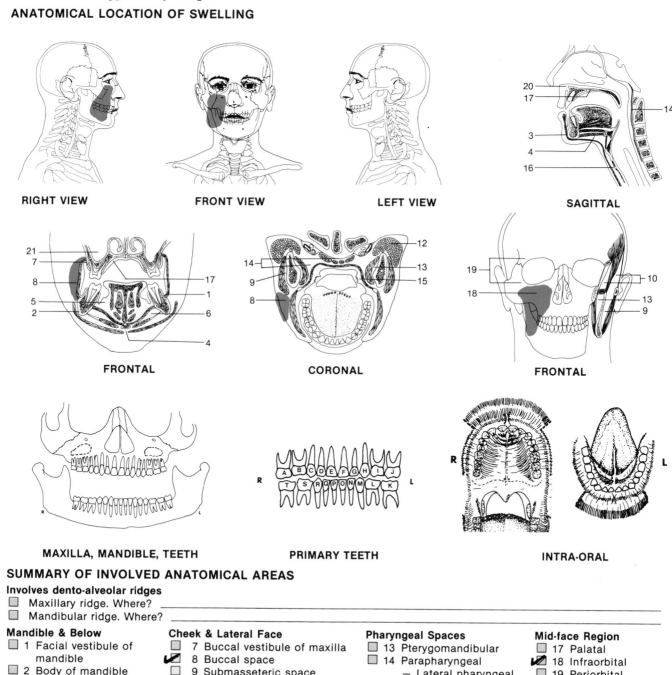

SUMMARY OF INVOLVED ANATOMICAL AREAS

Involves dento-alveolar ridges
- ☐ Maxillary ridge. Where? _____
- ☐ Mandibular ridge. Where? _____

Mandible & Below
- ☐ 1 Facial vestibule of mandible
- ☐ 2 Body of mandible
- ☐ 3 Mentalis space
- ☐ 4 Submental space
- ☐ 5 Sublingual space
- ☐ 6 Submandibular space

Cheek & Lateral Face
- ☐ 7 Buccal vestibule of maxilla
- ☑ 8 Buccal space
- ☐ 9 Submasseteric space
- ☐ 10 Deep Temporal space
- ☐ 10 Superficial Temporal
- ☐ 11 Infratemporal
- ☐ 12 Parotid space

Pharyngeal Spaces
- ☐ 13 Pterygomandibular
- ☐ 14 Parapharyngeal
    - – Lateral pharyngeal
    - – Retropharyngeal
- ☐ 15 Peritonsillar
- ☐ 16 Cervical Spaces

Mid-face Region
- ☐ 17 Palatal
- ☑ 18 Infraorbital
- ☐ 19 Periorbital
- ☑ 20 Base of upper lip
- ☐ 21 Maxillary sinus

How to Use the Checklist

The following steps should be used to minimize your time in determining the anatomical location of a swelling and to maximize efficient use of the anatomical drawings on the checklist.

Step 1. Visually estimate the extent of involved areas (both intra- and extraoral).

Step 2. Palpate the borders of the swelling to determine their relationship to underlying osseous landmarks. Soft tissue swelling will frequently obliterate normal tissue contours, thus palpation of osseous landmarks is essential to establishing the location of a swelling.

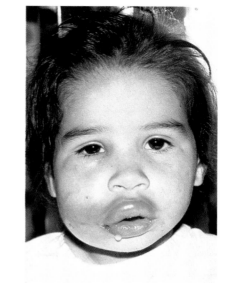

  EXAMPLE: Visual examination of the photograph to the right shows a swelling extending from the mandible inferiorly to the orbit superiorly in the right midface region. Palpation of osseous landmarks below the soft tissue reveals the swelling to extend from the inferior border of the mandible to the orbit and is anterior to the ascending ramus and zygomatic arch.

Step 3. Color the involved areas on the appropriate full-face diagrams in relation to the underlying osseous landmarks.

Step 4. Color the appropriate area(s) on the other anatomical diagrams. Some of the fascial spaces or areas are not shown in detail in the drawings provided. You should review the text in this unit if the area involved is not presented in sufficient detail.

Step 5. Use the number code system to assist you in naming the involved area(s). This number coding system was designed only to assist you in obtaining the names for anatomical areas that can be seen or palpated. You should carefully review a patient's other signs and symptoms to determine whether other areas are also involved.

  EXAMPLE: In the photograph on this page you can see extraoral involvement of the buccal space. In addition, patient has swelling below her right eye, thus indicating involvement of the infraorbital space as well. Both spaces should be colored and checked.

Step 6. Estimate the degree of risk associated with swellings of the involved areas. The significance of the color coding has been discussed on page 55. This color code refers to the severity of anatomical areas only, and does not take into account factors associated with patient health or the characteristics of any associated microorganisms.

  EXAMPLE: In a healthy patient, a yellow box for a buccal space infection means the patient can usually be managed on an out-patient basis from either your office or a specialist's office and followed on a daily basis. The presence of infraorbital swelling increases the seriousness of this infection (due to the risk of spread into the cavernous sinus). Very close monitoring is required and prompt referral to a specialist is necessary if serious signs develop. In a medically compromised patient, the degree of risk is greatly increased and the yellow boxes should be changed to red, indicating need for prompt referral to specialist and/or hospital.

Step 7. When radiographic data is obtained any abnormal areas should be added to the anatomical data checklist.

Using the checklist on page 96, you can see that we have colored the areas of involvement on the anatomical diagrams and identified the facial spaces or anatomical areas from the number codes on the diagrams. **Thus, this swelling involves the right buccal and infraorbital spaces and the degree of risk may be considered moderate to severe with a risk of spread to the cavernous sinus.**

POST-TEST — UNIT III

- Answer each of the following questions.
- Check your answers with the correct responses on page 103.
- If all questions are answered correctly, proceed to Unit IV, page 107.
- If you do not answer all questions correctly, read and study the content of this unit.

QUESTIONS

1. Name the anatomical areas or structures shown on the following illustrations.

a. *hard palate*
b. *submandibular*
c. *submental*
d. *max sinus*
e. *buccal vestible*
f. *masseter buccinator*
g. *sublingual*
h. *mylohyoid*

i. *digastric*
j. *platysma*
k. *carotid sheath*
l. *lat. parapharyngeal*
m. *pterygomandibular sp.*
n. *submasseter*
o. *masseter*
p. *buccal sp*

q. *parotid*
r. *facial n. ext carotid*
s. *ramus*
t. *med. pterygoid*
u. *peritonsillar*
v. *pterygopalatine*
w. *buccinator*

2. Match the number for each lymph node group shown on the illustration with its corresponding name.

_5_ a. inferior deep cervical
_2_ b. occipital
_1_ c. posterior auricular
_4_ d. posterior cervical
_6_ e. anterior auricular
_3_ f. superficial cervical

_9_ g. mental
_8_ h. buccal
_12_ i. jugulo-omohyoid
_7_ j. infraorbital
_10_ k. submental
_11_ l. submandibular

3. When evaluating lymph nodes, what two signs would you expect if your patient has an infection? _tenderness_ and _serous swelling_

4. A periodontal abscess involving the tissue between the mandibular central and lateral incisors would cause swelling of which lymph node(s)?_____
Submandibular mental submental

5. Infections involving which teeth can cause inflammation of the submandibular lymph node? (more than one choice is correct)
   a) maxillary molars   d) mandibular incisors
   b) mandibular molars   e) maxillary incisors
   c) mandibular canines

6. In this unit, infections involving fascial spaces are classified as to low, moderate or high risk. Describe the criteria for these classifications.

   Low-risk areas:_____

   _____

   Moderate-risk areas: _____

   _____

   High-risk areas: _____

   _____

7. Label the following fascial spaces according to the risk categories described in this unit. **L** = low-risk   **M** = moderate-risk   **H** = high-risk   **CS** = cavernous sinus risk

a. _H , CS_
b. _CS , A_
c. _L   M_
d. _L   M_
e. _M_
f. _M   H_
g. _L   M_
h. _A_
i. _M   H_
j. _M   A_
k. _M_
l. _M_

8. For the following fascial space infections, state the common odontogenic origin and name the fascial spaces into which these infections could directly spread.

Space	Odontogenic Origin	Spread
a. mandibular facial vestibule	_mand. inc._	_submentalis_
b. mentalis space	_mand. inc_	_submentalis_ _submandibular_
c. submandibular space	_mand post._	
d. sublingual space	_all_	_submandibular_

9. For the symptoms described below, identify the fascial space infection involved.

a. Severe trismus, very ill patient, bulging temporalis muscle
infratemporal _superior temporalis_

b. Severe trismus, deep-seated throbbing pain, little external swelling
submasseter _infratemporalis_

c. Moderate trismus, hard swelling below mandible, toxic appearance
submandibular

d. Severe dysphagia, elevation of tongue, no external swelling
sublingual

e. Severe dysphagia, swelling of lateral pharyngeal wall, no soft palate involvement
lateral

f. Acute pain, dysphagia, tense swelling of the tonsillar pillar, soft palate and uvular edema
peritonsillar

10. Infectons of which fascial spaces or anatomical areas can cause the following symptoms?

Trismus
super temp
deep temp
submasseter
submand.
pterygomand
parapharyngeal

Dysphagia
peritonsillar   _submandibular_
retro
lat
submental
sublingual

For each of the clinical cases presented on pages 100-102:
a. **Identify** the anatomical areas involved by coloring in the diagrams on the checklist.
b. Check the appropriate box.
c. Describe the degree of risk associated with each patient's problem.
d. Name the fascial spaces or areas where the infection may spread if not controlled.

Case #1 — *This 32-year-old female presented to your office complaining of pain and swelling on the right side of her face. She said the swelling began two days ago and that she had a severe toothache in her maxillary right first molar about a week ago. The toothache subsided but the pain and swelling developed on her face just after the tooth pain subsided.*

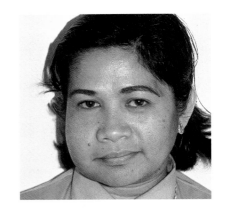

Examination revealed: *Temp 38.2°C; tender right cheek swelling which was redder and warmer than normal areas; normal mouth opening, no intraoral, lingual or pharyngeal swelling was seen. No tenderness over masseter, below inferior border of mandible, temporal area, around or below the eye. An area of fluctuance was palpable between the buccal mucosa and skin of the right cheek. The maxillary first molar was severely carious and non-vital. Periapical radiographs revealed no areas of radiolucency. All other data was non-contributory.*

ANATOMICAL LOCATION OF SWELLING

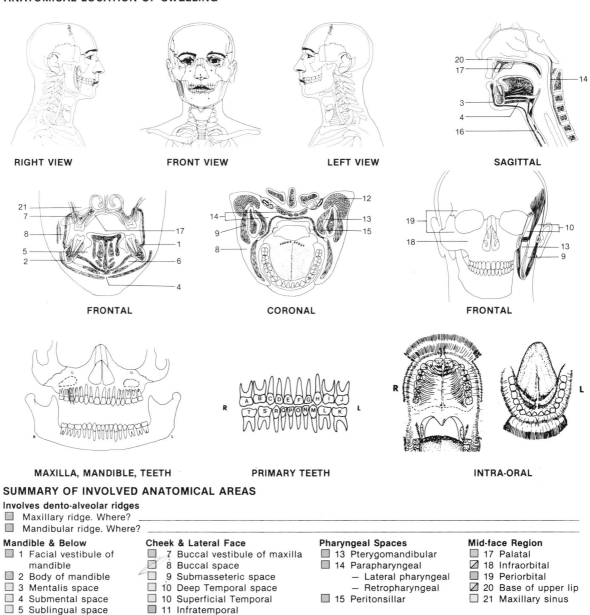

RIGHT VIEW   FRONT VIEW   LEFT VIEW   SAGITTAL

FRONTAL   CORONAL   FRONTAL

MAXILLA, MANDIBLE, TEETH   PRIMARY TEETH   INTRA-ORAL

SUMMARY OF INVOLVED ANATOMICAL AREAS

Involves dento-alveolar ridges
- ☐ Maxillary ridge. Where? _____
- ☐ Mandibular ridge. Where? _____

Mandible & Below	**Cheek & Lateral Face**	**Pharyngeal Spaces**	**Mid-face Region**
☐ 1 Facial vestibule of mandible	☐ 7 Buccal vestibule of maxilla	☐ 13 Pterygomandibular	☐ 17 Palatal
☐ 2 Body of mandible	☑ 8 Buccal space	☐ 14 Parapharyngeal	☑ 18 Infraorbital
☐ 3 Mentalis space	☐ 9 Submasseteric space	— Lateral pharyngeal	☐ 19 Periorbital
☐ 4 Submental space	☐ 10 Deep Temporal space	— Retropharyngeal	☑ 20 Base of upper lip
☐ 5 Sublingual space	☐ 10 Superficial Temporal	☐ 15 Peritonsillar	☐ 21 Maxillary sinus
☐ 6 Submandibular space	☐ 11 Infratemporal		
	☐ 12 Parotid space	☐ 16 Cervical Spaces	

Case #2 — *This 12-year-old male returned to your office five days after you extracted his cariously destroyed mandibular right first molar with the facial swelling as shown in the photograph. He said the swelling began yesterday and complains of pain, has some difficulty in swallowing and appears mildly toxic. He has no problems with respiration. At the time of extraction there was no soft tissue involvement but there was a 1.0 cm radiolucency at the apex of the involved tooth. At this time there is pain and a firm, non-fluctuant swelling below the right inferior border of the mandible extending from the angle of the mandible anteriorly to below the chin. Temperature = 39.5°C, B.P. = 120/80/80, Pulse rate = 78, Resp. rate = 18. There is no elevation of the tongue or swelling of the floor of the mouth nor is there any intraoral swelling in the posterior areas.*

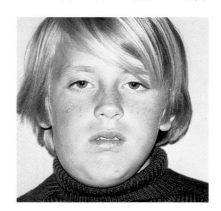

ANATOMICAL LOCATION OF SWELLING

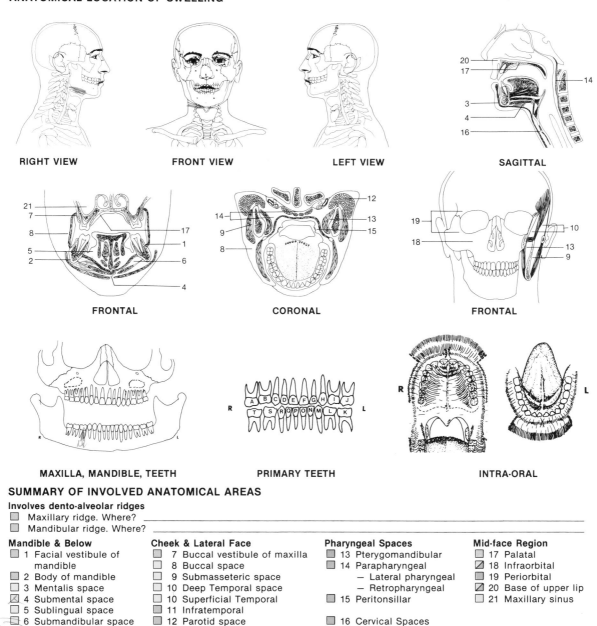

RIGHT VIEW   FRONT VIEW   LEFT VIEW   SAGITTAL

FRONTAL   CORONAL   FRONTAL

MAXILLA, MANDIBLE, TEETH   PRIMARY TEETH   INTRA-ORAL

SUMMARY OF INVOLVED ANATOMICAL AREAS

Involves dento-alveolar ridges
- ☐ Maxillary ridge. Where? _____
- ☐ Mandibular ridge. Where? _____

Mandible & Below	**Cheek & Lateral Face**	**Pharyngeal Spaces**	**Mid-face Region**
☐ 1 Facial vestibule of mandible	☐ 7 Buccal vestibule of maxilla	☐ 13 Pterygomandibular	☐ 17 Palatal
☐ 2 Body of mandible	☐ 8 Buccal space	☐ 14 Parapharyngeal	☒ 18 Infraorbital
☐ 3 Mentalis space	☐ 9 Submasseteric space	— Lateral pharyngeal	☐ 19 Periorbital
☒ 4 Submental space	☐ 10 Deep Temporal space	— Retropharyngeal	☒ 20 Base of upper lip
☐ 5 Sublingual space	☐ 10 Superficial Temporal	☐ 15 Peritonsillar	☐ 21 Maxillary sinus
☒ 6 Submandibular space	☐ 11 Infratemporal		
	☐ 12 Parotid space	☐ 16 Cervical Spaces	

Case #3 — This 18-year-old female returned to your office complaining of pain and facial swelling which has developed since you began root canal therapy of her right maxillary canine three days ago. At that time you instrumented the then non-vital canine, applied a medicated cotton pellet and sealed the orifice with temporary cement. At this time she has the following signs and symptoms: Temp. = 39.2°C; B.P. = 122/75/75; Pulse = 80; Resp. = 17; malaise; marked, firm facial swelling and redness of the midface region and alar of the nose, but no swelling of the eyebrow area. Her right eye was beginning to close. No fluctuance could be detected. Obvious bulging of the canine fossa was observed intraorally. There was no trismus or difficulty in swallowing or breathing.

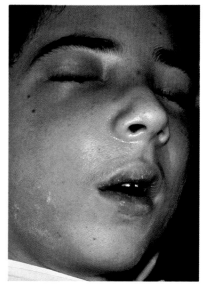

ANATOMICAL LOCATION OF SWELLING

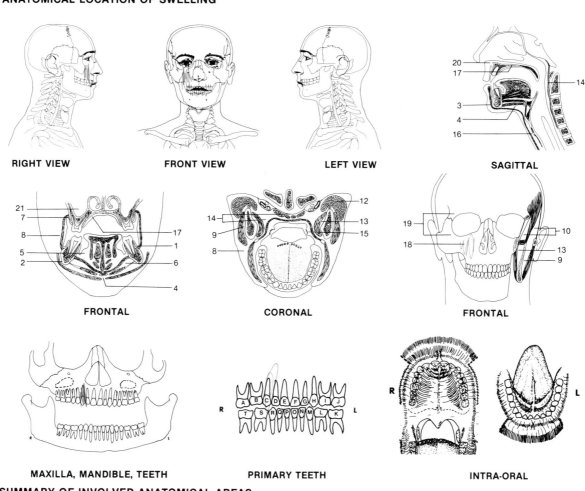

RIGHT VIEW   FRONT VIEW   LEFT VIEW   SAGITTAL

FRONTAL   CORONAL   FRONTAL

MAXILLA, MANDIBLE, TEETH   PRIMARY TEETH   INTRA-ORAL

SUMMARY OF INVOLVED ANATOMICAL AREAS

Involves dento-alveolar ridges
- ☐ Maxillary ridge. Where? _____
- ☐ Mandibular ridge. Where? _____

Mandible & Below	**Cheek & Lateral Face**	**Pharyngeal Spaces**	**Mid-face Region**
☐ 1 Facial vestibule of mandible	☐ 7 Buccal vestibule of maxilla	☐ 13 Pterygomandibular	☐ 17 Palatal
☐ 2 Body of mandible	☐ 8 Buccal space	☐ 14 Parapharyngeal	☑ 18 Infraorbital
☐ 3 Mentalis space	☐ 9 Submasseteric space	— Lateral pharyngeal	☐ 19 Periorbital
☐ 4 Submental space	☐ 10 Deep Temporal space	— Retropharyngeal	☑ 20 Base of upper lip
☐ 5 Sublingual space	☐ 10 Superficial Temporal	☐ 15 Peritonsillar	☐ 21 Maxillary sinus
☐ 6 Submandibular space	☐ 11 Infratemporal		
	☐ 12 Parotid space	☐ 16 Cervical Spaces	

POST-TEST ANSWERS — UNIT III

1. a. palate
   b. submandibular space
   c. submental space
   d. maxillary sinus
   e. maxillary alveolus
   f. buccinator muscle
   g. sublingual space
   h. mylohyoid muscle
   i. digastric muscle
   j. platysma muscle
   k. carotid sheath
   l. parapharyngeal space
   m. pterygomandibular space
   n. submasseteric space
   o. masseter muscle
   p. buccal space
   q. parotid gland
   r. external carotid artery
   s. ascending ramus
   t. pterygoid muscle
   u. peritonsillar space
   v. pterygomandibular raphe
   w. buccinator muscle

2. a. 5, inferior deep cervical
   b. 2, occipital
   c. 1, posterior auricular
   d. 4, posterior cervical
   e. 6, anterior auricular
   f. 3, superficial cervical
   g. 9, mental
   h. 8, buccal
   i. 12, jugulo omo-hyoid
   j. 7, infraorbital
   k. 10, submental
   l. 11, submandibular

3. swelling, tenderness

4. mental, submental submandibular

5. a. maxillary molars   b. mandibular molars   c. mandibular canines

6. see page 55.

7. a. periorbital - CS, H
   b. infraorbital - H/M, CS
   c. mentalis - M
   d. superficial temporal - M
   e. deep temporal - M
   f. pterygomandibular - H
   g. submasseteric - M
   h. parapharyngeal - H
   i. peritonsillar - H
   j. parotid - H
   k. submasseteric - M
   l. buccal - M

8. a. Any mandibular tooth
   b. mandibular incisors
   c. mandibular incisors, canines, premolars, mesial roots of first molars

   buccal space
   submental space
   submandibular space
   parapharyngeal space
   pterygomandibular space

9. a. Infratemporal space
   b. Submasseteric space
   c. Submandibular space
   d. Sublingual space
   e. Lateral pharyngeal space
   f. Peritonsillar space

10. Trismus — Submandibular, submasseteric, infratemporal, pterygomandibular, parapharyngeal

    Dysphagia — Submental, sublingual, submandibular, parapharyngeal, peritonsillar

Answers to Cases 1-3 are shown on pages 104-106.

Case #1 Discussion — This infection appears to involve the right buccal space only. Lack of tenderness over the masseter and lack of trismus indicate no submasseteric space involvement. Additionally, lack of swelling or tenderness in other areas indicates infection has also not involved any other areas. Since no intraoral swelling was apparent, this infection (originating from pulpal necrosis of the maxillary right first molar) tracked through the maxilla and exited into the buccal space of the cheek. This infection is of moderate risk and should be closely followed.

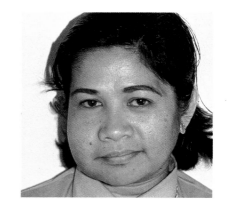

This infection could spread to the **submasseteric** space or to the **pterygomandibular, lateral pharyngeal, deep** or **superficial** temporal spaces if not closely followed. The presence of fluctuance indicates the likelihood of spread to other areas can be reduced if incision and drainage of the buccal space is performed and the dental source of the infection is controlled.

ANATOMICAL LOCATION OF SWELLING

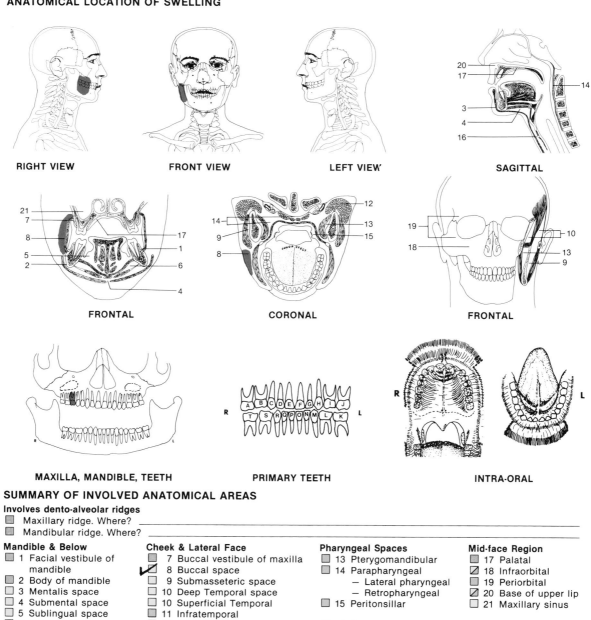

RIGHT VIEW   FRONT VIEW   LEFT VIEW'   SAGITTAL

FRONTAL   CORONAL   FRONTAL

MAXILLA, MANDIBLE, TEETH   PRIMARY TEETH   INTRA-ORAL

SUMMARY OF INVOLVED ANATOMICAL AREAS

Involves dento-alveolar ridges
☐ Maxillary ridge. Where? _____
☐ Mandibular ridge. Where? _____

Mandible & Below	Cheek & Lateral Face	Pharyngeal Spaces	Mid-face Region
☐ 1 Facial vestibule of mandible	☐ 7 Buccal vestibule of maxilla	☐ 13 Pterygomandibular	☐ 17 Palatal
☐ 2 Body of mandible	☑ 8 Buccal space	☐ 14 Parapharyngeal	☑ 18 Infraorbital
☐ 3 Mentalis space	☐ 9 Submasseteric space	– Lateral pharyngeal	☐ 19 Periorbital
☐ 4 Submental space	☐ 10 Deep Temporal space	– Retropharyngeal	☑ 20 Base of upper lip
☐ 5 Sublingual space	☐ 10 Superficial Temporal	☐ 15 Peritonsillar	☐ 21 Maxillary sinus
☐ 6 Submandibular space	☐ 11 Infratemporal		
	☐ 12 Parotid space	☐ 16 Cervical Spaces	

Case #2 Discussion — *This swelling appears primarily confined to the right submandibular space at this time, however early involvement of the submental space is evident under the chin. Other data indicates presence of a non-localized infection with signs of systemic involvement. The source of the infection is most likely the periapical lesion which penetrated the mandible into the submandibular space following extraction of the involved molar. Since this infection has developed rapidly, is not as yet localized (firm and non-fluctuant) and may involve both the submandibular and submental spaces, it must be considered **very serious** at this time. This infection could rapidly progress into Ludwig's angina, thus prompt, aggressive management is essential.*

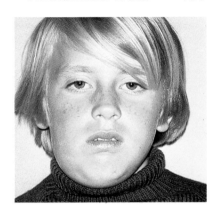

ANATOMICAL LOCATION OF SWELLING

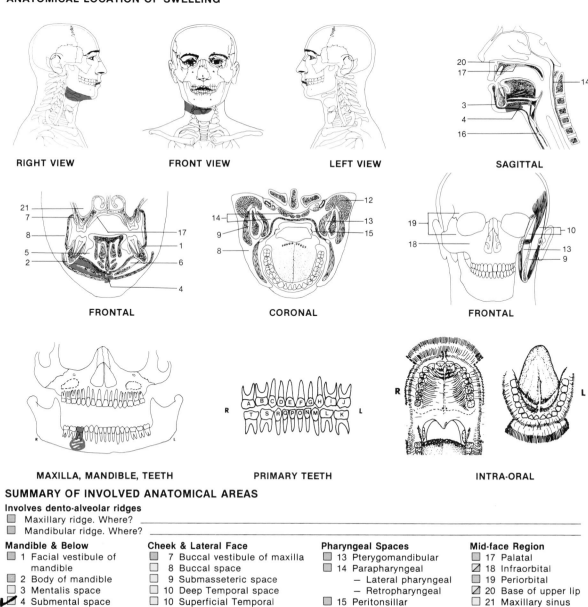

| RIGHT VIEW | FRONT VIEW | LEFT VIEW | SAGITTAL |

| FRONTAL | CORONAL | FRONTAL |

| MAXILLA, MANDIBLE, TEETH | PRIMARY TEETH | INTRA-ORAL |

SUMMARY OF INVOLVED ANATOMICAL AREAS

Involves dento-alveolar ridges
- ☐ Maxillary ridge. Where? _____
- ☐ Mandibular ridge. Where? _____

Mandible & Below	**Cheek & Lateral Face**	**Pharyngeal Spaces**	**Mid-face Region**
☐ 1 Facial vestibule of mandible	☐ 7 Buccal vestibule of maxilla	☐ 13 Pterygomandibular	☐ 17 Palatal
☐ 2 Body of mandible	☐ 8 Buccal space	☐ 14 Parapharyngeal	☑ 18 Infraorbital
☐ 3 Mentalis space	☐ 9 Submasseteric space	— Lateral pharyngeal	☐ 19 Periorbital
☑ 4 Submental space	☐ 10 Deep Temporal space	— Retropharyngeal	☑ 20 Base of upper lip
☐ 5 Sublingual space	☐ 10 Superficial Temporal	☐ 15 Peritonsillar	☐ 21 Maxillary sinus
☑ 6 Submandibular space	☐ 11 Infratemporal		
	☐ 12 Parotid space	☐ 16 Cervical Spaces	

Case #3 Discussion — *This swelling most likely originated from the pushing of microorganisms through the apex of the canine tooth into maxillary bone during endodontic instrumentation. Sealing of the canal prevented release of pressure and infection then penetrated into the infraorbital area (canine fossa).*

Currently an acute cellulitis is present in the **infraorbital** *area and spread to the periorbital area may occur. Prompt control of this serious infection is essential to prevent spread to the periorbital area or even to the cavernous sinus via venous drainage of this area. In addition, her fever and malaise indicate likely systemic involvement at this time. Daily monitoring of treatment is essential.*

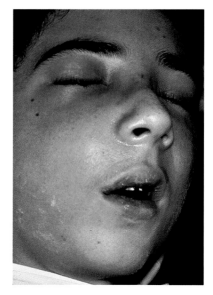

ANATOMICAL LOCATION OF SWELLING

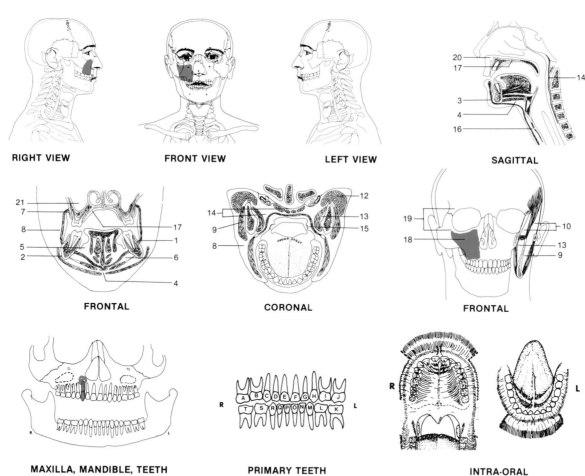

RIGHT VIEW   FRONT VIEW   LEFT VIEW   SAGITTAL

FRONTAL   CORONAL   FRONTAL

MAXILLA, MANDIBLE, TEETH   PRIMARY TEETH   INTRA-ORAL

SUMMARY OF INVOLVED ANATOMICAL AREAS

Involves dento-alveolar ridges
- ☐ Maxillary ridge. Where? _____
- ☐ Mandibular ridge. Where? _____

Mandible & Below	**Cheek & Lateral Face**	**Pharyngeal Spaces**	**Mid-face Region**
☐ 1 Facial vestibule of mandible	☐ 7 Buccal vestibule of maxilla	☐ 13 Pterygomandibular	☐ 17 Palatal
☐ 2 Body of mandible	☐ 8 Buccal space	☐ 14 Parapharyngeal	☑ 18 Infraorbital
☐ 3 Mentalis space	☐ 9 Submasseteric space	– Lateral pharyngeal	☐ 19 Periorbital
☐ 4 Submental space	☐ 10 Deep Temporal space	– Retropharyngeal	☑ 20 Base of upper lip
☐ 5 Sublingual space	☐ 10 Superficial Temporal	☐ 15 Peritonsillar	☐ 21 Maxillary sinus
☐ 6 Submandibular space	☐ 11 Infratemporal		
	☐ 12 Parotid space	☐ 16 Cervical Spaces	

UNIT IV
RADIOGRAPHIC DATA

OVERVIEW & OBJECTIVES

The purpose of this unit is to review how the basic principles of radiology are used in the diagnosis of oral and/or maxillofacial swellings. Emphasis is placed on the radiographic techniques commonly used by general dentists with a discussion of the specific advantages and disadvantages of periapical, occlusal, and panoramic views. Additional radiographic views used by specialists are reviewed, and special techniques such as bone scan with radioisotope studies and computerized tomography are included. Emphasis is also placed on how to record this data on the radiographic data checklist. Following completion of this unit you will:

1. Explain why diagnosis should **not** be made from radiographic data alone.

2. Name the three (3) radiographic views commonly used in general dentistry.

3. Describe the **advantages** and **disadvantages or limitations** of each of the following radiographic views:
   a. Periapical views
   b. Occlusal views
   c. Panoramic views

4. Name five (5) **additional radiographic views** which are used to view **maxillary and mandibular areas,** describe the orientation of the view, and name the anatomical structures that can be seen with these views.

5. Name **additional radiographic techniques** which can be used to view evidence of infection spread to the following:
   a. Neck   b. Lung, mediastinum, thorax   c. Condyle and ramus

6. Describe the role that **each** of the following radiographic views can play in the diagnosis of oral and/or maxillofacial infections:
   a. Lateral oblique
   b. Postero-Anterior (PA)
   c. Submentovertex (SMV)
   d. Anterior lateral face
   e. Water's (occipitomental)
   f. Cervical views (posterior-anterior and lateral)
   g. Chest views

7. Briefly describe the following **advanced radiographic techniques** and their application to the diagnosis of oral and/or maxillofacial infections.
   a. Bone scan with radioisotope studies
   b. Computerized tomography (C.T. Scan)

8. Name the radiographic view(s) which can be used to **view each of the following anatomical structures**:
   a. sinuses
   b. neck involvement
   c. lateral aspect of the maxilla
   d. mandibular symphysis
   e. lungs
   f. condyles
   g. angle of the mandible
   h. cortical plate of the mandibular ramus (3)
   i. thoracic involvement
   j. mandibular ramus
   k. inferior border of the mandible
   l. lateral view of sinuses

9. Given a description (historical, clinical, and/or anatomical data) for an oral or maxillofacial swelling and dental radiographs, determine the need for additional radiographs and name the additional radiographic view(s) that could be helpful.

10. Describe the three (3) steps you should follow when using the **radiographic data checklist** prior to making diagnostic decisions.

UNIT IV
RADIOGRAPHIC DATA

INTRODUCTION

Radiographic data can be essential in your diagnosis of many oral and/or maxillofacial swellings. Various radiographic views can give you clues as to the origin of a swelling and help you determine whether the swelling is associated with tooth structures (odontogenic origin).

NOTE: Radiographic data must never be used as the only data to diagnose the etiology of a swelling. Radiographs are not diagnostic but provide indirect evidence of pathologic processes. Radiographic data should be used in conjunction with historical data, clinical data and laboratory data to support your clinical diagnosis.

RADIOGRAPHIC VIEWS

Many radiographic techniques can be used in the diagnosis of head and neck swellings. We have divided these techniques into groups based upon the availability of techniques for a typical general dentist's office.

RADIOGRAPHIC VIEWS

TYPICAL DENTAL OFFICE VIEWS	VIEWS OBTAINED FROM A RADIOLOGIST		
	ADDITIONAL VIEWS		SPECIAL TECHNIQUES
• Periapical • Occlusal • Panoramic	• Lateral oblique • Postero-Anterior (PA) • Submentovertex (SMV) • Anterior Lateral Face	• Water's (occipitomental) • Cervical (neck) • Chest	• Radioisotope studies (bone scan) • Computerized tomography

The purpose of this unit is to review the basic radiographic techniques useful in the diagnosis of oral and/or maxillofacial swellings. **This unit is not intended to be a text in radiographic interpretation.**

*Describe why radiographic data **should not** be used as the only data to formulate your diagnosis.* not diagnostic, provides indirect evidence

DENTAL RADIOGRAPHIC VIEWS

The following radiographic views are commonly available in the office of a general dentist. These views should be considered your **first line of radiographic information** in the diagnosis of oral and/or maxillofacial swellings. Based upon the results of radiographic analysis and your clinical examination, **additional views** may be necessary. It is important for you to know the advantages and disadvantages for each of these radiographic views in order to collect accurate radiographic data without taking unnecessary radiographs.

Periapical Views

Periapical radiographic views may be valuable in the diagnosis of odontogenic infections.

Advantages — These views provide the **most detailed** information concerning the teeth and alveolar bone. They provide the highest degree of resolution for detecting changes in the apical region of the teeth and for visualizing alveolar bone loss associated with periodontal disease. Posterior maxillary views may partially show involvement of the maxillary sinus.

Disadvantages or limitations — The main disadvantages or limitations of periapical radiographs include:
- Patient with severe trismus may not be able to open his/her mouth wide enough for film placement.
- The size of film used and thus the area surveyed is small.
- The inability to view the following anatomical areas:

  inferior border of the mandible   **some portions of the palate**
  mandibular ramus & condyle   **upper parts of maxillary sinuses**
- Inability to observe the horizontal (mediolateral) dimension of a lesion.

Occlusal Views

Occlusal radiographic views should be used more frequently in the diagnosis of odontogenic infections. Occlusal views have the ability to show you a "top" view of the problem and augment the periapical views to give a three-dimensional view of many pathological processes.

Advantages — Occlusal views provide radiographic data from two areas not visible with periapical views:
- **Palatal bone** can be seen using a maxillary occlusal view
- **Periosteum** on the medial and lateral sides of the mandible can be seen using a mandibular occlusal view. **A view of the periosteal changes may be important evidence in distinguishing inflammation from neoplastic changes.**

Disadvantages or limitations — The disadvantages or limitations of the occlusal view are related to film size and angle of orientation and thus include:
- apices of posterior teeth are not clearly visible
- do not show mandibular ramus & condyle
- do not show inferior border of the mandible
- do not show vertical height of the lesion
- resolution is not as sharp as periapical views due to a longer cone-film distance and superimposition of osseous structures
- angulation may give you a distorted view of the lesion

Panoramic Views

In recent years, panoramic x-ray machines have become a component of many dental offices.

Advantages

- This technique provides **the best** overall survey of the entire mandible, maxilla, maxillary sinuses and other skeletal bones.
- In patients with **severe trismus** this may be the only dental radiograph obtainable because intraoral techniques are not possible.

Disadvantages or limitations — The major disadvantages or limitations of panoramic views include:

- lacks the resolution and detail attainable with periapical views
- interpretation is more difficult because of the artifacts generated by superimposition of multiple structures
- provides no information about the medio-lateral extension of the lesion
- frequent recalibration of the machine is necessary for consistent quality

SUMMARY OF DENTAL RADIOGRAPHIC VIEWS

In summary, periapical, occlusal and panoramic views are the primary diagnostic techniques used to collect initial radiographic data. **Table IV-1** shows a comparison of the anatomic areas seen on the three dental radiographic views.

Views	Overall Resolution	Teeth	Alveolar Bone	Medial & Lateral Periosteum	Ramus and Condyle	Maxillary Sinus	Angulation
Periapical	+ + +	+ + +	+ + +	O	O	+	Lateral
Occlusal	+ +	+ +	+ +	+ +	O	O	Occlusal
Panoramic	+	+ +	+ +	O	+ +	+ + +	Lateral

Table IV-1. Comparison of the anatomic areas surveyed by the three primary dental radiographic views. Overall resolution of these views is also compared. The number of (+) signs indicates the relative advantage of each view for each area. (O) indicates these structures are not shown in this view.

STUDY EXERCISES

1. The three (3) radiographic views most commonly used in dentistry are:
   a. _____PA_____ b. _____pan_____ c. _____occlusal_____

2. These views should be considered your "first _____line_____ of _____radiographic_____ information." Based upon the results of these radiographs and your clinical examination _____additional_____ views may be needed.

3. For each of the following statements, identify how each statement applies to each of the dental radiographic views. Circle "**A**" for advantage and "**D**" for disadvantage or limitation.

Statement	Periapical	Occlusal	Panoramic
a. Provides the most detailed view of root apex and surrounding alveolar bone.	(A) D	A (D)	A (D)
b. Provides the best overall view of entire mandible, maxilla, and maxillary sinus.	A (D)	A (D)	(A) (D)
c. Provides a mediolateral view of the mandible.	A (D)	(A) D	A (D)
d. Provides view of inferior border of the mandible.	A (D)	A (D)	(A) D
e. Provides view of ramus and condyle.	A (D)	A (D)	(A) D
f. Provides view of vertical size of a lesion.	(A) D	A (D)	(A) D
g. Can be obtained in cases of severe trismus.	A (D)	(A) D	(A) D
h. Provides good view of palatal bone.	A (D)	(A) D	A (D)

4. Three days after extraction of a maxillary third molar, your patient returns complaining of pain and a feeling of pressure in his cheek. You suspect a root fragment may have been dislodged into the maxillary sinus. What dental view would be useful to evaluate this? ___pan_____

5. On routine recall examination of a patient, you notice slight swelling of the lateral aspect of the mandible below the left second molar. The area is firm to palpation. You suspect the swelling is caused by increased cortical bone deposition. Would a dental radiographic view be useful? Yes _X_ No _____. Which?__pan_____

ANSWERS TO STUDY EXERCISES

1. a. periapical
   b. occlusal
   c. panoramic
2. First line of radiographic information, additional

3.

Statement	Periapical	Occlusal	Panoramic
a. Provides the most detailed view of root apex and surrounding alveolar bone.	A	D	D
b. Provides the best overall view of entire mandible, maxilla, and maxillary sinus.	D	D	A
c. Provides a mediolateral view of the mandible.	D	A	D
d. Provides view of inferior border of the mandible.	D	D	A
e. Provides view of ramus and condyle.	D	D	A
f. Provides view of vertical size of a lesion.	A	D	A
g. Can be obtained in cases of severe trismus.	D	A	A
h. Provides good view of palatal bone.	D	A	D

4. Panoramic
5. Yes. Mandibular occlusal.

ADDITIONAL RADIOGRAPHIC VIEWS

Additional radiographic views can be obtained from a medical radiologist or hospital. Generally these views are requested when the patient is referred to a specialist or hospital. While general dentists do not usually receive training in interpreting these views, you should know what views are available, what advantages they provide, and when they are indicated. The following views can be of value for viewing structures which cannot be seen in the usual dental views.

Lateral (Oblique) Jaw Projections

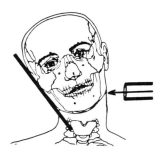

Lateral (oblique) jaw projections are primarily used to view structures in the mandible. The mandibular body, ramus, and condyle can be shown in lateral view. Because the patient's head and film plane are tilted about 15°, the side of the mandible closest to the film is relieved from superimposition by contralateral structures. The patient must protrude his/her chin to avoid superimposition from the cervical vertebrae in order to view the condyle and angle. This protrusion may be difficult for patients suffering from severe infections in posterior areas.

Postero-Anterior Mandibular Projection (PA)

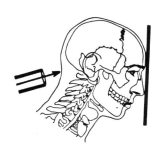

The **postero-anterior (PA) projection of the mandible** is unique in its ability to show the mediolateral aspects of the mandibular ramus and condyle. This view will allow you to visualize fractures of the condyles, rami, and posterior mandible from this orientation and also reveal any osseous changes associated with chronic infections of the pterygomandibular or submasseteric spaces.

Submentovertex (SMV) (Basilar) Projection

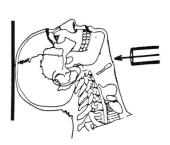

This view shows the skull in a supero-inferior projection and shows the foramen magnum, zygomatic arches, the base of the skull, and the mandibular ascending rami. This projection can be helpful in evaluation of moderate to serious infections by demonstrating involvement of the ascending rami or the soft tissue on the medial or lateral sides of the mandibular ascending rami.

Anterior Lateral Face Projection (ALF)

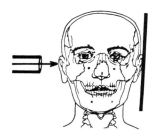

The **anterior lateral face projection** is an excellent view showing the antero-posterior dimension of the maxillary sinus. This view will show the antero-posterior location of lesions or objects in the maxillary sinuses, frontal sinuses, the sphenoid and ethmoid sinuses. This view also provides a lateral view of the parotid and infratemporal spaces. Superimposition of right and left sides of the maxilla, the mandible and teeth cause this view to be of little diagnostic value for viewing these structures.

Water's (Occipitomental) Projection

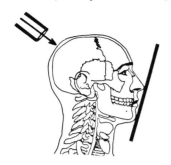

The **Water's (occipitomental) projection** is an extremely useful view to show the **maxillary, frontal** and most of the **ethmoid sinuses.** Increased opacity of the sinuses can indicate fluid in the sinuses (pus, cystic fluid, or blood) or neoplastic tissue growth. In addition, this view may be valuable in locating root tips, teeth, and/or foreign objects which have been displaced into the maxillary sinus.

Tomography

Tomography is a process by which radiographs can be taken at various depths in an anatomical structure. Therefore, any part of the head and neck can be serially viewed from multiple radiographic "slices" through a particular area. Although more time-consuming and more costly than standard radiographic views, tomographs can provide valuable information as to the depth and extent of many pathological changes at the expense of some decrease in clarity of detail.

Cervical (Neck) Views

The neck may be radiographically evaluated from a lateral view or a postero-anterior view.

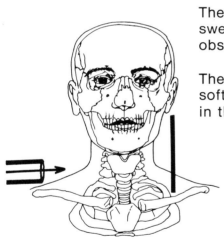

The **lateral view** may be helpful in the evaluation of soft tissue swellings in the retropharyngeal area. This view may also show obstruction of the airway.

The **postero-anterior view** can be used to view swellings in the soft tissues of the lateral neck. This view can show gas or fluid in the fascial planes of the neck tissue.

Chest View

A **postero-anterior chest view** may be helpful in the diagnosis and management of major dental infections involving the neck region because infections involving the fascial planes of the neck can easily extend into the mediastinum and involve the pericardium or the lungs. A chest view will reveal changes in the pericardial, pulmonary and/or mediastinal areas. Any patient with a dental infection which has spread to the chest area should be hospitalized.

Summary of Additional Radiographic Views

From the previous discussion you can see that several additional radiographic views can be used to demonstrate head and neck pathology which cannot be seen in the commonly used dental views. Additional views or projections are frequently used by specialists who have the training and experience to interpret the results. In addition, specialists are often equipped to obtain these radiographic views either in their offices or through a hospital or private radiology service. Most general practitioners of dentistry do not routinely use these views, nor have they had the necessary training in the interpretation of these additional views.

NOTE: If you are considering using these additional radiographic views, you should review your decision to refer or hospitalize your patient because the need for this information may in itself indicate the presence of a life-threatening problem requiring referral.

SUMMARY OF ADDITIONAL RADIOGRAPHIC VIEWS

VIEWS	STRUCTURES SHOWN IN VIEW
• LATERAL OBLIQUE (right & left view)	• View of entire mandibular ramus • Inferior border of mandible
• POSTERO-ANTERIOR (PA)	• Angle of the mandible • Mandibular symphysis • Changes in the cortex of the mandibular ramus
• SUBMENTOVERTEX (SMV)	• Cortical plate of the mandibular ramus • Sinuses
• ANTERIOR LATERAL FACE (ALF)	• True lateral view of maxilla • True lateral views of sphenoid, maxillary, and frontal sinuses
• WATER'S (occipitomental)	• Sinuses
• TOMOGRAPHY	• TMJ, condyles, ascending rami • Lateral or PA views
• CERVICAL (neck) RADIOGRAPHS	• Evaluation of neck involvement
• CHEST RADIOGRAPHS	• Evaluation of lung, mediastinal, and thoracic involvement

Table IV-2. Summary of additional radiographic views which are generally used by specialists to evaluate areas beyond the limits of dental radiographic views.

STUDY EXERCISES

Name five additional radiographic views which can be used to view maxillary and mandibular structures. a. _Lateral oblique_ b. _Submentovertex_
c. _Postero-antero_ d. _Antero lateral_ e. _Waters_

Tomograms are used to view the following structures: _TMJ_
and _condyles_

Which additional radiographic view could be used to evaluate possible neck involvement?
cervical radiographs

Which additional radiographic view could be used to demonstrate involvement of lung, mediastinum, and thorax? _chest radiographs_

ADVANCED RADIOGRAPHIC TECHNIQUES

Medical research has recently developed special techniques that can be used if the standard radiographic views do not yield sufficient data. Generally these techniques are not used by general dentists in routine practice unless they have received specialized training. You may encounter a situation in which reference to these techniques is made.

Bone scan with a radioisotope is a technique involving I.V. administration of radioactively labeled isotope which is taken up and deposited in the skeleton and then 8 hours later a scintillation screen is used to identify areas in the bony skeleton where increased or decreased blood flow is present.

Computerized tomography (C.T. scan) is a complex technique in which radiodensities from many angles are fed into a computer which in turn develops a computerized image of the area. The computerized image is then transferred onto radiographic film. This technique may be used to identify cranial involvement including such problems as brain abscesses, or brain tumors. It is also useful for locating abscesses in some fascial spaces and planes not easily seen by other methods.

Nuclear Magnetic Resonance (NMR) is a technique for creating images through the use of strong **magnetic** fields rather than x-rays. Small changes in magnetic field contour are detected, analyzed by a computer, and converted to observable images. This technique is extremely new and its potential for diagnostic use is yet to be realized.

STUDY EXERCISES

Two special radiographic techniques which may yield additional information are the ___RADIOISOTOPE___ scan and the ___COMPUTER TOMOGRAPHY___ scan. The ___COMPUTER TOMOGRAPHY___ is an image system produced by computer using tomographic views and may reveal ___BRAIN___ abscesses or ___BRAIN___ tumors.

The ___BONE___ scan technique utilizes radioactive isotopes to identify areas of altered blood flow in bone.

___NUCLEAR___ ___MAGNETIC___ ___RESONANCE___ is a new technique that uses strong magnetic fields instead of x-rays to produce images.

RECORDING RADIOGRAPHIC DATA

Prior to making a diagnosis involving radiographic data, you should first:
- record the radiographic views you have used on the radiographic data checklist
- record the radiographic findings from each view on the radiographic data checklist
- indicate the need for additional radiographs if the views you have taken do not include the entire lesion or area of involvement of the problem.

We have designed the following portion of the radiographic data checklist for recording this information.

RADIOGRAPHIC DATA

Views taken	Findings (record any abnormalities)	Additional Radiographic Views Needed
☐ Panoramic	_____	
☐ Periapical	_____	Results _____
☐ Occlusal	_____	_____
☐ Other	_____	_____

NOTE: The significance of radiographic data to diagnosis is not proportional to the space provided on the radiographic data checklist.

EXAMPLES OF "ADDITIONAL" RADIOGRAPHS USED IN THE DIAGNOSIS OF MAXILLO-FACIAL INFECTIONS

PA View of the Mandible

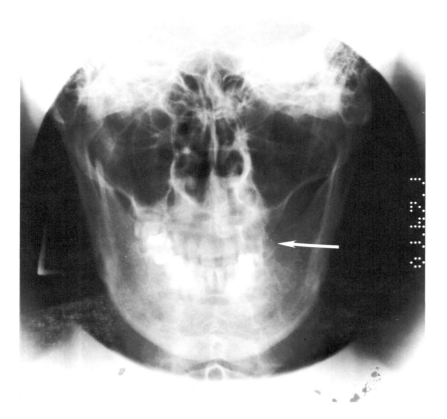

This P-A view of the mandible shows a medial enlargement and alterations in the trabecular pattern of the bone on the left side of the mandible near the base of the right ascending ramus. These changes resulted from a chronic, proliferative actinomycotic infection. The other radiographic view on this page and those on page 117 show additional views of this same case.

Lateral Oblique View of the Mandible

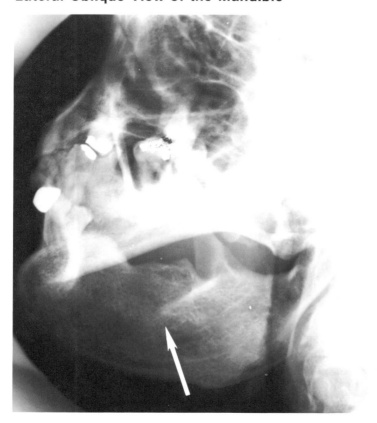

This is a lateral oblique view of the same condition as above. A loss of mineralization and changes in the trabecular pattern are seen in the body of the mandible in the area of the left mandibular angle.

Reverse Towne's View of Mandible

This Reverse Towne's projection is another "additional" radiographic view used to study the medial and lateral sides of the mandibular rami, condyles, and coronoid processes. In this example, new periosteal bone formation (1) can be seen. In addition, proliferative changes and changes in the trabecular pattern are seen in the bone at the base of the ascending ramus on the left side (patient's left). This problem resulted from a chronic, low-grade, actinomycotic infection. Also see page 116 for different radiographic views of this same problem.

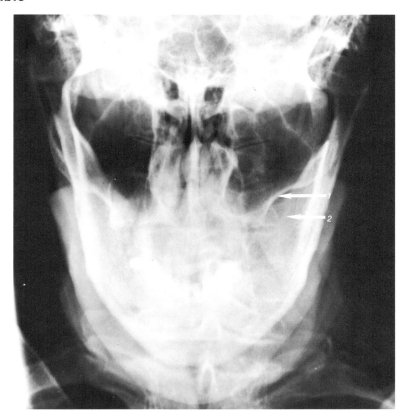

Submento-Vertex (SMV) View

In this example of a submento-vertex (SMV) view, an increase in the width (thickness) and an increase in radiopacity are seen on the right side in the area of the angle of the mandible. By tracing the outline of the left and right sides of the mandible, you can see the irregular pattern on the (patient's) right side. These radiographic changes resulted from a chronic, low-grade *actinomyces* infection.

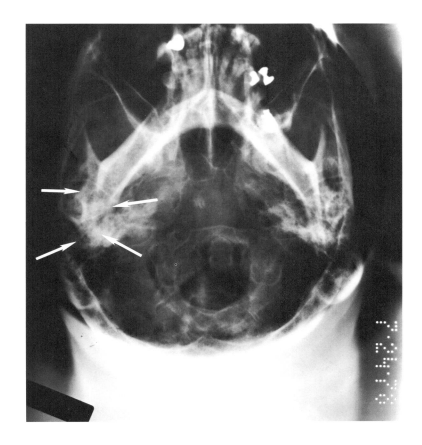

Bone Scan

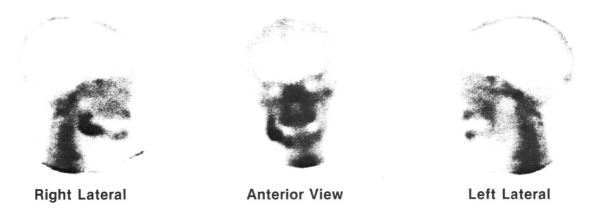

Right Lateral   **Anterior View**   **Left Lateral**

The above bone scan shows **increased uptake** of the radioactive isotope in the **area of the right mandibular angle** (dark area). This dark area was associated with a post-surgical infection in the angle region following an osteotomy procedure in the mandible.

Computerized Tomography (C.T. Scan)

This coronal view C.T. scan shows (1) a soft tissue swelling and (2) a fragment of non-vital bone, both associated with a chronic, post-surgical infection of the left mid-face (lateral face) region. You should compare the left and right sides to observe the soft tissue asymmetry and presence of the radiopaque foreign body (the bone fragment). The C.T. scan showed the fragment when conventional radiographs failed to reveal this small bony fragment.

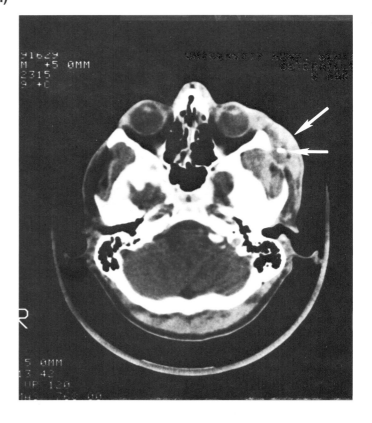

Tomograms of Right and Left Condyles

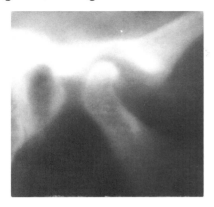

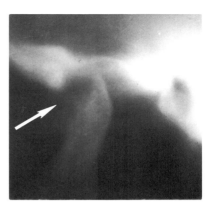

Right Side   **Left Side**

A tomogram of the normal condyle is seen on the right. The left condyle shows resorptive changes of the articular surface secondary to a staphylococcus infection caused by non-sterile injection into the TMJ.

Water's View

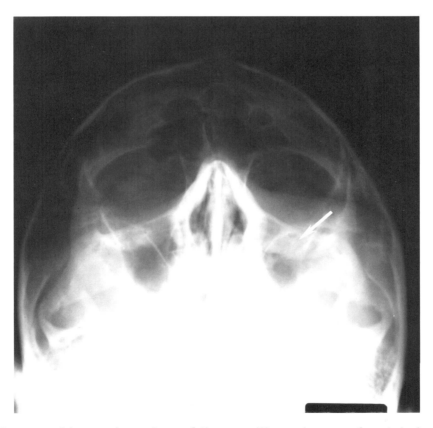

The Water's view provides a clear view of the maxillary sinuses, frontal sinus, orbital rim and the zygomas. In this radiograph, an area of increased radiopacity is seen in the left maxillary sinus. It represents an early inflammatory change in the sinus membrane secondary to a post-surgical infection in the area of the zygoma and posterior wall of the sinus (see C.T. example on page 118).

POST-TEST

- Answer each of the following questions.
- Compare your answers with the correct responses on page 122.
- If all questions are answered correctly, proceed to Unit V, page 124.
- If you do not answer all questions correctly, re-read and re-study the content of this Unit.

QUESTIONS

1. Explain why a diagnosis should not be made from radiographic data alone. _____
   ___NOT DIAGNOSTIC, PROVIDE INDIRECT EVIDENCE_____
   _____

2. Name three (3) radiographic views most commonly used in dentistry.
   a. ___PAN_____   b. ___PA_____   c. ___OCCLUSAL_____

3. For each of the following statements, identify how each statement relates to the advantages and disadvantages (limitations) of the three primary dental radiographic views. (You should have one answer for each view.)

	Periapical	Occlusal	Panoramic
a. Provides the most detailed view of root apices and surrounding alveolar bone.	(A) D	A (D)	A (D)
b. Provides the best overall view of the entire mandible, maxilla, and maxillary sinus.	A (D)	A (D)	(A) D
c. Provides a mediolateral view of the mandible.	A (D)	(A) D	A (D)
d. Provides a view of the inferior border of the mandible.	A (D)	A (D)	(A) D
e. Provides a view of the ramus and condyle.	A (D)	A (D)	(A) D
f. Provides a view of the vertical size of a lesion.	(A) D	A (D)	(A) D
g. Can be obtained in cases of severe trismus.	A (D)	A (D)	(A) D
h. Provides a good view of palatal bone.	A (D)	(A) D	A (D)

4. Name the "additional" radiographic view that shows the structures indicated on the right.

VIEWS	STRUCTURES SHOWN IN VIEW
a. ___LAT OBLIQUE_____	• View of entire mandibular ramus • Inferior border of mandible
b. ___POSTERO ANT._____	• Angle of the mandible • Mandibular symphysis • Changes in the cortex of the mandibular ramus
c. ___SUBMENTOVERTEX_____	• Cortical plate of the mandibular ramus • Sinuses
d. ___ANT LATERAL FACE_____	• True lateral view of maxilla • True lateral views of sphenoid, maxillary, and frontal sinuses
e. ___WATERS_____	• Sinuses
f. ___TOMOGRAPHY_____	• TMJ, condyles, ascending rami • Lateral or PA views
g. ___NECK_____	• Evaluation of neck involvement
h. ___CHEST_____	• Evaluation of lung, mediastinal, and thoracic involvement

5. *Name the* **advanced radiographic technique** *which is associated with each of the following statements.*
   a. *A* _Bone scan with Radioisotope_ *is a technique involving the use of a radioactive isotope which is taken up by areas in the skeleton and shows areas of increased or decreased blood flow.*
   b. *A* _Computerized Tomography_ *is a technique where the digitized radiodensities from many angles are first fed into a computer which, in turn, assembles the digitized data to form images on either a video monitor or film.*
   c. _Nuclear Magnetic Resonance_ *is a very new technique which measures small disruptions of a strong magnetic field, and converts this information into extremely detailed images.*

6. *Give the name (projection) for each of the following sketches.*

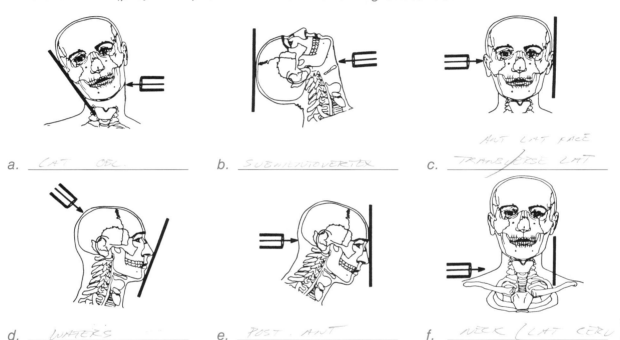

a. _CAT OCC._

b. _SUBMENTOVERTEX_

c. _ANT LAT FACE_ _TRANSVERSE LAT_

d. _WATERS_

e. _POST. ANT_

f. _NECK (LAT CERV)_

7. *What is the name of the imaging system that has produced the following?*

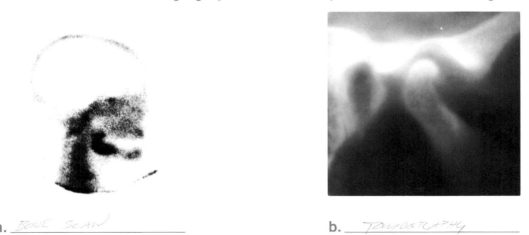

a. _BONE SCAN_

b. _TOMOGRAPHY_

*For each of the following clinical situations: a) Name the dental radiographic view(s) which should be considered (if none are appropriate write **NA**); b) give the additional view or advanced view which should be considered.*

8. *A 54-year-old female patient presents to your office with symptoms of dull pain in her right mid-face region. No intraoral or extraoral swelling is evident; however, she has a slight fever (99.8° F) and she says her upper right back teeth ache. Three months ago you extracted her maxillary right first molar and first premolar. One month ago you then placed a five-unit bridge in this area extending from the maxillary right second molar to the maxillary first premolar and canine.*

   a. Dental Views   **b. Additional Views**
   1) _PA_____   1) _WATER_____
   2) _PAN_____   2) _ALF_____
   3) _____   3) _____

9. *A 26-year-old female patient presents to your office with pain and extraoral swelling in the left lateral side of her face and in the submandibular area. You are unable to perform an intraoral exam because severe trismus has restricted her mouth opening (inter-incisor opening) to about 5 mm.*

   a. Dental Views   **b. Additional Views**
   1) _PAN_____   1) _LAT OBLIQUE_____
   2) _SMV_____   2) _____

POST-TEST ANSWERS

1. *Radiographs provide indirect evidence of pathologic processes. Diagnosis is derived from clinical data and confirmed with radiographic data.*

2. a. *Periapical*   b. *Occlusal*   c. *Panoramic*

3.

Statement	Periapical	Occlusal	Panoramic
a. Provides the most detailed view of root apex and surrounding alveolar bone.	A	D	D
b. Provides the best overall view of entire mandible, maxilla, and maxillary sinus.	D	D	A
c. Provides a mediolateral view of the mandible.	D	A	D
d. Provides view of inferior border of the mandible.	D	D	A
e. Provides view of ramus and condyle.	D	D	A
f. Provides view of vertical size of a lesion.	A	D	A
g. Can be obtained in cases of severe trismus.	D	A	A
h. Provides good view of palatal bone.	D	A	D

4. VIEWS	STRUCTURES SHOWN IN VIEW
a. Lateral oblique (right & left view)	• View of entire mandibular ramus
	• Inferior border of mandible
b. Postero-Anterior (PA)	• Angle of the mandible
	• Mandibular symphysis
	• Changes in the cortex of the mandibular ramus
c. Submentovertex (SMV)	• Cortical plate of the mandibular ramus
	• Sinuses
d. Anterior Lateral Face (ALF)	• True lateral view of maxilla
	• True lateral views of sphenoid, maxillary, and frontal sinuses
e. Water's (occipitomental)	• Sinuses
f. Tomography	• TMJ, condyles, ascending rami
	• Lateral or PA views
g. Cervical (neck) radiographs	• Evaluation of neck involvement
h. Chest radiographs	• Evaluation of lung, mediastinal, and thoracic involvement

5. a. Bone scan with radioisotope
   b. C.T. scan (computerized tomography)
   c. Nuclear Magnetic Resonance (N.M.R.)

6. a. Lateral oblique   d. Water's (Occipitomental)
   b. Submentovertex (SMV)   e. Postero-Anterior (PA)
   c. Anterior Lateral Face   f. Lateral Cervical

7. a. Bone scan with radioisotopes
   b. Tomogram

8. a. **Dental Views**   b. **Additional Views**
      1) Panoramic   1) Water's (Occipitomental) view
      2) Periapical   2) Anterior Lateral Face (ALF)

In this case, a generalized increase in radioopacity was seen in the right maxillary sinus and, in addition, a 3 mm root tip was seen. The above radiographic evidence helped to establish the presence of a dentally related maxillary sinus abscess. Referral to an oral and/or maxillofacial surgeon resulted in opening the sinus, removing the root tip and draining the sinus. Her bridge and remaining teeth were unaffected.

9. a. **Dental Views**   b. **Additional Views**
      1) Occlusal view   1) Lateral oblique view
      2) Panoramic view

UNIT V
LABORATORY DATA

OVERVIEW & OBJECTIVES

The purpose of this unit is for you to learn or review the various laboratory techniques used to establish the presence of infectious microorganism(s) and to observe the effects these microorganisms are having on your patient. In this unit you will learn what tests are available, when they should be used, how to collect a specimen for examination, and how to interpret the results. This unit also reviews basic microbiological concepts and how these concepts are related to diagnostic data collection. Following completion of this unit you will:

1. Explain why laboratory data can be essential in the diagnostic process of identifying the cause of oral and/or maxillofacial swellings.

2. Name the three (3) types of laboratory services which can be used, the tests performed by each, the type of specimen required, and the value of results to the diagnostic and treatment processes.

3. Name four (4) **hematology laboratory tests** which are often used in the diagnosis of oral and/or maxillofacial infections.

4. Given laboratory data for each of the following hematologic tests, describe the significance of these data and how they relate to the diagnosis of infections.
    a. WBC count   c. ESR
    b. WBC differential   d. Blood cultures

5. Name two (2) **histopathology laboratory tests** that can be used in the diagnosis of oral and/or maxillofacial infections.

6. Describe why **microbiological laboratory testing** and examination should always be considered in the diagnosis of any oral and/or maxillofacial swelling.

7. Describe the possible consequences of ignoring or delaying microbiological testing and examination when an oral and/or maxillofacial infection is present.

8. Define the following terms:
    a. Resident oral flora
    b. Transient oral flora

9. Name three (3) general characteristics of microorganisms which are important in the diagnosis and management of odontogenic infections.

10. Describe how **staining techniques** can be helpful in the diagnosis of infections.

11. Name five (5) ways in which the **gram stain** is a useful aid in the diagnosis and treatment of oral and/or maxillofacial infections.

12. Describe how gram stain results can be helpful to your tentative diagnosis and selection of initial antibiotic therapy.

13. Describe the indications for use of other staining techniques.

14. Describe the two (2) major classifications of microorganisms as to their **oxygen sensitivity** and the relative proportion of oral infections involving anaerobic microorganisms.

15. Describe four (4) reasons why the diagnosis and management of anaerobic oral and/or maxillofacial infections can be more difficult than for aerobic infections.

16. Describe how **antibiotic susceptibility and resistance** is determined.

17. Describe the ways microorganisms can become **resistant** to antibiotics.

18. Describe the advantages to your diagnosis and treatment provided by the laboratory **identification of the species** or group of microorganisms responsible for an infection.

19. Describe how a microbiology lab can provide you with a **"step-wise" flow of data** which will enable you to be more precise in diagnostic and treatment decisions while treating an oral and/or maxillofacial infection.

20. Describe why it is important to **identify** the **antibiotic(s)** a patient may have been taking prior to the onset of an infection.

21. Given a clinical example of an oral and/or maxillofacial infection, determine whether or not a specimen should be collected for culture and susceptibility testing.
    a. ideally
    b. practical guidelines

22. Describe two (2) main uses of culture information.

23. Name and describe the seven (7) **general principles** for collecting a specimen from an infectious swelling.

24. For each of the following problems associated with the culturing process, describe potential reasons for these results and potential solutions to these problems:
    a. Failure to obtain culture
    b. Failure to obtain laboratory growth
    c. Lab reports normal oral flora

25. Describe the criteria used for **selecting the best site** for culture specimen collection.

26. Given a clinical photograph and/or anatomical drawing of an oral and/or maxillofacial infection, determine whether an **intraoral** or **extraoral** route for specimen collection should be selected.

27. Name the anatomical areas or fascial spaces that **should not be cultured** by a general dentist unless he/she has had specialized training and clinical experience.

28. Name three (3) **intraoral methods** for collecting a culture specimen.

29. Describe how each of the seven (7) **steps of culturing** are performed during **culturing from an infected tooth**.

30. Describe how each of the seven (7) steps of culturing are performed during **intraoral transmucosal aspiration**.

31. Describe why the **use of cotton swabs is not recommended** for collection of a culture specimen from an incised swelling.

32. Describe the technique for **intraoral tissue biopsy** as a culturing technique and the types of information that can be derived by this technique.

33. Describe the indications for using **extraoral specimen** collection methods.

34. Name the three (3) extraoral methods for specimen collection.

35. Describe the seven (7) steps of specimen collection for **extraoral transcutaneous aspiration**.

36. Describe why the collection of a culture specimen from extraoral incision and drainage or extraoral tissue biopsy is often not used by general dentists.

37. Given **any** clinical situation involving an oral and/or maxillofacial swelling requiring the collection of laboratory data, **identify** and **describe** the **laboratory tests** needed and describe the limitations of each test.

UNIT V
LABORATORY DATA

INTRODUCTION

Thus far in the data collection process, you have been able to obtain important information through questioning and clinical examination of your patient. While this information is extremely valuable, it will not provide you with information about changes occurring in your patient at the physiological or cellular level, nor will clinical examination provide you with any information as to the identity or antibiotic susceptibility of the causative microorganism(s).

Any diagnosis not based upon laboratory identification of the causative organisms, their antibiotic susceptibility, or laboratory information about the changes occurring in a patient's body as a result of the pathologic process is only an **initial** or **presumptive diagnosis based upon incomplete information.** Far too frequently dental practitioners fail to utilize laboratory data in their diagnosis and management of oral infections only to find the infection does not respond to initial treatment. The additional time required to obtain this information after initial treatment has failed can put a patient's life in jeopardy.

The purpose of this unit is to describe the various kinds of laboratory data that can be obtained, to explain how to collect specimens, and how to interpret the significance of the results, as well as provide guidelines as to when various lab tests are needed. We will also review the fundamental principles of oral microbiology as related to suppurative oral infections.

NOTE: Laboratory data will allow you to make a more definitive diagnosis earlier in the diagnostic and management process. Because the time required to perform these studies can be up to 6 days, initial treatment cannot be postponed. However, when results are obtained, you can alter your treatment as needed.

The three major types of laboratory services which can be used in the diagnosis and treatment of oral infections include the following:
- **HEMATOLOGIC STUDIES**
- **HISTOPATHOLOGIC EXAMINATION**
- **MICROBIOLOGICAL EXAMINATION & TESTING**

Table V-1 summarizes various laboratory tests that can be useful in both the initial and definitive diagnostic processes.

SUMMARY OF LABORATORY TESTS

TYPE OF LABORATORY	TESTS	VALUE OF RESULTS	TYPE OF SPECIMEN
HEMATOLOGY	• WBC count • WBC differential • ESR	• Verify presence of infection with systemic involvement	Venous blood sample collected under sterile conditions is needed
	• Blood cultures	• Verify bacteria and/or septicemia	
Immunology	• T-cell activity	• Determine increased or decreased T-cell numbers and activities	Venous blood sample
	• Complement activity	• Detect complement disorders often associated with neoplastic processes.	
	• Immunodeficiency tests	• Identify immuno-incompetence	
HISTOPATHOLOGY	• Histologic examination • Special stains	• Determine histological structure of tissue • Establish presence of microbes in tissue if culturing is unsuccessful	Tissue specimen collected aseptically
MICROBIOLOGY	• Gram stain	• Immediate data describing gram stain response of organisms and whether single or multiple microorganisms are involved	Sample of suppuration collected aseptically
	• Special stains	• Identification of TB, *actinomyces*, yeasts, *corynebacterium* and other microorganisms	
	• Culture and antibiotic susceptibility	• Identification of species and determination of antibiotic susceptibility	Specimen of pus collected under anaerobic conditions
	• Culture tissue specimen	• Culture of microbes that are difficult to culture from suppuration	Tissue specimen collected aseptically

Table V-1. Summary of laboratory tests that can be used in the diagnosis and management of oral and/or maxillofacial swellings.

HEMATOLOGIC STUDIES

Hematology tests are performed on a sample of your patient's blood. Hematologic or blood tests can be an important diagnostic aid in determining the presence of an infection and the degree of systemic involvement. The relevant tests when an infection is suspected include:

- **WBC** — White blood cell count
- **WBC Differential** — % of different white blood cell types present
- **ESR** — Erythrocyte sedimentation rate
- **Blood cultures** — Detect presence of viable bacteria in the blood stream
- **Immunological tests** — Identify immunological disorders

- **White Blood Cell Count (WBC) & Differential**

  The most diagnostically useful hematologic screening test for infections is the WBC and differential. The WBC and differential may be used in making an **initial diagnosis** and also during treatment **to monitor the degree of resolution** of the infection. In most infections involving the head and neck **an increase in the WBC count occurs within a relatively short time (24-48 hours) after the onset of an infection. The normal range** WBC is **7,000 ± 3,000 WBC/mm³**. During an infection the WBC count may rise to **10,000 or above.**

NOTE: **Normal WBC count for individuals varies considerably. If your patient has had an examination by his/her physician recently, you should contact that office to find the patient's normal WBC levels for comparison.**

- **Differential**

  The **differential** or **ratio of white blood cell types** is also highly significant in diagnosis of infections. We will discuss these changes in relationship to the various types of white blood cells and summarize this discussion in **Table V-2.**

  ### Polymorphonuclear Neutrophils
  With a rise in WBC count to 10,000/mm^3 during an acute infection the predominant increase occurs in the polymorphonuclear neutrophils (polys). This increase is due to the increased delivery of these cells to the site of injury or infection. To compensate for the utilization of the polys (neutrophils) at the site of the infection, there is an increase in the production of neutrophils in the myelogenous tissues. Therefore, **immature cells** which are precursor forms of the neutrophils (myelocytes and promyelocytes) increase in the marrow and a release of metamyelocytes or "stab forms" is seen in the circulating blood. This movement toward circulation of immature forms has been termed a "shift to the left."

  ### Monocytes
  An increase in monocytes may be seen in tuberculosis, bacterial endocarditis, protozoal and rickettsial infections, Hodgkin's disease, osteomyelitis, or infectious mononucleosis.

  ### Eosinophils
  An increase in eosinophils can be seen in parasitic infections or allergic manifestations. However, bacterial infections will not cause any change in these values.

HEMATOLOGIC TEST	NORMAL VALUES	CHANGES DURING INFECTION
WBC COUNT	7,000 ($\pm$ 3,000/mm^3)	**Rises above 10,000/mmfl with bacterial infections* (See note above)**
DIFFERENTIAL		
Polymorphonuclear neutrophils (PMN)	60-70%	• **Numbers greatly increased in acute bacterial infection. No increase in viral infections.**
Lymphocytes	20-30%	• **No change in acute bacterial infection. Usually increases in viral infections.**
Monocytes	4-5%	• **Increased in some infections.**
Eosinophils	1%	• **Little change in bacterial infection.**
Basophils	0.5%	• **Little change in acute infection.**

Table V-2. Summary of changes in WBC count and differential resulting from microbial infection.

- **ESR (Erythrocyte Sedimentation Rate)**

  ESR (erythrocyte sedimentation rate) may be used as a screening test for an abnormality in the globulin fraction of the blood. One such abnormality associated with an inflammatory process is the globulin-fibrinogen disturbances.

  In this test, venous blood, treated with an anticoagulant, is allowed to stand undisturbed for one hour. The distance from the top of the plasma to the red cell column is measured. Normal and abnormal ranges are as follows:

SEX	NORMAL ESR	CHANGE IN ESR DURING INFECTIONS
Men	0-15 mm/hr	30-70 mm/hr
Women	0-20 mm/hr	30-70 mm/hr

Table V-3. Normal ESR values and how they change during an acute infection.

The results of ESR tests must be interpreted somewhat lightly because other systemic conditions such as severe anemia, myeloma and systemic lupus erythematosis can also cause an increase in ESR values. However, if these conditions are not involved, ESR testing can be useful in confirming an infection.

- **Blood Cultures**

  Venous blood may be mixed with broth and cultured for blood-born microorganisms. Blood cultures can be especially valuable in the diagnosis of an uncontrolled odontogenic infection which has progressed to septicemia or bacterial endocarditis. Blood cultures should be considered for a patient with a temperature above 39°C.

  If blood cultures are to be used, blood specimens must be collected under strict aseptic conditions to prevent contamination with normal skin flora. In cases where body temperature changes follow a consistent pattern, the best time to obtain a blood culture is when the temperature is just beginning to elevate.

- **Immunological tests** are available to detect defects in a patient's immunological system. The following immunologic studies are available:

  Test for T-cell activity
  Test for complement activity
  Test for immunodeficiency

  Immunologic testing is seldom used in managing dental infections. Usually dental infections are controlled by the use of surgical procedures and antibiotic therapy. If an infection persists after established treatment methods have failed, you should refer the problem to a dental specialist. Occasionally dental specialists will also consult with a specialist in infectious diseases who, in turn, may request immunological tests.

  As a general practitioner, you should not order these tests unless you have had experience in interpreting their results.

Recording Hematologic Data

Once you have determined the need for hematologic tests, you should check the "yes" box in the **laboratory data** section of the **checklist** and indicate which test(s) you have ordered. You can either draw the blood specimen yourself (if you have the facilities and training to do so) or refer this service to an appropriate hematologic laboratory.

LABORATORY DATA

Yes	No	
☑	☐	Culture material available at this time
☐	☑	STAT Gram stain indicated
☐	☑	Specimen collected for micro lab
☐	☑	Specimen collected for histopathologic exam
✔	☐	Hematology studies needed. Which? *WBC & ESR*

You should then summarize the results of hematologic examination or tests in the space provided for **summary of laboratory data.**

SUMMARY OF LABORATORY DATA

HEMATOLOGY LAB

☐ WBC count *17,000*
☐ WBC Differential:

Polys	*86* %	Eosinophils	*1* %
Lymphocytes	*14* %	Basophils	___ %
Monocytes	___ %	Immature?	*5%*

ESR ___ *60* ___ mm/hr
Blood Culture *none*

HISTOPATHOLOGIC EXAMINATION

A histopathology laboratory specializes in the examination of tissue specimens on both the gross and microscopic levels. Histopathological examination of a tissue specimen from a swelling may help distinguish non-infectious diseases from infectious processes and also establish the presence of microorganisms in tissue when standard culturing techniques fail to yield sufficient information for diagnosis.

Tissue examination procedures used by histopathology laboratories which can be of assistance in the diagnosis of oral and/or maxillofacial swellings include:
- Gross examination of the specimen
- Microscopic examination to determine cell types and histological structure
- Use of special stains to demonstrate the presence of microorganisms in a tissue specimen

Indications for Histopathological Studies

Generally you would consider histological studies as a backup to microbiological testing. These studies are particularly useful when you suspect a **chronic infection** is caused by the following microorganisms:
- ***Actinomyces*** (cervicofacial actinomycosis)
- ***Mycobacterium*** tuberculosis (TB)
- Fungal infections such as
   Monillia (candidiasis, monilliasis)
   Aspergillis
   Mucor (Mucor mycosis)
   Cryptococus neoformans

Most frequently, tissue specimens from purulent bacterial infections **show mixed flora.** This information can be helpful in planning definitive therapy.

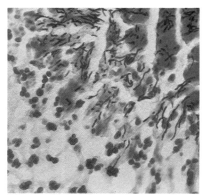 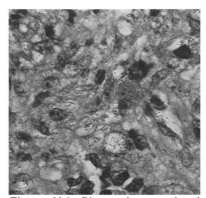 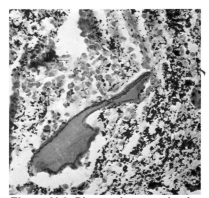

Figure V-1. Photomicrograph of *Actinomyces* seen in a tissue specimen from a mandibular third molar extraction site.

Figure V-2. Photomicrograph of *Mycobacterium species* in a tissue specimen.

Figure V-3. Photomicrograph of a mixed bacterial flora in bone. Large red area is necrotic bone.

NOTE: You may also use histopathologic studies if you believe an infection to be associated with an underlying neoplastic process.

Obtaining A Specimen

When obtaining a specimen for histological study, you should follow standard biopsy procedures as described in **Principles of Biopsy** by T. H. Morton, Jr., et al (Stoma Press, 1983). A tissue specimen is removed and promptly fixed in formalin. You should complete a laboratory request form and indicate your clinical suspicion of the presence of infectious microorganism(s). A description of associated clinical signs and symptoms and radiographs of the involved area should be included.

If culturing of the tissue is also planned, a specimen should be collected aseptically and should NOT be fixed in formalin prior to aseptic transfer to culture media. Formalin fixation will preclude microbiological culture studies.

Some general dentists who regularly perform biopsy procedures may elect to perform this procedure and obtain the pathologist's report prior to making a referral decision. Other general dentists may elect to refer this entire process to a specialist.

You would be well advised to select a histopathology laboratory which has the services of an oral pathologist or pathologist trained in the examination of oral tissues.

Obtaining Histopathological Data

A histopathology laboratory usually requires about 3 days to fix, stain, section and examine the specimen. This entire process frequently takes 6-7 days if specimen and report are mailed. Verbal communication with the pathologist can shorten this time by 1-2 days.

Recording Histopathological Data

If you decide histopathological data is needed you should check the appropriate box in the **laboratory data checklist** and record a summary of the pathologist's report in the space provided in the **summary of laboratory data**. An example of a summary extracted from the pathologist's report is shown below.

LABORATORY DATA

Yes No
- ☐ ☐ Culture material available at this time
- ☐ ☐ STAT Gram stain indicated
- ☐ ☐ Specimen collected for micro lab
- ☑ ☐ Specimen collected for histopathologic exam
- ☐ ☐ Hematology studies needed. Which? _____

SUMMARY OF LABORATORY DATA

HISTOPATHOLOGY LAB
Tissue specimen analysis _____
Tissue contained intensly inflammed connective tissue and polymorphonuclear neutrophiles (polys), Gram (+) cocci and Gram (-) bacteria were also present

STUDY EXERCISES

Hematologic tests require a sample of venous _blood_ . *If **blood cultures** are to be done, the specimen must be collected under* _aseptic_ *conditions.*

The most useful tests for determining systemic involvement of an infection are the _WBC_ *total cell count and* _Diff_ . *These tests may also be used to monitor the degree of* _resolution_ *for an infection. The normal value for* **total WBC count** *is* _7_ ,000 ± _3_ ,000. *This value may vary from individual to individual. You may be able to obtain the normal WBC count for a particular patient by calling his/her* _physician_ . *A WBC count above* _10_ ,000 *is usually an indication of systemic infection. The **WBC differential** is also helpful in establishing the presence of an* _infection_ . *During acute infections,* _PMN_ *counts rise disproportionally and more* _immature_ *forms are seen. Counts for* _lymphocyte_ , _monocyte_ , _eosinophils_ , *and* _basophils_ *are usually unaffected for bacterial infections, however, increases in* _PMN_ *are seen in leukemia and increases in* _lymphocyte_ *are often seen with systemic viral infections.*

***ESR** is an abbreviation for* _ERYTHROCYTE_ _SEDMENTATION_ _RATE_ . *Abnormal ESR rates can indicate systemic* _infection_ *if other pathological processes are ruled out.*

***Blood cultures** are used to determine the presence of viable* _microbes_ *in blood and indicate septicemia (or transient bacteremia).*

*Three **immunological tests** that may be used by specialists in infectious diseases are* _T cell_ , _complement_ , *and immuno* _deficiency_ .

Histopathologic examination is used to confirm the presence of *microbes* in tissue. This procedure is most useful in diagnosing *chronic* infections caused by *Actinomyces*, *Mycobacterium*, and *Fungal*. Specimens for histopathologic examination must be collected using *standard biopsy* technique and (must/must not) *must not* be fixed in formalin if culturing from tissue specimens is desired.

*Describe the significance of the following **hematologic data** to establishing the presence of infection.*

Case #1-A

HEMATOLOGY LAB
☐ WBC count *18,000*
☐ WBC Differential:
Polys *95* %   Eosinophils *2* %
Lymphocytes *15* %   Basophils *.5* %
Monocytes *5* %   Immature? ___
ESR_____mm/hr
Blood Culture _____

Brief history: This patient is diabetic, febrile (101°F), and has an acute anterior submental non-fluctuant swelling resulting from pulpal necrosis of his mandibular left central incisor. Blood studies were initiated to form a baseline for evaluation of host defense status and future monitoring.
Significance of hematological data: _____
↑ in count & PMN's indicate inf.

Case #1-B

HEMATOLOGY LAB
☐ WBC count *12,000*
☐ WBC Differential:
Polys *80* %   Eosinophils *2* %
Lymphocytes *15* %   Basophils *.5* %
Monocytes *5* %   Immature? ___
ESR_____mm/hr
Blood Culture _____

Brief history: Same patient as above, but 72 hours later. Initially, antibiotics were given, infection localized, extra-oral incision and drainage performed (drain removed yesterday), and the involved tooth was endodontically treated. Body temperature is now normal.
Significance of hematological data: _____
↓ in count
↓ lymph
↑ poly

*Given the following clinical description of the specimen and its **brief case history description** and the subsequent **histopathology report**: a) summarize the histopathology report on the checklist and b) describe the significance of this information to establishing the presence of an infective process.*

Case #3

Clinical description and history of the specimen (provided by the dentist):
This tissue specimen was obtained from a mandibular left second molar extraction site which developed a proliferation of red, highly vascular tissue 7 days following the extraction of this tooth. A periapical radiograph (duplicate enclosed) showed an unremarkable extraction socket.

Histopathology Report:
Section contains edmatous granulation tissue associated with an intense acute inflammatory cell infiltrate. Portions of the granulation tissue are covered by stratified squamous epithelium exhibiting extensive inflammatory hyperplasia and focal degeneration. In one area within the granulation tissue, there is an amorphous collection of bacteria which, when Gram stained, revealed mixed Gram (+) and Gram (−) and areas of calcification consistent with organized dental plaque and calculus.

HISTOPATHOLOGY LAB
Tissue specimen analysis ___
Edmatous granulation tissue due to acute inflammation from plaque & calc. in extraction site

Significance: _____

Discussion of Cases:

Case #1-A: Significance of hematological data: The data indicated presence of acute infection producing systemic signs of increased numbers of polys (neutrophiles) and release of immature neutrophiles.

Case #1-B: Significance of hematological data: Reduction in WBC count and differential indicate control of systemic involvement and confirm that the infection is under control. No further blood studies are necessary if patient's condition continues to improve.

Case #2:

HISTOPATHOLOGY LAB
Tissue specimen analysis _____.

Epulis granulomatosis due to acute inflammation from the presence of dental plaque and calculus in the extraction site

Confirms presence of foreign body reaction & bacteria

Significance of histopathology report: This report establishes the presence of a mixed infection and acute inflammatory hyperplasia in the extraction socket. This infection was initiated by the presence of dental plaque and calculus which was most likely deposited in the extraction site at the time of surgery. Inadequate debridement of the surgical site permitted the microorganisms in this material to proliferate in the blood clot and disrupt the epithelialization of the extraction socket.

MICROBIOLOGICAL DATA

The purpose of this section is to review the major characteristics of microorganisms which cause oral and/or maxillofacial infections. In addition, we will review methods for collecting specimens from infections, methods for transporting the specimens to the microbiology laboratory, and recording the results of laboratory analysis.

Since the initial inflammatory response to invasive microorganisms is a general response, it is not possible to assess the specific characteristics of the involved species from the clinical appearance of the infection without the help of a microbiology laboratory.

The Value of Microbiological Data

Microbiological data can be of assistance both in diagnosing the cause of an oral and/or maxillofacial swelling and in selection of appropriate treatment methods. In general terms, microbiological studies can provide clinicians with valuable information by:
- **verifying the presence of microorganisms in the swelling**
- **identifying the microorganism(s) present**
- **establishing the relative numbers and dominant species in mixed infections**
- **providing guidance for antibiotic selection**
- **confirming the resolution of an infection.**

Thus, microbiological data supports and expands your clinical findings. The **sooner** you have specific information about the microorganisms responsible for an infection, the **sooner** you will be able to **select alternative treatment methods if initial treatment fails to resolve the problem.**

Oral Flora and Infections

The microorganisms found in the oral cavity comprise a population of microbes coexisting in a complex ecological environment. The mouth harbors a characteristic **resident** flora which is usually unique to each individual and different from the flora of other body areas (e.g., skin, intestine, etc.).

In addition to its resident oral flora, the oral cavity is constantly subjected to invasion by microorganisms from the surrounding environment. Some environmental microorganisms may be integrated with the resident population while others may reside only temporarily in the mouth and are referred to as **transient flora.** When managing an oral infection you must consider both **resident** and **transient** flora as possible causative agents.

Within the oral cavity **three major ecological niches (econiches)** are recognized. Each niche provides an environment which favors the growth of certain microorganisms while discouraging the growth of others. These niches include the **buccal mucosa**, the **tongue** and the **areas around the teeth. Saliva** is considered as only a washing medium and may contain species from any of the econiches. The flora of the **tongue** and **buccal mucosa** can be associated with **needle track, suture track,** or other **wound-related infections.**

The flora around the **teeth** presents a complex econiche involving the microorganisms of **dental plaque** both **above** the gingival sulcus (**supragingival plaque**) and **in** the gingival sulcus (**subgingival plaque**). The microorganisms living in these two environments are responsible for the majority of dental infections (caries, periodontal disease, pericoronitis, etc.). Individuals who practice **good oral hygiene** have fewer microorganisms in this econiche than do individuals who allow a buildup of dental plaque through poor oral hygiene practices. In addition, the predominant species of organisms present will vary.

Areas of localized inflammation resulting from accumulation of dental plaque disrupt the normal epithelial layer of gingival tissues, thus facilitating the entry of plaque flora into surrounding tissues and the bloodstream. In addition, persons with poor oral hygiene are more likely to develop lung infections from the inhalation of oral flora.

NOTE: **Persons with poor oral hygiene are more likely to develop infections of teeth (caries, pulpal necrosis), oral soft tissue (periodontal disease, periodontal abscesses, pericoronitis) and oral infections resulting from invasive dental procedures (surgery, anesthetic injection, curettage, etc.). Ectopic infections of the lungs, bloodstream, and brain are also more likely to occur in patients with poor oral hygiene.**

The anaerobic environment of the **supragingival area** can be altered by use of toothbrush, dental floss, and coronal polishing of teeth. The anaerobic environment of the **subgingival area** can be altered by use of dental floss (shallow pockets), perio aids, and corrective periodontal (and osseous) surgery. Ultimately the extraction of teeth may be necessary to eliminate local infections in patients who cannot control periodontal disease. **Elective surgery** in this area should be delayed until infections are resolved or at least until large amounts of plaque are removed.

NOTE: **Almost any species of microorganism which inhabits or is introduced into the mouth can be involved in an infection if provided access to underlying tissues. Thus the removal of heavy plaque accumulation and the use of oral antiseptic rinses is recommended prior to dental treatment (especially surgery) to reduce the incidence of post-treatment infections.**

For many years it was believed that oral infections were predominantly caused by aerobic or facultative microorganisms and were mostly single species infections with only an occasional infection caused by multiple species. Recent developments in anaerobic culture techniques and research by oral microbiologists **have dramatically changed these earlier beliefs.** At this time we have indisputable evidence that:

- **Anaerobic microorganisms are involved in 75-90% of all periapical abscesses** and are involved in many other oral infections.
- **Most oral infections involve more than one species of microorganism.** Frequently as many as 4-6 different species may be recovered from acute abscesses including **both anaerobic and facultative aerobic species.**

These findings help to explain why previously used treatment methods have failed to resolve many oral infections, and definitely increases the usefulness of microbiological data in the management of oral and/or maxillofacial infections.

Some infections are caused by a single species of microorganism. The pathological process involves the interaction between the patient's body defense system and the specific characteristics of each microorganism. With previously available clinical and laboratory culturing techniques, most dental infections were thought to involve *Streptococcus* species. Since about 98% of this group are susceptible to penicillin therapy, this antibiotic became the drug of choice for treating oral infections. Many general practitioners saw no need to initially obtain Gram stain or culture and antibiotic susceptibility data unless the infection failed to resolve. This approach, while still followed for many mild to moderate infections, can compromise treatment by specialists since this information is often needed to manage serious infections.

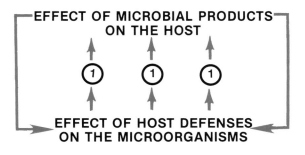

Figure V-4. Infections from a single species of microorganism are regulated by the interactions between host defenses and the microbe.

Many infections are caused by more than one species of microorganism. Mixed infections present a much more complicated pathological picture. **First,** each of the involved species has effects on the other species involved. Thus, an ecological interaction exists between species creating predominant and less dominant organisms. **Secondly,** this ecological group of microorganisms is influenced by the status of the host defenses and, conversely, the host defenses are influenced by the **combined effects** of the various microbial species.

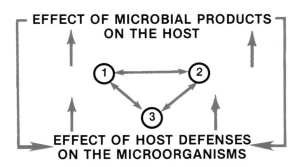

Figure V-5. Infections from multiple species of microorganisms are regulated by the interactions between microbial species as well as host defenses. This interaction is much more complex than simple species infections.

Our current understanding of the variables that control or regulate the ecology of mixed infections is extremely limited. Therefore, our knowledge of the specific effects of host defense mechanisms and therapeutic agents on mixed infections is also quite limited.

Microbiological data can play a significant role in the management of moderate fascial space infections. Generally speaking, therapy directed toward the predominant species will alter mixed flora infections such that the patient's defenses can gain control over the remaining organisms. However, this is not always the case. Occasionally, elimination of the predominant species by one antibiotic will allow another species which is not susceptible to this antibiotic to flourish. The following brief discussion of specific microbial characteristics is presented in order to demonstrate the clinical significance of microbiological principles as applied to the diagnosis and treatment of oral and/or maxillofacial infections.

STUDY EXERCISES

Microbiological data can be of assistance when diagnosing maxillofacial swellings. This data can provide information verifying the presence of __microorganisms__ in the swelling, __identifying__ the microorganism(s) present, establishing the relative numbers and dominant species in mixed infections, providing guidance in __antibody__ selection confirming the __cause__ of an infection.

Anaerobic microorganisms are involved in about __75-90__% of periapical abscesses.

Most oral infections involve (one/more than one) __more than one__ species of microorganism.

Describe the difference between resident and transient oral flora. ____ __transient is temporary__ ____

Three microbial econiches in the oral cavity are: 1)__buccal mucosa__, 2)__tongue__, 3) area around the __teeth__. Dental plaque is divided into __supra__ gingival and __sub__ gingival econiches. Poor oral hygiene promotes build-up of __bacterial plaque__, which in turn predisposes patients to infections of the __periodontia__, oral soft __tissue__, and __teeth__ and are more likely to develop infections of oral tissues following __invasive__ treatment. Ectopic infections of the ____ can occur from inhalation of oral flora. Accumulation of dental plaque produces __infection__ of gingival tissue and causes loss of the epithelial layer of this tissue, which facilitates entry of microorganisms into the __blood__ stream and increases the probability of __bacterial endocarditis__ infections and infections of other body areas.

Infections from a single species of microorganism are regulated by interactions between __microbial products__ and the __host__. Infections from multiple species of microorganisms are regulated by the interactions between __microbial products__ as well as __host__ __defense__.

GENERAL CHARACTERISTICS OF MICROORGANISMS

The general characteristics of microorganisms inhabiting the oral cavity vary widely from species to species, and knowledge of these characteristics can be significant to your diagnosis and management of oral and/or maxillofacial infections. The general microbial characteristics which are identified through routine laboratory analysis of a specimen from an infection include:

- **Staining characteristics** (Gram stain and other diagnostic stains)
- **Oxygen sensitivity** (aerobic, facultatively aerobic, and anaerobic)
- **Antibiotic susceptibility**

In addition, microorganisms **can be identified** as to groups present and even to genus and species if necessary.

• Staining Characteristics

The morphological characteristics of many microorganisms can be readily observed by the use of various staining techniques. **Simple staining** techniques such as methylene blue can be used to identify the presence of bacteria in pus and/or tissue. **Differential staining** techniques can be used to show differences between microbial cell types or components. Differential staining techniques are widely used by microbiology laboratories to **provide initial screening data** and **species identification data** to the clinician as a basis for both initial and definitive therapy decisions.

Gram Stain

Clinically, the most useful diagnostic staining technique is the **Gram stain.** With this technique, microorganisms can be classified into the broad categories of **Gram positive (+)** or **Gram negative (−)** organisms and within these categories the particular **shape** of the organism (cocci, rods, or other) can also be determined. The Gram stain can provide immediate and useful information to help you:
  • Establish the presence of microorganisms
  • Identify the morphological and Gram stain classification of the involved organisms
  • Select initial antibiotic
  • Gain information about the causative microorganism(s) even if future cultures are negative
  • Verify that future culturing data contain the same groupings that are present in the initial stain (Did the lab lose some species?)

Through years of clinical practice the Gram stain has proven helpful in identifying **single species** or **mixed species infections** and in selection of an antibiotic or antibiotics before identification of species and antibiotic susceptibility can be performed in the laboratory.

> **EXAMPLE:** If you find Gram (+) cocci occurring in chains, your initial diagnosis would implicate a streptococcal infection. Since penicillin is usually the antibiotic of choice for Gram (+) streptococci, you would most likely prescribe penicillin if an antibiotic is indicated. However, if these Gram (+) cocci are not in chains, the causative organism may be *Staphylococci,* which often produce penicillinase. In this case penicillin would not be the antibiotic of choice.

The term **STAT** is used in ordering a Gram stain from your clinical microbiology laboratory when **the results are needed immediately.** This procedure will take about 15-20 minutes plus the time needed to transport the specimen to the laboratory. Some dental practitioners perform STAT Gram stain in their offices rather than using an outside laboratory.

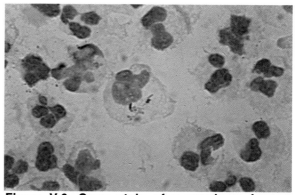

Figure V-6. Gram stain of a specimen from a chronic periapical abscess. Gram (+) and Gram (−) bacteria can be seen either inside or on the surface of the white blood cell near the center of this photograph.

STAT Gram Stain Results
☐ Single specie ☑ Mixed ☐ No microbes present
☐ Gram (+) cocci *4+ staph* ☐ Gram (−) cocci *2+*
☐ Gram (+) rods _____ ☐ Gram (−) rods _____
☐ Other _____

Other Staining Techniques

Other differential staining techniques can be used to identify pathogenic microorganisms. These techniques can be used when initial treatment proves inadequate or when an unusual microorganism is initially suspected. Usually a general dentist will refer management of these unusual cases to a specialist who will then seek additional laboratory data to identify the problem in more detail. If your clinical evidence indicates the possibility of an unusual organism, the laboratory must be informed of this to provide the appropriate culture and staining techniques. If you are unfamiliar with the management of these special infections you should refer your patient to the appropriate specialist.

EXAMPLES OF SPECIAL STAINING TECHNIQUES

Staining Technique	Used to Identify
Acid-fast (Ziehl-Neelsen)	*Mycobacteria (T.B.)*
Kinyoun (Carbolfuchsin acid fast)	*Mycobacteria (T.B.)*
Wet mounts	Fungi
Giemsa stain	Rickettsia, Clamydia
Fluorescing Antibody	*Haemophilus influenzae,* Neisseria gonorrhea, Streptococcal groups

Table V-4. Examples of special staining techniques used for definitive diagnosis.

These special stains are not routinely performed unless requested or you state that you are clinically suspicious that the infection is not due to the usual oral flora.

STUDY EXERCISES

Clinically, the most useful diagnostic staining technique is the __Gram__ *stain. This technique allows you to classify the causative organisms as either* __G +__ *or* __G +__ *as well as determine the particular* __shape__ *of the organisms.*

The Gram stain can provide useful information for you to:
a. Establish the presence of __microorganism__ *.*
b. Establish __the__ *identification of some or all of the involved microorganisms.*
c. Select an initial __antibody__ *for treatment.*
d. Gain information even if __cultures__ *fails to yield results.*
e. Tell if the lab has __miss__ *some of the microorganisms during culturing.*

A Gram stain will enable you to make a more precise initial __choice__ *and a more rational selection of an* __bacterial__ *antibiotic.*

The term STAT Gram stain means _____ *and usually requires* __15__ *to* __20__ *minutes plus the time required to* __transport__ *the specimen to the* __lab__ *.*

When might you request one of the special staining techniques be used for an oral infection? __when suspect unusual__

A patient presents to your office with pericoronitis associated with his mandibular right third molar. Your initial antibiotic treatment is penicillin 500 mg qid. When the patient returns 3 days later, he has a fever of 39°C and advanced buccal swelling. Would Gram staining have helped in initial management of this patient's problem? (Yes/No) __yes__ *Why?* __identifies bacteria present__ *What can you do at this point to help assure your antibiotic selection is more effective?* __make a better selection__

• OXYGEN SENSITIVITY

Different species of microorganisms vary with regard to their ability to tolerate available oxygen. At one end of the spectrum are those species which require oxygen for survival (**aerobes**), and at the other extreme are those species which cannot survive in the presence of oxygen (**anaerobes**). **Facultative aerobes** can survive with or without oxygen. Many species found in the oral cavity are anaerobic. In recent years, specimen collection methods and laboratory culture techniques have been developed to identify anaerobic oral microorganisms. A highly significant number of oral and maxillofacial infections (75-90%) are caused by anaerobic species or by combinations of both aerobic and anaerobic organisms. The management of any oral infection can be more difficult if an anaerobic organism is involved because:

- Collecting a specimen of anaerobic microorganisms and transporting it to the laboratory is more difficult.
- The time required by the laboratory to grow and identify some anaerobic species (up to 6 days) is longer than that required for aerobes.

NOTE: Because anaerobic species play such a significant role in oral infections, your overall management strategy must accommodate for the increased problems associated with collection, preservation and cultivation of these microorganisms.

As mentioned earlier, the numbers and species of microorganisms which live in the econiche around the teeth and gingival sulcus depend to a large extent on the level of oral hygiene practiced by your patients. As dental plaque is allowed to accumulate, this environment is transformed from predominantly aerobic to an environment which favors proliferation of anaerobic microorganisms. Additionally, as the gingival sulcus is deepened through chronic inflammation, the microbial flora of the sulcus becomes progressively more abundant and more anaerobic.

Oral infections can develop from mixtures of aerobic, facultative, and anaerobic flora at any stage in this environmental transition. Thus, oral infections vary widely in the composition of involved species. **If your technique for collecting a specimen for examination does not preserve anaerobic species, then the value of laboratory studies is severely compromised.**

During the process of abscess formation, oxygen levels decrease to anaerobic conditions. Drainage of the abscess (an essential key to infection management) will result in increased oxygen levels in the tissue and thus aid in eliminating anaerobic microorganisms.

STUDY EXERCISES

Microbial species which require oxygen for survival are called ___aerobes___ .
Those that are killed by the presence of oxygen are called ___anaerobes___ .
___facultative___ ___aerobes___ *are microbes which survive with or without oxygen. As many as* __75__-__90__ *% of oral and/or maxillofacial infections may involve* ___anaerobic___ *microorganisms.*

The management of an infection involving anaerobic microorganisms can be more difficult because:
- _____lab studies value compromise_____
- _____oral infection vary_____

• ANTIBIOTIC SUSCEPTIBILITY AND RESISTANCE

Microorganisms also have a variety of reactions to specific antibiotic agents and to the specific dosage of each antibiotic. Although strong inferences can be made from staining techniques such as Gram stain, determination of specific antibiotic sensitivity can only be determined through laboratory study. **Figure V-7** shows an example of an **antibiotic sensitivity test** for bacteria obtained from an oral infection. The size of the zone of no bacterial growth around the antibiotic disks is an indicator of bacterial susceptibility to the antibiotic.

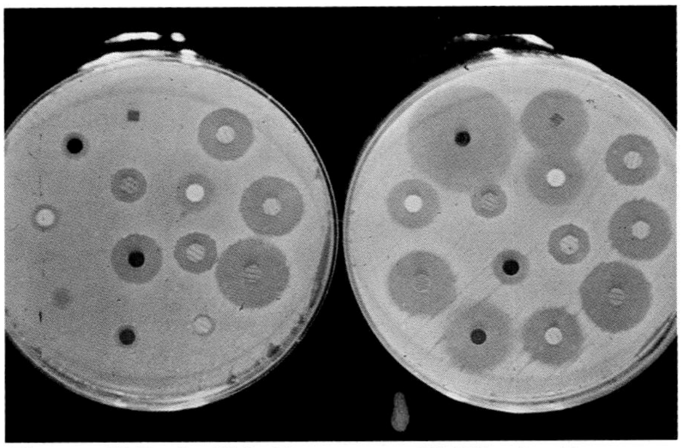

Figure V-7. Antibiotic susceptibility testing can assist you in choosing an appropriate antibiotic. The culture dishes shown are the results of antibiotic susceptibility tests on cultures obtained from different odontogenic infections. Notice the differences in the antibiotic susceptibilities of these two examples.

Types of Antibiotic Resistance

The susceptibility of a particular species (or strain) of microorganism to a specific antibiotic is dependent upon the individual characteristics of the microorganism. Microorganisms may have **natural (mutational) resistance** or gain **acquired (transferred) resistance** to specific antibiotics.

Natural (Mutational) Resistance

Some species of microorganisms are totally unaffected by certain antibiotics due to their structure and genetic composition. It has been shown that many microorganisms are resistant to specific antimicrobial agents without prior contact with the agent. This natural **resistance** is believed to be derived from a random, spontaneous mutation of microbial genes and **is not** related to the presence of the antibiotic agent. Mutations occur at the rate of $1:10^7$ to $1:10^9$ cell divisions. Two types of mutations are seen:
1. **"Single-step"** mutation event causing total resistance
2. **"Multiple-step"** mutations causing a progressive increase in the **minimal inhibitory concentration (MIC)**.

While clinicians have little control over the single-step random mutations which cause total resistance, the clinical use of large doses (higher blood levels) of antibiotics will destroy the "multiple-step" mutants before complete resistance is reached. Long-term and/or low-dose regimes will encourage development of "multiple-step" resistant mutants.

The clinical use of antibiotics does not "create" new resistant microorganisms but does promote those microorganisms which are already resistant to the specific antibiotic.

Acquired (Transferred) Resistance

Acquired (or transferred) antibiotic resistance may occur by three mechanisms:
- **Genetic Transformation** — involves uptake of DNA containing genes for antibiotic resistance. This method has little clinical significance.
- **Viral Transduction** — involves transfer of DNA from cell to cell by bacteriophage (viral) infection.
- **Conjugation** — involves the transfer of **plasmids** containing the genetic code for antibiotic resistance during the union of two bacterial cells. Plasmid transferred DNA can then be integrated into the recipient bacteria's genetic structure and passed on during subsequent cell divisions. Plasmids have been shown to transfer genetic resistance to up to ten antibiotics (tetracycline, streptomycin, gentamicin, kanamycin, chloramphenicol, neomycin and sulfonamides) and involve both Gram (−) and Gram (+) bacteria.

NOTE: Due to these acquired antibiotic resistance mechanisms and the overuse of antibiotics, selection of appropriate antibiotics based upon Gram stain categories is becoming less reliable. This reduces the probability of success for your initially selected antibiotic and increases the necessity to obtain culture and susceptibility data in order to determine appropriate antibiotic therapy.

Bacteriocidal and Bacteriostatic Antibiotics

Bacteriocidal antibiotics result in the death of bacterial cells. **Bacteriostatic** antibiotics inhibit multiplication of bacteria but do not kill the bacteria. While **bacteriocidal** agents kill the susceptible microorganisms, bacteriostatic agents hold susceptible microorganisms "in check" and allow body defenses to localize and remove the infection. Premature withdrawal of bacteriostatic agents may produce a rebound of the infection once blood levels have fallen below the minimal inhibitory concentration (MIC). Combining bacteriocidal agents with bacteriostatic agents can negate the activity of bacteriocidal agents and promote infection rebound (e.g. combining penicillin and tetracycline can be both ineffective and a waste of money for your patients).

NOTE: Your patient's medical history should be carefully reviewed to detect a history (especially current or recent) of antibiotic use. This information can be useful in selecting an initial antibiotic. This information should also be transmitted to your microbiology lab with any cultures submitted.

The potential for **antibiotic resistant microorganisms** must never be overlooked. Patients who are taking antibiotics for other medical problems may develop oral flora which are resistant to the usual drug of choice at the usual dosages. You must take this into consideration when selecting drugs of choice and/or dosages of choice from standard reference sources. When selecting an initial antibiotic you should avoid prescribing any antibiotic which your patient has been taking. Laboratory data on antibiotic sensitivity will be of additional help to you when the data are received, especially if the infection persists following initial treatment.

We will discuss the therapeutic use of antibiotics in the management of oral and/or maxillofacial infections later in this book.

Minimal Inhibitory Concentration (MIC)

Microbial resistance to antibiotics can be accurately measured *in vitro* through determination of the **minimal inhibitory concentration (MIC)** which is the lowest concentration of the antimicrobial agent that will inhibit visible microbial growth after overnight incubation. Unfortunately, the direct application of *in vitro* MIC data to the *in vivo* clinical management of infections is currently minimal.

You should, however, be aware of the concept of MIC, and, as the scientific link between MIC and the pharmacokinetics of antibiotic activities improves, modifications in the "currently accepted" antibiotic regimens may be necessary. At present, however, you should follow the "accepted" regimens for each antibiotic and avoid "faddish proclamations" or arbitrarily reducing dosages or durations.

SPECIES IDENTIFICATION

In clinical situations where the use of antibiotics is indicated, identification of the involved species may be essential. Identifying the causative microorganism(s) will enable you to select the proper antibiotic(s) and effective dosage(s). It will also provide useful information about the usual clinical course of such infections.

NOTE: The more experience you obtain through knowledge of the microbiology of oral infections the better you will be able to correlate the patterns of clinical pathology with particular species of microorganisms. This will enhance your ability to make appropriate initial management decisions with each new infection.

SUMMARY OF MICROORGANISMS ISOLATED FROM ORAL AND MAXILLOFACIAL INFECTIONS

GRAM (+) COCCI
 AEROBES
  Streptococcus mitior
  Streptococcus salivarius
  Streptococcus mutans
  Streptococcus pneumoniae
  Streptococcus pyogenes
  Streptococcus faecalis
  Streptococcus sanguis
  Streptococcus intermedius
  Staphylococcus epidermidis
  Staphylococcus aureus
 ANAEROBIC SPECIES
  Peptostreptococcus species
  Peptostreptococcus anaerobis
  Peptostreptococcus micros
  Peptococcus species

GRAM (−) COCCI
 AEROBES
  Neisseria species
  Candida albicans
 ANAEROBES
  Veillonella paruvia

GRAM (+) RODS
 AEROBES
  Lactobaccilus species
 ANAEROBES
  Bifidobacterium species
  Lactobacillus species
  Enbacterium species
  Actinomyces species
  Actinomyces israelii

GRAM (−) RODS
 AEROBES
  Klebsiella-Enterobacter species
  Escherichia coli
 ANAEROBES
  Bacteroides species
  Bacteroides fragilis
  Bacteroides melanogenicus group
  Bacteroides corrodens
  Bacteroides oralis
  Fusobacterium species
  Fusobacterium nucleatum
  Leptotrichia buccalis

Figure VI-8. Summary of microorganisms isolated from oral and maxillofacial infections. Frequently the organisms occur in mixed infections.

While the identification of microorganisms involved in an oral and/or maxillofacial infection may be essential to the final resolution of the infection, the **time required** to obtain definitive species identification and antibiotic susceptibility may **exceed the time required** for the clinical resolution of the infection.

Your microbiology laboratory can, however, provide valuable information **prior to** definitive species identification. Through an ongoing relationship with your laboratory (frequently beginning with the patient's initial visit) the lab can supply you with progressively more information as their results are obtained. This information can enable you to be **more precise** in your diagnosis and **more accurate** in your selection of antibiotics. The following discussion describes the staging of information you should expect from your lab progressing to the ideal of definitive species identification with antibiotic susceptibility data. You should discuss these steps with your lab in advance of submitting a specimen from an acute infection.

- **Verify the presence of microorganisms in an aspirate specimen from a swelling (or blood specimen).** Usually this step is combined with the next step but may involve special stains.
   Time Required: About 20 minutes (from receipt of specimen)

- **Perform Gram stain to categorize microorganisms and allow initial selection of an antibiotic(s) to be based on generalized Gram stain susceptibility charts.** (See antibiotic therapy in Unit VIII).
   Time Required: About 20 minutes (from receipt of specimen)

This step will group microorganism(s) into categories but **will not distinguish** between **dead or viable microorganisms** or between **aerobic or anaerobic species** (see page 137).

- **Determine the overall antibiotic susceptibility of all microorganisms (single or mixed species) present in the specimen.** This technique involves streaking the specimen onto appropriate media, applying antibiotic disks, followed by **both aerobic and anaerobic incubation.**

   Time Required: 24-48 hours (may require up to 7-10 days for slow-growing anaerobes)

   When **applied to mixed infections**, this technique is subject to many errors including:
   - Distortion of the numbers and proportion of the mixed species involved.
   - Data for fast-growing species will be reported first. Generally, aerobes grow faster than anaerobes.

   However, this information can be helpful in **verifying** your initial choice of antibiotics and **is better than no information** at all. Advise your lab to do this if they have previously reported "mixed oral flora" or "normal oral flora" and did not continue with species identification and antibiotic susceptibility data tests.

   If the infection **is not controlled**, continuing microbiological studies is essential. Your initial antibiotic may have been ineffective, there may have been a shift in flora produced by the selective pressure from the initial antibiotic (**verify with new Gram stain and culture**) or a more thorough analysis of host defense status may be necessary.

   If a mild to moderate infection **is "controlled"** within 48 hours (2 days), then you may call the lab and tell them to discontinue detailed analysis if this will save the patient money.

- **Determine the group or species of microorganism(s) involved.** This technique involves **streaking for isolation** (results in 24-48 hours) followed by growth in **differential** media (24-48 hours) and inoculation of plates for **antibiotic susceptibility** (24-48 hours). This series of tests must be done under both aerobic and anaerobic conditions. Anaerobic tests may require 7-10 days for each step, thus the time period required is quite variable and often greatly exceeds the rate of clinical resolution.

   Time Required: 2-14 days

   Since most oral infections involve mixed flora and contain both aerobic and anaerobic microorganisms, completion of a detailed analysis of the causative agents may require extensive laboratory work and incur considerable expense to your patient. However, this expense is a small price to pay if initial treatment proves ineffective in controlling infections and definitive data is not available when needed.

   An alternative is to only study the predominant species in the infection. This approach is valid for many infections; however, if the flora shifts (due to antiboitic pressure) you will not have meaningful data for future decisions.

   Laboratory analysis should be initiated from the start and may be discontinued if initial treatment is effective.

Summary

This review of general microbial characteristics and guidelines for species identification represents a simplified (perhaps over-simplified) approach to a difficult and often confusing area. If you routinely treat moderately serious infections, you should devote significant effort to **understanding the microbiology of oral and/or maxillofacial infections** and working out a **smooth system of communication** with your clinical microbiology lab.

NOTE: Ideally you should choose a lab which can manage anaerobes and has personnel experienced with oral flora (hopefully an oral microbiologist).

In many instances, clinical microbiology labs lack **adequate training or knowledge** in the specialized area of oral infections and you may be called upon to provide your lab with instructions on how to manage your specimens and how to report their findings.

OBTAINING A SPECIMEN FOR MICROBIOLOGICAL EXAMINATION

"Taking a culture" is a clinical phrase frequently used to describe **the process of obtaining a specimen for microbiological examination** of the **staining characteristics** and **species identification** of the microorganisms that could be associated with an oral or maxillofacial swelling. **"Culture and susceptibility" (sensitivity)**, abbreviated as C&S, implies determination of the antibiotic susceptibility of the involved microorganisms.

NOTE: The only way you can obtain definitive information about the microorganisms responsible for an infection is through culturing and microbiologic examination.

Culturing (C&S) provides you with supportive information which can make your clinical diagnosis more accurate and thus your treatment more specific.

LABORATORY DATA

Yes No
- ☑ ☐ Culture material available at this time
- ☐ ☑ STAT Gram stain indicated
- ☐ ☑ Specimen collected for micro lab
- ☐ ☑ Specimen collected for histopathologic exam
- ☐ ☑ Hematology studies needed. Which? _____

STAT Gram Stain Results
- ☐ Single specie ☐ Mixed   ☐ No microbes present
- ☐ Gram (+) cocci _____   ☐ Gram (−) cocci _____
- ☐ Gram (+) rods _____   ☐ Gram (−) rods _____
- ☐ Other _____

WHEN TO CULTURE

Ideally, **cultures should be taken from any oral or maxillofacial infection**. However, clinical practice has shown that the majority of **minor oral infections** can be resolved without this information through use of standard treatment methods. **The question that arises with this approach is "what do I do if my initial standard treatment methods fail and I lack specific information upon which to base future treatment."** The additional time required to obtain laboratory information can be critical to the well being of your patient.

A practical answer to this dilemma of when to culture may be summarized by the guidelines shown in **Table V-6.**

TO CULTURE OR NOT TO CULTURE

Culture IS essential if:	Initial culture IS NOT essential if:
• **Infection has spread to fascial planes of the head and/or neck.**	• **Infection is small and confined to the alveolar ridge and adjacent soft tissue (i.e., periodontal and endodontic abscess).**
• **Initial treatment has failed to resolve the problem.**	• **Infection has established drainage through the alveolar ridge and no vestibular or fascial spaces are involved.**
• **Patient has a serious medical compromise affecting host resistance factors.**	• **Infection (such as pericoronitis) is contaminated with intraoral flora.**
• **Patient shows signs of systemic toxicity or systemic spread.**	• **Infection has little potential of spread to critical fascial spaces.**

Table V-6. Summary of guidelines for deciding whether culturing of infectious material is indicated.

NOTE: If culturing is initially indicated but no specimen can be obtained, you should initiate treatment and collect a specimen as soon as suppurative material (pus) is available.

NOTE: The preceding recommendations must be viewed as guidelines only. You must evaluate each patient with an infection on an individual basis and make the decision to culture or not. Within practical limits, it is better to over-utilize culturing than to risk not having this information available when initial treatment methods fail to resolve an infection.

VALUES OF INFORMATION OBTAINED FROM A MICROBIOLOGICAL LAB

Information obtained from direct examination or culturing of a specimen obtained from a swelling can be quite useful in both initial and definitive treatment decisions. **Table V-7** summarizes the primary uses of culture information.

USEFULNESS OF INFORMATION FROM A MICROBIOLOGICAL LABORATORY

SERVICE	VALUE OF RESULTS
STAINING TECHNIQUES	
Gram Stain	• Immediate results • Verify presence and morphology of infectious microorganisms • Determine if infection is single species or mixed species • Estimate of relative numbers involved in mixed infections • May assist in determination of correct initial antibiotic • May not detect small Gram (−) microorganisms (frequently anaerobes)
Other Stains	• Identify unusual microorganisms (usually performed if initial treatment fails)
SPECIES IDENTIFICATION	• Determine identity of causative agent(s) • Determine if anaerobes are present • Provide basic understanding of the effects of the species on the patient • Requires 2-7 days
ANTIBIOTIC SUSCEPTIBILITY	• Established through *in vitro* testing — reduces guessing • Requires 2-14 days

Table V-7. Summary of the value of culture information in the diagnosis and treatment of odontogenic infections.

Many clinical microbiology laboratories **are not accustomed to dealing with specimens from oral infections containing anaerobic microbes.** They will often report "**mixed normal oral flora**" (even though you have followed correct specimen collection procedures), and **fail to perform antibiotic susceptibility tests**. You should request that they do susceptibility testing with predominant species. Additionally, a clinical microbiological laboratory's routine may not include saving culture plates in anaerobic conditions for several days in order to detect slow-growing microorganisms.

STUDY EXERCISES

Culturing is the term used to describe the process of obtaining a _____*specimen*_____ for _____*microbiological*_____ examination. Culture analysis can provide you with information about:

 a. _____*staining*_____ characteristics
 b. _____*species*_____ identification
 c. _____*antibody*_____ susceptibility

Describe four situations in which a culture is essential for proper patient management.
 a. Infection has spread to _____*facial spaces*_____
 b. _____*initial tx*_____ has failed.
 c. Patient has serious _____*medical*_____ _____*compromises*_____ affecting host resistance factors.
 d. Patient shows signs of systemic _____*toxemia*_____ or _____*systemic spread*_____.

The only way you can obtain definitive information about causative microorganisms is through _____*culture*_____ and _____*staining*_____.

GENERAL PRINCIPLES FOR COLLECTING A SPECIMEN

Collecting a specimen of infected material for examination and culturing can be difficult and the results frustrating to interpret. Improperly collected specimens can yield negative or misleading results which, in turn, may lead to misdiagnosis, prolonged infective states, or unnecessary use of antimicrobial drugs.

You should always consider the following seven (7) guidelines in order to collect a specimen which will be most reflective of the infective process and thus maximize the value of the information obtained.

- **The specimen collected should be material that is most representative of the infective process.** The specimen can be pus, saline aspirate, or a small piece of involved tissue. For example, culturing a small fragment of bone obtained from an osteomyelitis may reflect the infective process better than purulent exudate expressed into the oral cavity and recovered on a cotton swab.

- **Avoid contamination of specimen by patient's own flora.** This principle is particularly important for odontogenic infections where salivary contamination is extremely common and can provide misleading information. A small amount of oral contaminant will produce a rich growth of organisms in the nutrient culture media. The culture will yield a diverse mixture of organisms which may not accurately reflect the flora of the lesion.

- **Collect specimen under conditions that will preserve anaerobic microorganisms.** Up to 75% of odontogenic infections are caused by anaerobes. Improper collection technique can destroy these species, thus delaying an accurate definitive diagnosis and prompt definitive treatment. You should obtain a specimen via aspiration rather than using a cotton swab after incising tissue.

- **Obtain sufficient material for adequate examination.** The smaller the sample collected the less chance you have of obtaining a representative sample and adequate growth in culture media. In the early stages of odontogenic infections, it may be difficult to obtain adequate amounts of suppurative material for culturing. However, some material is better than none.

- **Collect specimen prior to antimicrobial therapy.** The specimen should be collected prior to antimicrobial therapy if possible because the growth-retarding properties of antimicrobial drugs may affect the specimen. Changes in the ecological factors of the infective organisms caused by antimicrobial drugs may also change or mask the true infective organism.

- **Use proper containers and transport media.** Obviously, sterile containers and appropriate physiologic conditions in transporting containers are important in supporting organisms until they can be cultured. For example, exposing anaerobic organisms to room air for short periods will destroy the organisms. Therefore, it is crucial to place the collected specimen in an anaerobic container for transport. Transport medium should not contain nutrients that would permit disproportionate growth of fast-growing species during delays in transport or cultivation.

- **Prompt transport of specimen to laboratory is essential.** Delay in delivery and culturing decreases the survival of organisms and minimizes the success of the culturing process. You should deliver the collected specimen promptly to the diagnostic lab.

The most common causes of problems associated with the collection of a specimen for laboratory examination and reasons why the laboratory report may not provide useful information are summarized in **Table V-8:**

MOST COMMON PROBLEMS ASSOCIATED WITH THE CULTURING PROCESS

PROBLEMS	SOLUTION TO PROBLEMS
FAILURE TO OBTAIN CULTURE MATERIAL	
• Premature attempt to collect specimen	• Submit sterile saline solution injected and withdrawn from involved area • Wait until fluctuance develops
• Incorrect placement of needle for collection of specimen	• Reassess site of aspiration • Verify presence of fluctuance
FAILURE TO OBTAIN LABORATORY GROWTH	
• Failure to preserve anaerobes during specimen collection	• No viable organisms were present. Results are valid • Use anaerobic collection methods
• Failure to preserve vitality during transit to laboratory	• Use anaerobic transport methods • Transport specimen more rapidly to laboratory
• Failure of laboratory to correctly manage specimen	• Contact laboratory to discuss their management of the specimen. Verify their procedure to manage anaerobes
LAB REPORTS NORMAL ORAL FLORA	
• Salivary contamination of specimen	• Review your collection technique. Collect new specimen under more aseptic conditions • Remember that most odontogenic infections arise from "normal oral flora"
• Laboratory did not perform detailed identification	• Inform lab of need to be more specific as to dominant species and to do antibiotic susceptibility tests on those

Table V-8. Summary of the most common problems associated with the culturing of infectious material from an infectious swelling.

With the above background information in mind, we will next review the basic techniques for collecting a specimen for culturing.

STUDY EXERCISES

Seven general guidelines you should follow when obtaining a culture specimen include:
1. *Collect material that is most* ___represent___ *of the infective process.*
2. *Avoid contamination by the patient's* ___oral___ ___flora___.
3. *Collect specimen under conditions that will preserve* ___anaerobes___ *microorganisms.*
4. *Obtain sufficient material for analysis.*
5. *Collect specimen prior to* ___antibiotic___ *therapy.*
6. *Use proper containers and* ___transport___ ___media___.
7. *Transport specimen to laboratory promptly.*

What should you do if you are unable to obtain culture material from an infection site?

_____

_____

If your laboratory reports that a culture you submitted contains a mixture of normal oral flora, what error in specimen collection technique may be the cause? ___Sent sterilyzed saline injected & withdrawn___

If the laboratory is unable to obtain growth from a culture specimen, what are three possible errors in collection technique which may have caused this? 1. ___failure to preserve anaerobes___ 2. ___failed to preserve vitality___
3. ___Lab fail to manage___
Which type of organism is more likely to present this problem ___anaerobe___ *(anaerobic/aerobic)?*

SELECTION OF THE SAMPLING SITE

Selection of the specific site or location for specimen collection can influence your ability to obtain an adequate specimen. The general guidelines for site selection are:
- The most fluctuant area should be sampled.
- The most direct route to the abscess should be used.

The optimum sampling site may be either **intraoral** or **extraoral** depending upon the proximity of the infection to the oral mucosa or skin surface. **Table V-9** summarizes the most common site for collecting specimens from the various fascial spaces or areas of the head and neck and rates the relative degree of difficulty for specimen collection from each space or area. Extraoral specimen collection is classified as difficult due to the lack of experience general dentists have with these techniques.

SITE SELECTION FOR ASPIRATION

SPACES WITH INTRAORAL ACCESS		SPACES WITH EXTRAORAL ACCESS	
LESS DIFFICULT	MORE DIFFICULT	LESS DIFFICULT	MORE DIFFICULT
Buccal Vestibules	Lateral Pharyngeal (+,*)	Submental Space	Parotid Space
Mental Space	Retropharyngeal (+,*)	Submandibular Space	Periorbital Space
Body of Mandible	Pterygomandibular (+,*)	Mentalis Space	Fascial Planes of the Neck
Palatal Space	Sublingual (*)		
Base of Upper Lip	Submandibular (+,*)		
Infraorbital	Submasseteric Space (*)		
Buccal Space	Temporal Spaces		
Sublingual	Infratemporal (+,*)		

+ Use of the extraoral route may be necessary if access through intraoral route is impaired due to trismus.

* Generally, you will have identified the anatomical location of any infection in this area and tentatively made a decision to refer difficult fascial space infections before considering collection of specimens from these areas.

Table V-9. Most frequent route for collecting abscess specimens from swellings of various fascial spaces of the head and neck.

STUDY EXERCISES

Spaces which are usually accessible for intraoral drainage may require extraoral drainage if access is limited due to ___trismus___.

When selecting a sampling site for obtaining a culture specimen you should consider:
a. The most ___fluctuant___ area of swelling.
b. The most ___direct___ route of access.

For the diagrams below, name the numbered spaces and state whether specimen collection from an infection of this space should be via intraoral or extraoral access. Also state the relative degree of difficulty for specimen collection via this route.

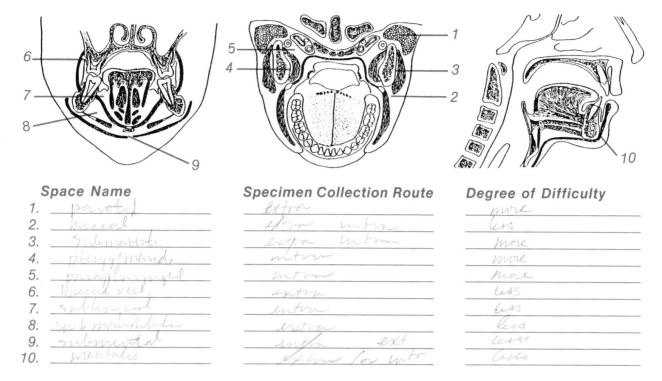

	Space Name	Specimen Collection Route	Degree of Difficulty
1.	parotid	extra	more
2.	buccal	extra intra	less
3.	submasseteric	extra intra	more
4.	pterygomandib.	intra	more
5.	parapharyngeal	intra	more
6.	buccal vest.	intra	less
7.	sublingual	intra	less
8.	submandib.	extra	less
9.	submental	intra ext	less
10.	mentalis	extra /or intr	less

ANSWERS:

	Space Name	Specimen Collection Route	Degree of Difficulty
1.	Parotid	Extraoral	More difficult
2.	Buccal	Intraoral	Less difficult
3.	Submasseteric	Intraoral	More difficult
4.	Pterygomandibular	Intraoral	More difficult
5.	Parapharyngeal	Intraoral	More difficult
6.	Buccal vestibule	Intraoral	Less difficult
7.	Sublingual	Intraoral	More or less difficult
8.	Submandibular	Extraoral	Less difficult
9.	Submental	Extraoral	Less difficult
10.	Mentalis	Intra or extraoral	Less difficult

THE PROCESS FOR OBTAINING A SPECIMEN

The process for obtaining any specimen for microbiological examination will involve the following steps:

1. Pain control
2. Site preparation
3. Collection of specimen
4. Transport to laboratory

Since the value of the laboratory data is dependent upon the specimen received from you, it is essential that your collection technique does not introduce extraneous contamination into the specimen nor lead to the death of anaerobic species.

We will discuss specific techniques for both intraoral and extraoral specimen collection.

□ INTRAORAL COLLECTION METHODS

The following methods are commonly used for specimen collection:

- Collect from infected tooth
- Transmucosal aspiration
- Tissue biopsy

• Collect From Infected Tooth

The collection of a specimen from an infected tooth can be a useful technique. This will only be applicable to teeth in which the pulp chamber has not been exposed to oral flora. The specific details of this are frequently discussed in endodontic texts and thus will only be summarized here (see **Table V-10**).

STEP	PROCESS OR TECHNIQUE
Pain control	Block anesthesia (Never inject anaesthetic and/or epinephrine into the infected tissue).
Isolation of site	Single tooth rubber dam.
Site preparation	Disinfect tooth with Betadine or Zephiran prior to gaining access to pulp.
Collection of specimen . . .	1. Sterile paper points, or needle aspirate of pus.
	2. Flush with small volume of sterile saline and aspirate with needle. Remove air from syringe, cap, send to lab.
Use of transport media . . .	Tryptocase soy with 0.1% agar for paper points.
Transport to lab	1. Transport media to lab ASAP
	2. Transport syringe to lab ASAP (within 20 minutes)

Table V-10. Summary of procedures for collecting a microbial specimen from an infected tooth.

The value of cultures obtained from root canal drainage can vary depending upon:

- **The degree of severity of the infection.** Abscesses which are confined to alveolar ridges will generally resolve through initial treatment methods and a definitive diagnosis is only needed when initial treatment methods fail.

- **Your ability to obtain cultures in a sterile environment free from previous salivary contamination.** Extensive carious breakdown of teeth which extends into pulp chamber will cause salivary contamination, thus compromising the value of laboratory data.

The technique of collecting specimens from the root canals using sterile paper points has inherent limitations. First, **sensitive anaerobes can be killed** during the transfer of the paper point from the root canal to the transport medium. In addition, the growth-supporting characteristics of the **transport medium can select for some species while depressing growth of other species**. The clinical value of this technique has been debated for many years.

STUDY EXERCISES

Three techniques commonly used for intraoral specimen collection are:
1. _____transmucosal_____ aspiration
2. Collect from an infected _____tooth_____
3. _____tissue_____ _____biopsy_____

It may be difficult to collect an uncontaminated specimen from an infected tooth because of extensive _____caries_____ and _____saliva_____ contamination.

• Transmucosal Aspiration

Transmucosal aspiration is a method for collecting a specimen with the use of a needle which obtains access to the abscess through the oral mucosa. When the most direct access to an infected area is from an intraoral route, then transmucosal aspiration is the technique of choice. Areas where this technique is most useful are listed in **Table V-9** on page 148.

The technique of transmucosal aspiration is summarized in **Table V-11.**

STEP	PROCESS OR TECHNIQUE
Pain control	Local block anesthesia or topical anesthesia. Mucosal infiltration around but not into area of inflammation. Adequate anesthesia will be difficult.
Isolation of site	Dry mucosa and prevent contact by other oral structures (tongue, cheek).
Site preparation	Decontaminate mucosa at needle entry site with an iodine-based antiseptic (Betadine®). Use a quaternary amonium solution if patient is allergic to iodine.
Collection of specimen . . .	Aspirate infective material transmucosally using disposable syringe with an 18 g needle of adequate length to penetrate to the depth of the infection.
	If no material is obtained, a small amount (.25-.50 cc) of sterile saline can be slowly instilled (drop by drop) into the infected area and immediately aspirated.
	If aspirated material is obtained, remove needle, express all air from syringe, aseptically seal the tip of syringe hub with a sterile rubber stopper to prevent contamination.
Use of transport media . . .	Generally none used. Seal syringe and place sterile rubber stopper over needle tip.
Transport to lab	Transfer specimen promptly to lab (within 20 min.).

Table V-11. Summary of procedures for collecting a microbial specimen by intraoral transmucosal aspiration.

The value of cultures obtained by transmucosal aspiration will vary according to your techniques of isolation, site preparation, collection technique, use of anaerobic transport media and how rapidly you can transport the specimen to the lab.

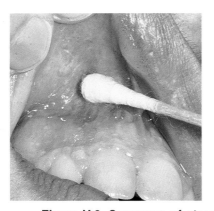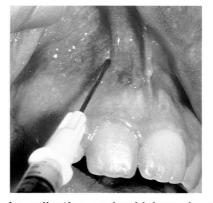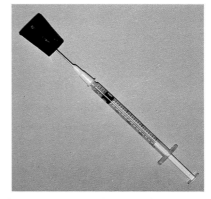

Figure V-8. Sequence of steps for collecting a microbial specimen by transmucosal aspiration.

NOTE: Use of a cotton swab to collect a specimen from an incised swelling is NOT accepted as the best method to collect a specimen. Use of this technique will lead to the death of anaerobic microorganisms before they reach the laboratory which, in turn, can seriously affect laboratory results.

- **Tissue Biopsy for Culturing**

A piece of tissue may also be removed and cultured if other collection techniques fail to yield sufficient numbers of microorganisms. **Culturing of a tissue specimen is especially useful for:**
- Identification of delicate anaerobic microorganisms
- Establishing the presence of microorganisms in a local cellulitis when no suppuration can be obtained.

This technique may be performed as part of your initial data collection process or as part of incision and drainage procedures. **Do not fix the specimen in formalin. Place directly into transport media.**

NOTE: Tissue biopsy for culturing must be performed under aseptic conditions and contamination by saliva and/or other oral flora avoided.

STEP	PROCESS OR TECHNIQUE
Pain control	Block anesthesia, mucosal infiltration away from area of inflammation, topical anesthesia.
Isolation of site	Same as for transmucosal aspiration.
Site preparation	Same as for transmucosal aspiration.
Collection of specimen . . .	Use excisional biopsy, punch biopsy or needle biopsy techniques using careful aseptic techniques.
Transport media	Place into transport media. Do not fix in formalin.
Transport to lab	Same as for transmucosal aspiration.

Table V-12. Summary of procedures for collecting an intraoral tissue specimen for microbiological culturing and examination.

STUDY EXERCISES

When there is direct intraoral access to an infected area, the technique of choice for obtaining a specimen is use of an ___sterile syringe___, not a cotton ___swab___.

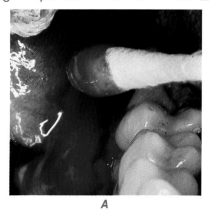

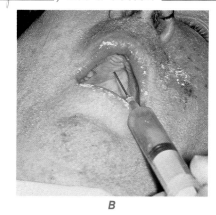

A

B

Which picture above illustrates the recommended technique for collecting an intraoral specimen, A or B? ___B___ What problem will you encounter by using the incorrect technique? ___loss of viable sample___

Describe the recommended technique for transmucosal aspiration.

Pain control: ___Block___ *or* ___topical___ *anesthesia*

Isolation: *Dry* ___area___ *and prevent contact with other intraoral tissue.*

Site Preparation: *Decontaminate with* ___Betadine___ *or* ___zephiran___.

Collection of Specimen: *Aspirate with disposable syringe with* ___18___ *gauge needle.*

If no aspirate is obtained, ___inject sterile saline + withdraw___.

Tissue biopsy can be used to identify ___anaerobes___ *in the* ___biopsy___ *and establish* ___presence of microbes___. *DO NOT* ___fix___ *the specimen in* ___formalin___ *because this will kill the microorganisms.*

☐ EXTRAORAL COLLECTION METHODS

Extraoral specimen collection is indicated if swelling is close to the skin surface or inaccessible from intraoral sites. The extraoral route may be necessary if intraoral access is limited due to trismus. Many general dentists have little involvement with the extraoral techniques for collecting specimens. Generally, infections requiring extraoral procedures are best referred to specialists who are experienced with extraoral anatomy and procedures for extraoral incision and drainage. Usually, infections requiring extraoral procedures are moderate to serious life-threatening problems that require close medical supervision. The following techniques for obtaining a specimen using an extraoral approach will be discussed:

- **Transcutaneous aspiration**
- **Extraoral tissue biopsy**

NOTE: Collecting a specimen of suppurative material by aspiration or cotton swab FOLLOWING incision and drainage may be acceptable for Gram staining, but not for culturing. Once suppuration is exposed to air, fragile anaerobic microorganisms can be killed, thus culture results would not be representative of the actual infection.

- **Transcutaneous Aspiration**

Extraoral transcutaneous aspiration is the method of choice for obtaining a specimen from swellings that are close to the skin surface or are too remote for intraoral techniques. Specimens are collected with the use of a needle which obtains access to the abscess through the skin. This technique is the same as that used for transmucosal aspiration. **Table V-9** on page 148 summarizes the areas in which extraoral specimen collection is indicated.

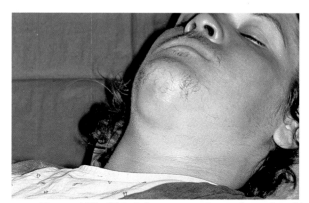 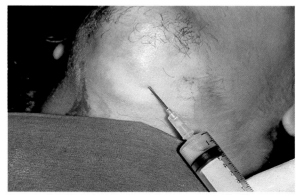

Figure V-9. Obtaining a specimen for microbiological examination by transcutaneous aspiration.

- **Extraoral Tissue Biopsy**

Collection of a tissue specimen and subsequent culturing of the tissue can be performed if necessary. Care must be taken to **avoid microbial contamination** from either cutaneous flora or poor aseptic surgical techniques.

NOTE: Usually extraoral tissue biopsy is performed by a specialist because most general dentists have not had training in extraoral surgical procedures.

STUDY EXERCISES

Generally infections requiring ___transcutaneous___ *procedures for specimen collection should be referred to a specialist. Usually these infections are moderate to serious* ___life___-___threatening___ *problems and require close* ___medical___ ___supervision___. *In addition, many general practitioners have not had training and experience in* ___extraoral___ *procedures for collecting specimens.*

Extraoral specimen collection *is indicated if: 1) the swelling is near the* ___cutaneous___ *surface, 2) the swelling is not accessible via* ___intraoral___ *routes, and 3)* ___opening___ *limits intraoral access.*

Two techniques used for **extra-oral** *collection are: 1) trans-*___cutaneous___ ___aspiration___ *and 2) extraoral tissue* ___biopsy___

INDICATING NEED FOR MICROBIOLOGICAL DATA

The following space has been provided on the **laboratory data** checklist for indicating the need for microbiological laboratory studies and the results of STAT Gram stains.

Yes	No	
☑	☐	Culture material available at this time
☐	☑	STAT Gram stain indicated
☐	☑	Specimen collected for micro lab
☐	☑	Specimen collected for histopathologic exam
☐	☑	Hematology studies needed. Which? _____

We have color coded the "yes/no" columns to emphasize the need for microbiological testing and the significance of this information or lack of information to your diagnosis and management strategy. General principles expressed by this color-coded system include:

- Non-localized acute infections (acute cellulitis) are a higher risk to your patients than localized infections.
- Definitive diagnosis must be delayed until culture specimen can be obtained, thus prolonging use of non-specific initial treatment methods.
- If culture material is available but you do not obtain a Gram stain then your initial diagnosis is less accurate than it could be and during initial treatment you are more likely to select an inappropriate antibiotic.
- Given that culture material is available and the infection involves fascial spaces, if you do not obtain a specimen for microbiological studies, you have precluded obtaining a timely definitive diagnosis and thus cannot promptly institute definitive antibiotic therapy if your initial treatment is unsuccessful.

RECORDING MICROBIOLOGICAL DATA

You should record laboratory results on the checklist as soon they are available. STAT Gram stain results can be used in your initial diagnosis and treatment, while culture data generally is not available for several days after initial treatment has begun.

Summary of Laboratory Data
MICROBIOLOGY LAB
☐ Single species   ☐ Mixed   ☐ None
Predominant species: _____
_____
_____
☐ Aerobic   ☐ Anaerobic
Antibiotic Sensitivity:
    1st choice_____
    2nd choice _____
    3rd choice_____

STAT Gram Stain Results
☐ Single specie   ☐ Mixed   ☐ No microbes present
☐ Gram (+) cocci _____   ☐ Gram (−) cocci _____
☐ Gram (+) rods _____   ☐ Gram (−) rods _____
☐ Other _____

POST-TEST — UNIT V

- Answer each of the following questions.
- Check your answers with the correct responses on pages 162-164.
- If all questions are answered correctly, proceed to page 165 to begin the section on diagnosis.
- If you do not answer all questions correctly, read and study the content of this unit.

QUESTIONS

In each of the following questions, more than one choice may be correct.

1. Which of the following statements is/are **true** regarding the usefulness of laboratory data to the diagnosis and treatment of oral and/or maxillofacial swellings?
   a. Laboratory data should be collected for **all** swellings
   b. Clinical data is generally sufficient to allow you to evaluate the effects of a swelling on the host
   c. Laboratory data should be used only if your initial treatment fails
   d. Initially obtaining laboratory data may enable you to change treatment methods more rapidly if initial treatment does not resolve your patient's problem
   e. None of the above statements are true

2. Which of the following laboratory tests are usually performed by a **hematology laboratory?**
   a. Antibiotic susceptibility testing
   b. Gram stain of abscess specimen
   c. Microscopic examination of a tissue specimen
   d. WBC count and differential
   e. Blood cultures

3. Which of the following laboratory tests are usually performed by a **microbiology laboratory?**
   a. Culture microorganisms from a tissue specimen
   b. Establish presence of microorganisms in a tissue specimen
   c. Gram stains
   d. Determine antibiotic susceptibility of microorganisms
   e. Erythrocyte sedimentation rate (ESR)

4. Which of the following statements is/are **true** for white blood cell count (WBC) and differential?
   a. This is the most useful hematological test for establishing the presence of infection
   b. A WBC of 8,000/mm^3 indicates an infection is not present
   c. In the differential, polymorphonuclear leukocytes may be increased and show/release immature forms (shift to the left)
   d. Lymphocytes are increased in acute bacterial infections
   e. Eosinophils are increased in acute bacterial infections

5. Which of the following statements is/are **true** for erythrocyte sedimentation rates?
   a. Is a diagnostic test for confirming the presence of infection
   b. This test involves centrifuging of a blood specimen
   c. Normal values are 0-15 mm/hr. for men and 0-20 mm/hr. for women
   d. During an infection ESR values may increase to 30-70 mm/hr.
   e. Conditions such as severe anemia, myeloma, and systemic Lupus erythematosis can also cause an increase in ESR values

6. Which of the following statements is/are **true** for blood cultures and immunological tests?
   a. Blood cultures are indicated for patients with body temperatures above 39°C
   b. A specimen used for blood cultures must be aseptically collected
   c. Tests for T-cell activity are routinely used in the diagnosis of dental infections
   d. Tests for complement activity are used routinely in diagnosis of dental infections
   e. Immunological tests are occasionally used by specialists in infectious disease when consulted by dental specialist during the management of persistent infections

7. Which of the following statements is/are **true** for the histopathologic examination of a tissue specimen?
   a. Will help distinguish between neoplastic lesions and lesions resulting from infectious microorganisms
   b. May identify microorganisms in tissue if culture techniques are unsuccessful
   c. Are especially useful in identification of **actinomyces, mycobacterium,** and fungi
   d. Tissue specimens for microscopic examination are promptly fixed in formalin
   e. Tissue specimens for culturing are **not** fixed in formalin and must be aseptically transferred to culture media

8. How should the following **hematological** data be interpreted?

   a.   b.   c.

   HEMATOLOGY LAB
   ☐ WBC count 9,000/mm³
   ☐ WBC Differential:
   Polys 65 %   Eosinophils 1 %
   Lymphocytes 25 %   Basophils 0.5 %
   Monocytes 5 %   Immature? few
   ESR   15 mm/hr
   Blood Culture negative

   HEMATOLOGY LAB
   ☐ WBC count 120,000/mm³
   ☐ WBC Differential:
   Polys 6 %   Eosinophils 1 %
   Lymphocytes 92 %   Basophils 0.5 %
   Monocytes 1 %   Immature? many
   ESR negative mm/hr
   Blood Culture negative

   HEMATOLOGY LAB
   ☐ WBC count 13,000/mm³
   ☐ WBC Differential:
   Polys 80 %   Eosinophils 1 %
   Lymphocytes 20 %   Basophils 0.5 %
   Monocytes 3 %   Immature? slight
   ESR 60 mm/hr
   Blood Culture positive

9. Which of the following **histopathological** data would indicate the presence of an infection?

   a. Dk   b. leukemia   c. yes

   HISTOPATHOLOGY LAB
   Tissue specimen analysis tissue consists of hard and soft tissue. The hard tissue consists of irregular spicules of non-vital bone surrounded by granulation tissue containing an intense acute & chronic cell infiltrate. Focal accumulations of PMN's are seen surrounding amorphous aggregates which reveal Gram (+) and Gram (-) structures.

   HISTOPATHOLOGY LAB
   Tissue specimen analysis the specimen consists of numerous PMN's surrounding islands of irregularly stained material which reveals Gram (+) filamentous forms.

   HISTOPATHOLOGY LAB
   Tissue specimen analysis tissue consists of islands, cords and strands of poorly differentiated epithelial cells in a fibrous connective tissue stroma. A mild to moderate chronic inflammatory cell infiltrate is observed.

10. Which of the following statements is/are **true** regarding the value of microbiological data to the diagnosis and treatment of oral and/or maxillofacial infections?
    a. Can verify the presence of microorganism(s) in a swelling
    b. Can identify specific microorganisms involved in an infection
    c. Can establish relative numbers and dominant species of microorganisms involved in an infection
    d. Can provide guidance for antibiotic selection
    e. Can aid in confirming the resolution of an infection

11. The flora of the oral cavity is:
    a. Unique to this location
    b. Composed of resident and transient flora
    c. Divided into 3 recognized eco-nitches including buccal mucosa, tongue, and area around the teeth
    d. Composed of both aerobic and anaerobic species
    e. Influenced by the level of oral hygiene

12. Which of the following statements is/are **true**?
    a. Some oral infections are caused by a single species of aerobic microorganisms
    b. Many oral infections are caused by multiple microbial species, some of which may be aerobic and others anaerobic
    c. Single species infections are the result of the balance of effects of the microorganism upon the host and the effects of host defenses on the single species
    d. Mixed infections are the result of the interactions between the species involved as well as the overall effect of the various species on host defense system and the effect of host defenses on each of the various species involved
    e. With mixed infections, an antibiotic may kill the dominant organism but allow a less-dominant organism which is not susceptible to the antibiotic to become dominant

13. The Gram stain is
    a. A simple staining technique used to show presence of microorganisms
    b. A differential staining technique used to separate and identify microorganisms by their reaction to this staining technique and by the shape of the organism
    c. A valuable aid to the selection of an appropriate antibiotic
    d. A valuable technique for obtaining information about microorganisms even if culturing is unsuccessful
    e. Used to verify that future culturing data contains the same microbial groupings that are present in the initial stain

14. Which of the following statements are **true** for infections involving anaerobic microorganisms?
    a. About 75 to 90% of all oral infections involve anaerobes (either alone or in combination with aerobes)
    b. Collecting a specimen for anaerobic culturing can be more difficult
    c. The time required to grow some anaerobic microorganisms in the laboratory is longer than for most aerobic species
    d. Failure to use an anaerobic technique for collecting a specimen from an oral infection can compromise the value of laboratory studies
    e. Drainage of anaerobic infections can increase the oxygen levels (remove anaerobic environment) and thus lead to the death of anaerobes

15. Describe the relationship between oral hygiene and the qualitative and quantitative presence of anaerobic oral flora around the teeth, _____
    _____ ↑ oral hygiene   ↓ oral flora _____
    _____
    _____

16. Name two (2) ways by which a microorganism previously susceptible to an antibiotic can acquire antibiotic resistance.
    a. _____ natural mutation _____
    b. _____ acquired mutation _____

17. Define the following terms as applied to the effects of antibiotics on microbial cells.
    a. Bacteriocidal: ___Kills___

    b. Bacteriostatic: ___maintains levels___

18. Explain why antibiotic susceptibility tests performed in the laboratory are not necessarily directly transferrable to patient treatment. ___host factors___
    ___— excretion, filtration or alteration___
    ___affect conc.___

19. Describe the practical approach to species identification that should be used by the microbiological laboratory to best serve the clinician in the management of oral infections. ___Gram stain, antibody susceptibility___
    ___and anaerobic culture___

20. For each of the following clinical situations, indicate the need for culturing by matching the numbers to the right with each of the lettered statements:
    a. __2__ Infection is small and confined to alveolar ridge
    b. __1__ Infection has spread to the fascial planes of the head or neck (and fluctuance is present)
    c. __1__ Patient shows signs of systemic toxicity
    d. __2__ Infection (pericoronitis) is contaminated with oral flora
    e. __2__ Infection has established drainage through the alveolar ridge and no vestibular or fascial spaces are involved
    f. __1__ Patient has serious medical compromises affecting his host resistance factors

    1. Culture essential
    2. Initial culture is **not** essential

21. Name the seven (7) general principles for collecting a specimen for microbiological examination:
    a. ___avoid contamination___
    b. ___representative sample___
    c. ___transfer to lab quickly___
    d. ___keep in anaerobic condition___
    e. ___transfer by correct means___
    f. ___collect prior to antibody tx___
    g. ___obtain adequate sample___

22. A common problem associated with the culturing process is failure to obtain a culture specimen. Name two (2) reasons for this and describe what you could do to overcome each problem.

    Problem
    a. ___not in great enough #___
    b. ___incorrect need position___

    Solutions
    1. ___wait___
    2. ___inject & withdraw saline solution___
    3. ___verify fluctuance___
    4. ___reassess site___

23. Another problem in culturing is that the lab is unable to grow any microorganisms. What could be the problems and how can they be overcome?

Problem

a. _not collected anaerobically_
b. _not transport anaerobually_
c. _lab failure_

Solutions

1. _use anaerobic methods_
2. _"   "   collections_
3. _transport rapidly_
4. _✓ lab_

24. Another problem in culturing is that the lab reports normal oral flora. What could be the problems and how can they be overcome?

Problem

a. _contaminated_
b. _lab didn't i.d. correctly_

Solutions

1. _review collection_
2. _remember mixed flora_
3. _discuss with lab_

25. For the following fascial spaces, name the space and state the route for specimen collection using the following numbered categories: **1** = intraoral, easily performed. **2** = intraoral, more difficult. **3** = extraoral, generally referral

Space — Route and difficulty

a. Space #8 ___3___ ___1___
b. Space #5 ___1___ ___1___
c. Space #6 ___2___ ___2___
d. Space #4 ___3___ ___3___
e. Space #12 ___3___ ___3___
f. Space #14 ___2___ ___2___
g. Space #13 ___1___ ___2___
h. Space #9 ___2___ ___2___

26. Name three (3) intraoral methods for collecting a specimen for microbiological examination.

a. _aspiration_
b. _infected tooth_
c. _biopsy_

27. Describe the process for intraoral transmucosal aspiration:

Pain control: _____

Isolation of aspiration site: _____

Site preparation: _Betadine_ _____

Collection of specimen: _____

Use of transport medium: _____

Transport to lab: _____

28. Explain why use of cotton swabs is generally considered an unacceptable method for collecting a specimen for microbiological culturing. _contamination_
   and not anaerobic

29. Name two (2) extraoral methods used to collect a specimen for microbiological laboratory culturing.
   a. _aspiration_
   b. _biopsy_

30. Given the following description of an oral and maxillofacial infection, determine the need for microbiological analysis of a specimen and describe the method and route of specimen collection:

   Chief Complaint: A 56-year-old male presents to your office with pain and swelling of the right buccal space and infraorbital area.

   History of Chief Complaint:
   His problem began 3 days ago with a severe toothache in the area of his maxillary right second premolar. The toothache subsided and was replaced by facial swelling. He received no previous treatment for this condition and no factors were present which either improved or exacerbated this condition. There was no history of local trauma. He had been advised by another dentist (six months previously) of caries in both his maxillary and mandibular teeth, however he could not remember which teeth were involved.

   Past Medical Factors:
   A review of past medical factors revealed that the patient has mild diabetes controlled by diet. His nutritional status is currently adequate, as are his psychological and family and social factors.

   Clinical Examination:
   Clinical examination showed no serious general signs. Vital signs: Temp. = 100.4°F, BP = 165/85/83, Pulse 78 and regular, Resp. Rate = 17.

   Extraoral Examination:
   Extraoral examination reveals tender and enlarged right buccal and submandibular lymph nodes and swelling confined to the buccal space and infraorbital area. No involvement of the periorbital area is currently present.

   Intraoral Examination:
   Intraoral examination reveals a slight fluctuant swelling of the maxillary right buccal vestibule adjacent to the right second premolar. A large carious lesion is seen in the maxillary right second premolar.

   Radiographic Examination:
   A periapical radiograph reveals caries extending into the pulp chamber of the maxillary right second premolar and disruption of the lamina dura at the apex of this tooth.

   a. Need for culturing __×__Yes ____No
   b. Description of method and route: _____
      _____ extra oral aspiration into buccal space _____
      _____
      _____
      _____
      _____
      _____

31. *A 24-year-old female presents with an acute swelling at the base of her upper lip. She has recently had root canal therapy in her maxillary central incisor. You believed the infection to be dentally related and treated it with penicillin. Four days later, the infection was not improved. At this time you received the following laboratory information. Summarize the data in the* summary of laboratory data *section of the checklist and evaluate the data in comparison with your initial diagnosis and treatment.*

Histopathology Report: None requested.

Hematology Report:
WBC = 16,450/mm³
Neutrophils = 85% (80% segs, 5% stabs)
Lymphocytes = 14%
Eosinophils = 1%

Microbiology Report:

Source of Specimen:									Date and Time Received:							

Collected: Date_____ Time_____ a.m./p.m.   Ordered by:_____
Specimen Description: _____

Gram Stain:_____WBC_____Epithel. Cells   Comments:
++++ _____Gram Positive Cocci
++ _____Gram Positive Rods
++ _____Gram Negative Cocci
++++ _____Gram Negative Rods

Colony Count (Colonies/ml.)   ZN Stain:

	Penicillin G	Ampicillin	Methicillin	Cephalothin	Tetracycline	Chloramphenicol	Erythromycin	Streptomycin	Kanamycin	Polymyxin	Thiosulphil	Nitrofurantoin	Clindamycin	Gentamicin	Carbenicillin	
Staphylococci Coag+	R	R	S	S	T	S	S									
Klebsiella	R	R	R	S	S	S	R									

Code: ++++ — Profuse   ++ — Scanty   S — Sensitive   R — Resistant   Patient's Name:
      +++ — Moderate   + — Very Scanty   I — Intermediate Sensitivity   Date Reported:

Summary of Laboratory Data

MICROBIOLOGY LAB
☐ Single species ☑ Mixed ☐ None
Predominant species: _____
Staph
Kleb
☐ Aerobic ☐ Anaerobic
Antibiotic Sensitivity:
  1st choice_cephalothin_
  2nd choice_chloramphenicol_
  3rd choice_____

HEMATOLOGY LAB
☐ WBC count _16,450_
☐ WBC Differential:
Polys _85_% Eosinophils _1_%
Lymphocytes_14_% Basophils ____%
Monocytes ____% Immature? ____
ESR_____mm/hr
Blood Culture _____
_____
_____

HISTOPATHOLOGY LAB
Tissue specimen analysis _____
_____
_____
_____
_____
_____

Analysis: _infection gone cephalothin_
_____
_____
_____
_____
_____
_____
_____
_____

ANSWERS TO POST-TEST

1. *d*

2. *d, e*

3. *a, c, d*

4. *a, c*

5. *a, c, d, e*

6. *a, b, e*

7. *a, b, c, d, e*

8. a. *Normal hematologic profile.*
   b. *Not representative of an infection process but is very typical of acute lymphocytic leukemia.*
   c. *Typical hematologic profile of an acute infective process.*

9. a. *Osteomyelitis with mixed bacterial infections*
   b. *Actinomycosis*
   c. *Malignancy (carcinoma)*

10. *a, b, c, d, e*

11. *a, b, c, d, e*

12. *a, b, c, d, e*

13. *b, c, d, e*

14. *a, b, c, d, e*

15. *A person who practices good oral hygiene in the area of the teeth will have little accumulation of dental plaque both supragingivally and subgingivally. As the level of hygiene decreases, plaque levels increase and an anaerobic environment increases. Inflammation of gingival tissue is also associated with plaque accumulation. In deep gingival pockets oxygen demand exceeds availability, thus increasing anaerobic conditions and favoring proliferation of anaerobic species previously supressed. Thus, an increase in total cell numbers and an increase in anaerobic species present is associated with poor oral hygiene levels.*

16. a. *Spontaneous mutation*
    b. *Acquisition of a plasmid containing genetic material coding for antibiotic resistance*

17. a. *Bacteriocidal — antibiotic leads to the death of the cell, or renders the cell incapable of reproduction*
    b. *Bacteriostatic — Temporarily prevents cell from multiplying but is reversible once antibiotic is removed*

18. *Laboratory tests deal with known concentrations of antibiotics but a patient's absorption and rates of clearance (excretion, filtration, or alteration) affect the blood levels. In addition, one has little control over the actual concentration at an abscess site because circulation through fibrous encapsulation is variable, as are the effects of pus on the antibiotic.*

19. *The microbiology lab can be of great assistance to the clinician by providing immediate Gram stain results, a preliminary report on predominant species within 24-48 hours (both aerobes and anaerobes), a report of antibiotic sensitivity for predominant species within 4 days, and continuing to incubate anaerobic cultures for 7-10 days to detect presence of slow-growing anaerobes.*

20.   a. *2.*   b. *1.*   c. *2.*   d. *1.*   e. *2.*   f. *1.*

21. a. Specimen should be representative of the infective process
    b. Avoid contamination with oral flora
    c. Collect specimen under conditions that will preserve anaerobes
    d. Obtain sufficient material for adequate examination
    e. Collect specimen prior to beginning antibiotic therapy
    f. Use proper containers and/or transport media
    g. Transport specimen promptly to the lab

22. a. Premature attempt to culture

    b. Incorrect needle placement

    1. Inject sterile saline and withdraw into syringe
    2. Verify presence of fluctuance
    3. Reassess aspiration site
    4. Wait for fluctuance to develop

23. a. Failure to preserve anaerobes during collection
    b. Failure to transport anaerobically
    c. Failure of lab to correctly manage specimen

    1. Use anaerobic collection methods
    2. Use anaerobic transport media
    3. Transport specimen more rapidly to lab
    4. Contact lab to discuss their anaerobic techniques

24. a. Specimen contaminated with saliva

    1. Review collection technique and collect new specimen free from oral flora
    2. Remember that most infections are from mixed oral flora

    b. Lab did not perform detailed identification

    1. Inform lab to be more specific as to dominant species and do antibiotic suceptibility tests on those microorganisms

25. a. Buccal space — 1-intraoral, easy access
    b. Sublingual space — 1-intraoral, easy access
    c. Submandibular space — 2-intraoral more difficult (or 3-extraoral, more difficult)
    d. Submental space — 3-extraoral, more difficult
    e. Parotid space — 3-extraoral, more difficult
    f. Parapharyngeal space — 2-intraoral, more difficult
    g. Pterygomandibular space — 2-intraoral, more difficult
    h. Submasseteric space — 2-intraoral, more difficult

26. a. Collect from infected tooth
    b. Transmucosal aspiration
    c. Tissue biopsy for culturing

27. See page 151.

28. Use of cotton swabs will lead to the death of anaerobes.

29. a. Transcutaneous aspiration
    b. Extraoral tissue biopsy

30. a. **Need for culturing:** Yes
    This infection involves multiple anatomic spaces (buccal vestibule, buccal space and infraorbital space). The history of diet-controlled diabetes indicates that the patient could become seriously compromised if adequate diet cannot be maintained because phagocytic leucocyte activity may be reduced. Antibiotic susceptibility data should be available as soon as possible if the infection does not improve following initial treatment. This patient should be closely monitored or promptly referred to a specialist.

b. **Description of method and route:** *Intraoral transmucosal aspiration of a specimen of pus should be performed by inserting the needle into the margin of the vestibular swelling and also into the infraorbital area. Anaerobically seal the needle by inserting it into a sterile rubber stopper and transport syringe to the lab within 10-15 minutes.*

31. *You should have summarized the laboratory data as follows:*

Summary of Laboratory Data

MICROBIOLOGY LAB	HEMATOLOGY LAB	HISTOPATHOLOGY LAB
☐ Single species ☒ Mixed ☐ None	☐ WBC count *16,450/mm³*	Tissue specimen analysis _____
Predominant species: _____	☐ WBC Differential:	
Staphylococci Coag⁺	Polys *85* % Eosinophils *1* %	*none*
Klebsiella	Lymphocytes *14* % Basophils ___%	
☐ Aerobic ☐ Anaerobic	Monocytes ___% Immature? *5%*	
Antibiotic Sensitivity:	ESR *not done* mm/hr	
1st choice *cephalothin*	Blood Culture *not done*	
2nd choice *chloramphenicol*		
3rd choice _____		

Analysis: *The hematology report suggests the presence of an infection due to elevated WBC count and the presence of stabs (immature polys) (or shift to the left). The microbiology report establishes presence of a* **mixed** *infection with* **coagulase (+) staphylococci** *and* **klebsiella** *as the dominant microorganisms. Both of these organisms are resistant to penicillin, thus an alternative antibiotic is now indicated. In addition, four (4) morphological types were seen in Gram stain and only two species were recovered in culture. In all probability, anaerobic species were lost in the lab since both organisms identified are aerobic (see pages 142-143). You should contact your microbiological laboratory and discuss their methods for managing specimens from oral infections.*

DIAGNOSIS

The next two units of this book focus on the process of diagnosing the causes of oral and/or maxillofacial infections. **Diagnosis is an intermediate process which links data collection with treatment** as shown in the flow diagram below.

MANAGEMENT SYSTEM FOR ORAL AND MAXILLOFACIAL SWELLINGS

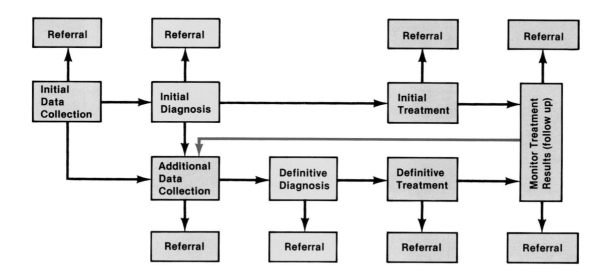

Unit VI — Review of Oral and/or Maxillofacial Infections — This unit reviews many of the diseases causing swellings of the oral and/or maxillofacial area. The pathogenesis and typical signs and symptoms are reviewed to enable you to make the diagnostic decisions discussed in the next unit.

Unit VII — Diagnostic Decisions — This unit presents a system for establishing a diagnosis of the cause of swellings and describing the overall seriousness of the problem.

The diagnostic process relies upon your careful collection of signs and symptoms (data) and your knowledge of pathological conditions which can produce these signs and symptoms.

Some patients may present to a dentist with oral infections so advanced that even the best of care cannot reverse their condition, and other patients may not respond to appropriate management. However, death from infections may result from inadequate initial diagnosis, inadequate initial treatment, delays in appropriate treatment, and/or delays in timely referral.

Serious delays in treating non-infectious swellings or non-odontogenic infections frequently result from a general dentist's erroneous assumption that the problem is an odontogenic infection.

UNIT VI
CAUSES OF ORAL AND/OR MAXILLOFACIAL SWELLINGS

OVERVIEW AND OBJECTIVES

The purpose of this unit is to review many of the causes of oral and/or maxillofacial infections. Since all oral and/or maxillofacial swellings are not the result of microbial infection, we will also briefly summarize the signs and symptoms of non-microbial swellings to assist you in diagnostic decisions (discussed in the next unit). Routes of microbial invasion and routes of infection spread are discussed as are the general characteristics of infections involving the **soft tissues**, **periosteum**, and **hard tissues** of the head and neck region. Dentally related infections (odontogenic and those that can result as a consequence of dental treatment) are distinguished from infections not of dental origin (non-odontogenic infections). We have also included a category of **infections of special significance** to stress the early diagnosis and referral of these problems. Following completion of this unit you will:

1. List four (4) general causes for oral and/or maxillofacial swellings of **non-microbial** origin and name an example in each category.
2. Given a list of signs and symptoms associated with an oral and/or maxillofacial swelling, identify those that are associated with **non-microbial** etiologies.
3. Descrive five (5) **routes of microbial invasion** by which microorganisms can gain entry into the tissues of the oral and/or maxillofacial area and name one example of an infection which begins by each route.
4. Describe the sequence of events which generally take place when microorganisms gain entry into soft tissues. This discussion should include a description of:
   a. **cellulitis**
   b. **stage of infiltration**
   c. **abscess formation**
   d. **fistula**
5. Describe how microorganisms can gain entry into the potential space between the periosteum and cortical bone.
6. Describe the reaction of periosteum to inflammation.
7. Compare and contrast the terms **periostitis** and **subperiosteal abscess**.
8. Compare and contrast the terms **osteitis** and **osteomyelitis**.
9. Define the following terms:
   a. **odontogenic infection**
   b. **non-odontogenic infection**
   c. **dentally related non-odontogenic infection**
10. Name five (5) dentally related **soft tissue infections** and identify which of these are **odontogenic** and which are **non-odontogenic**.
11. Name three (3) infections involving **periosteum**.
12. Name four (4) infections involving **hard tissues**.
13. Name four (4) infections which we have classified as **infections of special significance**.
14. Name six (6) infections of **non-dental origin** which could involve the tissues of the oral and maxillofacial area.
15. Define the term **periodontal abscess** and describe its pathogenesis, signs and symptoms, and radiographic appearance.
16. Define the terms **chronic and acute pericoronitis** (pericoronal abscess) and describe the pathogenesis, signs and symptoms, and radiographic appearance.
17. Define the terms **chronic and acute periapical alveolar abscess** and describe the pathogenesis, signs and symptoms, and radiographic appearance.
18. Name four (4) types of post-surgical infections and describe how these infections are produced.

19. Name three (3) forms of **post-injection infections** and describe how these infections develop.
20. Given any clinical example of a dentally related **soft tissue infection**, a review of historical data, clinical data, and radiographic data, identify the symptom complex name for the problem.
21. Given relevant patient data describing **non-dental soft tissue infections**, distinguish these infections from dentally related infections and identify the specific etiology for the non-dental soft tissue infection.
22. Given relevant patient data describing an **infection of periosteum**, classify the type of infection and describe its pathogenesis.
23. Given relevant patient data describing an infection of **hard tissue** classify the type of infection and describe its pathogenesis.
24. Describe the basis for classifying the following as infections of special significance:
    a. **acute cellulitis**
    b. **Ludwig's angina**
    c. **cavernous sinus thrombosis**
    d. **osteoradionecrosis**
25. Given relevant patient data describing any of the **infections of special significance**, identify the type of infection and describe the pathogenesis and potential consequences of the infection.

UNIT VI
REVIEW OF ORAL & MAXILLOFACIAL INFECTIONS

Introduction
Swellings of Non-Microbial Origin
Routes of Microbial Invasion
Spread of Oral Infections
Tissue Involvement
  Soft tissue infections
  Infections of periosteum
  Infections of hard tissue
Classification by Origin
Oral and/or Maxillofacial Infections
  Dentally Related Soft Tissue Infections
    Periodontal abscess
    Pericoronitis
    Periapical abscess
    Post-surgical infections
    Maxillary sinusitis
  Non-Dental Soft Tissue Infections
    Peritonsillar infections

Salivary gland infections
Superficial skin infections
Ear infections
Infections of Periosteum
  Post-surgical subperiosteal abscess
  Post-injection
  Periostitis
Infections of Hard Tissue
  Acute alveolar osteitis
  Osteomyelitis
  Osteitis
  Osteoradionecrosis
Infections of Special Significance
  Acute cellulitis
  Ludwig's angina
  Osteoradionecrosis
  Cavernous sinus thrombosis

INTRODUCTION

The purpose of this unit is to review various clinical conditions (sign and symptom complexes) which result from microbial invasion (infection) of oral and/or maxillofacial structures.

These sign and symptom complexes have received common names (such as pericoronitis, pyogenic osteomyelitis, etc.) which facilitate diagnosis and assist you in determining appropriate treatment methods. While primarily focusing on conditions (infections) arising from teeth or tooth-related structures (odontogenic infections) we will also discuss infections arising from other structures of the oral and maxillofacial area (non-odontogenic infections) since these conditions can be confused with odontogenic infections if your data collection is insufficient or your diagnosis is made in haste. Since swellings (a common sign of infection) of the oral and maxillofacial area can also be of non-microbial origin, we will briefly dicuss non-microbial causes of swellings.

NOTE: **When diagnosing the cause of any oral and/or maxillofacial swelling you must not prematurely assume a microbial origin (infection) nor prematurely assume an infection to be of dental (odontogenic) origin.**

SWELLINGS OF NON-MICROBIAL ORIGIN

Non-microbial causes of oral and/or maxillofacial swellings include:

- Facial or tissue trauma (such as hematomas and post-surgical edema)
- Growth of neoplastic tissues (benign or malignant)
- Developmental abnormalities (such as cysts)
- Immunological disorders (such as angioneurotic edema)

A complete discussion of swellings of non-microbial origin is beyond the scope of this book; however, a summary of the various signs and symptoms of non-microbial swellings is provided here to assist you in distinguishing these problems from those of microbial origin. (See **Table VI-1**.)

SUMMARY OF SIGNS AND SYMPTOMS
FOR SWELLINGS OF NON-MICROBIAL ORIGIN

TRAUMA
- Recent trauma
- Bruising, ecchymosis, hematoma
- Swelling tender to palpation
- Fractured teeth, bone
- Active bleeding
- Malocclusion
- Absence of transmitted mobility
- Loss of function of mandible
- Paresthesia
- Shock
- Little change in vital signs

NEOPLASTIC SWELLINGS
- Slower growing
- Absence of inflammation (unless secondary infection)
- Hard, firm, indurated
- Minimal edema
- Normal vital signs
- Paresthesia (intrabony)
- Ulcers or open lesions with minimal inflammation
- Non-tender enlarged lymph nodes (may have slight tenderness)

DEVELOPMENTAL SWELLINGS
- Congenital abnormalities
- Process associated with growth & maturation
- No signs of inflammation
- No changes in vital signs

IMMUNOLOGICAL DISORDERS
- Allergic related angioedema
- Usually no changes in vital signs except tachycardia with allergic reactions

Table VI-1. Summary of the signs and symptoms associated with non-infectious swellings. You should notice that the classical signs of inflammation are generally lacking from this list.

ROUTES OF MICROBIAL INVASION

Most species of microorganisms comprising the oral flora, whether resident or transient, are capable of causing infections and developing into abscesses if provided access to underlying tissues. The various routes by which microorganisms can gain entry to oral tissues include:

- **Isolation of microorganisms in an enclosed space or pouch** — Abscess formation can occur from the entrapment of microorganisms in a closed space or pouch. Typical examples of infections which are caused by this process include **periodontal abscesses** and **pericoronal abscesses.**

- **Progressive tooth decay with invasion of the dental pulp** — Progressive tooth decay can result in exposure of the dental pulp to oral flora. Many species of microorganisms can then invade pulp tissue, spread to periapical areas causing **periapical abscesses** and then spread into surrounding soft tissue or bone.

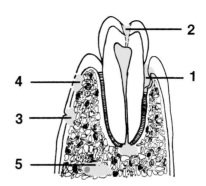

Figure VI-1. Routes of microbial invasion into oral and maxillofacial tissues: 1) isolation of microbes in an enclosed pouch, 2) progressive tooth decay with invasion of dental pulp, 3) introduction of host flora into deeper tissues, 4) breakdown of host tissues, 5) hematogenous spread from another site of infection.

- **Introduction of host flora into deeper tissues by trauma** — Injury to oral soft tissue is a common cause of oral infections. Although these infections are not considered odontogenic in origin, they can frequently result from trauma associated with dental procedures. Typical examples include: **wounds, needle-track infections,** and **post-surgical infections** resulting from the entrapment of contaminated surgical debris under surgical flaps.

- **Breakdown of host tissues** — Certain disease processes such as **diabetes, long-term starvation, vitamin deficiencies** and **radiation therapy** of the head and neck can cause oral mucosa to lose its normal ability to restrict the entry of oral microorganisms. While infections resulting from these disease processes are not considered odontogenic in origin, they can be initiated by dental procedures. An example of this route of infection is seen in post-extraction osteoradionecrosis.

- **Hematogenous spread from another site of infection** — This mode of spread is relatively rare; however, it does occur and should be differentiated from an odontogenic infection. Tuberculosis of the jaws could be an example of hematogenous spread from another site of infection.

SPREAD OF ORAL AND/OR MAXILLOFACIAL INFECTIONS

Any infection, regardless of its initial cause, has the potential for spread to adjacent areas or tissues. The diagram to the right illustrates the spread of infection to oral tissues and/or maxillofacial tissues from **external sources** (skin and oral cavity), the **bloodstream** (red) and from **adjacent tissues** (soft tissues, periosteum, hard tissues). Ultimately your diagnosis will include a statement of involved tissues and your treatment methods will be directed toward relieving the problems associated with each tissue. Errors in diagnosis and treatment can be minimized by reviewing the relationships as diagramed. Remember — oral and/or maxillofacial infections can result from non-dental as well as dental origins.

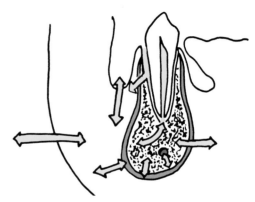

Figure VI-2. Summary of the spread of oral and/or maxillofacial infections.

TISSUE INVOLVEMENT

The body's primary reaction to microbial infection is **initiation of the inflammatory response**. This response produces different clinical signs and symptoms in various tissues and treatment methods will also vary with the tissues involved. Thus a brief review of specific tissue reactions to microbial infection should assist you in understanding the pathobiology of the individual infections discussed in this unit and assist you in diagnosing and treating these problems.

- **Soft Tissue Infections**

  Soft tissue infections of the oral and maxillofacial area present with a similar clinical pattern, regardless of their origin. A review of the course of soft tissue infections can be helpful.

  The term **cellulitis** is used to describe an early phase of infection and indicates an infection of a spreading nature. **The term cellulitis implies a diffuse inflammation of soft tissue which is not circumscribed or confined to one area, and which is free to spread through the tissue spaces along the fascial planes.** Cellulitis is characterized by leucocytic infiltration, capillary dilation, and rapidly multiplying bacteria. This process is believed to result from the production of hyaluronidase and fibrinolysins by the microorganisms (such as beta hemolytic streptococci) and causes a breakdown of the connective tissue. **The clinical manifestations of cellulitis are pain, tenderness, redness (erythema) and diffuse edema.**

  As the body defenses are mobilized to combat the infection, a cellulitis progresses into the **stage of infiltration.** An **infiltrate** is a firm, brawny, painful swelling of the involved soft tissue. If superficial tissues are involved the skin becomes inflamed (occasionally to the extent of becoming purple). If the infection spreads along deeper tissue planes, the overlying skin may remain of normal color. In this stage of the infection, suppuration (pus) is histologically present, but is not localized to a specific area.

  With further infiltration of polymorphonuclear leukocytes and lymphocytes an **abscess** develops. In this stage the infection is localized and contains suppuration (pus) which can accumulate in large quantities and through increased pressure extend the infection into adjacent tissues along fascial planes or (by direct extension) through muscle, skin, or mucosa.

  Once a localized abscess establishes a **fistula** (opening) in skin or mucosa, drainage of the infection can occur and the risk of tissue extension diminishes.

- **Infections of Periosteum**

Periosteal infections can result from **extension of infections** from either soft tissue or bone, or can result from **direct infection** from needle tracks or entrapment of post-surgical debris under full-thickness flaps. The term **periostitis refers to inflammation of the periosteum** while the term **periosteal abscess describes accumulation of suppuration** (pus) between the periosteum and cortical bone.

The periosteum is histologically composed of an outer layer of **fibrous tissue** and inner layers of **preosteoblasts** and **osteoblasts**. It has a good blood supply from the surrounding soft tissue which also branches into cortical bone. Periosteum is attached to bone via Sharpey's fibers. This attachment is relatively loose in young people but becomes more firm in adults. Periosteum can be detached from bone by: **mechanical** (surgery or trauma) **means**; by the **accumulation of inflammatory exudate or suppuration** between the periosteum and cortical bone; or by the expansion of bone from a **neoplastic process**. Once detached, the periosteum responds by increased osteoblastic activity and new bone is formed adjacent to the periosteum. Bone formation must proceed for several days to weeks to form sufficient amounts to be radiographically visible. When new bone is radiographically visible it appears as a thin layer (egg shell) of bone distinct from cortical bone. Since formation of new bone is the standard biological reaction of periosteum when it **lacks underlying cortical bone**, you should carefully evaluate the underlying cause of this reaction. **Do not prematurely assume the cause to be inflammatory.**

Chronic inflammation of the periosteum often produces layers of bone deposition which appear in an "onion-skin" or layered pattern. If a chronic subperiosteal infection is allowed to progress, an **osteitis** and even **osteomyelitis** of underlying bone may result. Following elimination of the cause of inflammation, this new bone will resorb and normal bony architecture will be re-established.

Acute infections of periosteum can also produce detachment of the periosteum from the buildup of suppuration. Frequently, however, proteolytic enzymes from bacteria or suppuration will erode the periosteum, allowing drainage into soft tissue before new bone formation occurs. Acute subperiosteal infections may also erode into underlying bone causing osteitis and osteomyelitis.

Inflammation and/or infection of the periosteum most frequently occurs on the buccal, lingual, and inferior border of the mandible. Thus, periapical radiographs will usually not show new bone formation. **Occlusal radiographs** will show bone formation on buccal and lingual sides and other **additional radiographs** are necessary to show bone formation in other areas of the mandible (see **Unit IV — Radiographic Data**).

- **Infections of Hard tissues**

Infections involving trabecular (medullary) and/or cortical bone are considered infections of hard tissue.

The term **osteitis** refers to the inflammation of bone and is somewhat analogous to cellulitis. In osteitis, microorganisms are present in the bone and an inflammatory response is established; however, edema and/or pus accumulation does not result in bone destruction. An **osteitis** may result from a **periapical abscess** which passes through hard tissue and periosteum into soft tissue, from **inflammation of exposed bone** following tooth extraction (acute alveolar osteitis and fibrinolytic alveolar osteitis [or dry socket]), or from a chronic, low-grade, microbial irritation of trabecular bone. **Chronic osteitis** may result in bone resorption, however this slow process does not result in sequestrum formation. Elimination of the cause of osteitis usually results in remineralization of bone, which often appears more dense than surrounding bone. Osteitis may progress to osteomyelitis if an exaggerated inflammatory response results.

The term **osteomyelitis** is a clinical term used to describe inflammation of bone resulting in the death of bone tissue with subsequent demineralization and formation of **sequestra**. Regardless of the source of inflammation (microbial, chemical, or physical) the resulting edema and/or pus accumulation in the Haversian network produces localized areas of ischemia and death of bone tissue. In this book we will confine our discussion to **pyogenic osteomyelitis** (caused by pus-producing microorganisms, usually bacteria), **actinomycotic osteomyelitis** (caused by Actinomyces species) and **osteoradionecrosis** (occurring following radiation therapy).

Osteoradionecrosis is a special condition in which **previously irradiated bone** has become more susceptible to death and degeneration from microbial invasion or other causes of inflammation (e.g. surgery).

CLASSIFICATION OF INFECTIONS BY ORIGIN

The origin of oral and/or maxillofacial infections can be categorized into the following **two** general groups:

Odontogenic infections are those infections arising from microbial invasion of teeth or tooth-related structures which have spread to involve adjacent tissues and/or the bloodstream. Odontogenic infections commonly result from microbial growth in the **dental pulp, periodontal sulcus** and/or the **pericoronal sulcus.**

Non-odontogenic infections are infections arising in or from the oral and maxillofacial area which are **not** related to the teeth or tooth-related structures. Non-odontogenic maxillofacial infections can be associated with infections of **skin, mucous membranes, ear, sinuses, salivary glands,** and **tonsils**. These infections may result from:
- **Microbial invasion of skin, mucous membranes, salivary glands, tonsils, ears, etc.**
- **Infection of injuries to oral and/or maxillofacial structures**
- **Secondary infection of cancer sites**
- **Diseases transmitted to susceptible hosts**
- **Oral manifestations of systemic diseases**

Many non-odontogenic infections (**post-surgical, post-injection, superficial skin, ear,** etc.) are discussed in this book because they often produce clinical signs and symptoms similar to odontogenic infections.

For the purposes of this book, we will consider **infections resulting from dental treatment** under the category of **dentally related infections**. While these infections are by definition **non-odontogenic** (since they do not arise from teeth or tooth-related structures), they may develop as a consequence of treating **odontogenic** problems.

NOTE: In many instances you will be able to identify the original route of entry for an oral and/or maxillofacial infection while in others you will not. Determining the route of entry can be of help in both diagnosing and treating the problem and avoiding unnecessary or ineffective treatment.

STUDY EXERCISES

1. The term non-infectious swelling refers to a swelling which develops from non microbial causes *such as* facial trauma   neoplasms   development immune disorders *while infectious swellings result from* bacteria *.*

2. Name or describe five (5) routes by which oral flora can invade oral structures:
   a. enclosed space   c. blood   e. trauma
   b. tooth decay   d. host breakdown

3. When an infection becomes localized and accumulates suppuration it is called a/an _____*Abcess*_____ .

_____*cellulitis*_____ is the term used for an early stage of infection characterized by diffuse inflammation.

A firm, brawny swelling of soft tissue is termed _____*infiltrate*_____ .

4. Define the following terms:
   a. Cellulitis: *diffuse inflammation of soft tissue*
   b. Stage of infiltration: *body mobilizes to fight infection*
   c. Abscess: *infection localizes & contains pus*
   d. Fistula: *opening in skin or mucosa*
   e. Periostitis: *inflammation of periodontium*
   f. Subperiosteal abscess: *abcess under the periosteum*
   g. Osteitis: *inflammation of bone*
   h. Osteomyelitis: *reaction of bone to inflammation — demineralization*
   i. Osteoradionecrosis: *necrosis of bone after radiation tx*
   j. Odontogenic infection: *infection due to teeth*
   k. Non-odontogenic infection: *not due to teeth*

ORAL AND/OR MAXILLOFACIAL INFECTIONS

In the following section of this unit we will discuss several oral and/or maxillofacial infections (sign and symptom complexes) which have been named (somewhat inconsistently) by origin (e.g. dentoalveolar abscess), area of involvement (e.g. pericoronitis), location (e.g. subperiosteal abscess), or pathologic process (e.g. acute cellulitis).

While we have divided these infections into categories of **soft tissue, periosteal,** and **hard tissue**, you should remember that the use of these common names **may not** adequately describe the origin, severity, areas of tissue involvement or pathologic processes involved.

We have also developed a category for **infections of special significance** to emphasize the **extreme seriousness** of these problems. Management of these infections usually requires the assistance of physicians or oral and maxillofacial surgeons in a hospital facility. **All** of these infections can result from a variety of primary sources and **early diagnosis** and **prompt management** are essential.

The following infections will be discussed:

Soft Tissue (dentally related)
- ☐ Periodontal Abscess
- ☐ Pericoronal Abscess
- ☐ Dento-Alveolar Abscess
- ☐ Post-surgical Infection
- ☐ Post-injection Infection
- ☐ Maxillary Sinusitis
- ☐ Other _____
- _____

Periosteum
- ☐ Subperiosteal abscess
- ☐ Post-Injection
- ☐ Periostitis

Hard Tissue
- ☐ Acute alveolar osteitis (dry socket)
- ☐ Osteitis
- ☐ Osteomyelitis
- ☐ Osteoradionecrosis

Special sigificance
- ☐ Acute cellulitis
- ☐ Ludwig's angina
- ☐ Osteo-radionecrosis
- ☐ Cavernous sinus thrombosis

Soft tissue (non-dental)
- ☐ Maxillary sinusitis
- ☐ Peritonsillar abscess
- ☐ Salivary gland infection
- ☐ Ear infection
- ☐ Superficial skin infection
- ☐ Superficial mucosal infection
- ☐ Other _____

DENTALLY RELATED SOFT TISSUE INFECTIONS

Dentally related soft tissue infections which are **odontogenic** in origin or which can **result from dental treatment** are summarized to the right. We will briefly review the definition, pathogenesis, signs and symptoms, and radiographic appearance of these infections.

Soft Tissue (dentally related)
- ☐ Periodontal Abscess
- ☐ Pericoronal Abscess
- ☐ Dento-Alveolar Abscess
- ☐ Post-surgical Infection
- ☐ Post-injection Infection
- ☐ Maxillary Sinusitis
- ☐ Other _____

☐ Periodontal Abscess

Definition: A periodontal abscess is an abscess which develops in the gingival sulcus and arises from the microbial flora of the sulcus.

Pathogenesis

A periodontal abscess begins in the gingival sulcus. In a deep pocket, this abscess proliferates and can cause pronounced swelling if drainage cannot occur. Osseous involvement does not generally occur in acute cases; however, osteoclastic activity can often be seen in chronic infections.

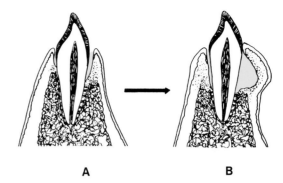

A   B

Figure VI-3. The stages in the development of a periodontal abscess. A. Inflammation of marginal gingiva and formation of periodontal pocket, B. pus formation in pocket which cannot drain.

Signs and Symptoms

The following signs and symptoms are commonly associated with periodontal abscesses.
- **A deeper than normal periodontal pocket** is usually present.
- **The gingiva will be red and frequently swollen.**
- **Swelling is usually seen on lingual, labial, buccal or palatal gingiva or mucosa.**
- **Probing the sulcus of the affected tooth usually results in purulent drainage.**
- **Pain** is usually localized to gingiva and alveolus.

Periodontal abscesses can be either **acute** which arise rapidly, produce a large, red, and painful swelling, or more **chronic** which generally shows little swelling, less to no color change, and is less painful.

NOTE: Chronic periodontal abscesses can be more difficult to diagnose than acute periodontal abscesses because the signs and symptoms are often subtle and hard to distinguish from the surrounding tissue. Periodontal probing is essential to a diagnosis of chronic periodontal abscesses.

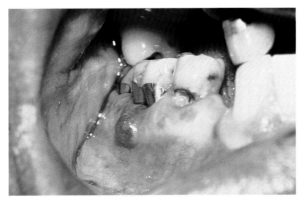

Figure VI-4. An acute periodontal abscess producing expansion of alveolar mucosa.

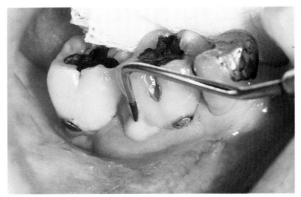

Figure VI-5. A chronic periodontal abscess showing profuse pus when probed.

Radiographic Appearance

Acute periodontal abscesses may not cause overt radiographic changes. However, a **chronic periodontal abscess may accelerate the alveolar bone loss** associated with periodontal disease. Bone loss accompanying a chronic periodontal abscess may become radiographically apparent after two to three months. Periodontal bone loss on the lingual or facial sides of the tooth may not be radiographically detectable due to the superimposition of root structure.

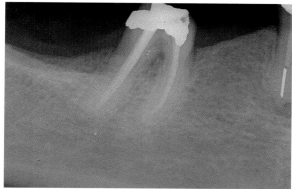

Figure VI-6. Radiographic appearance of an acute periodontal abscess. This radiograph shows no signs of bone loss.

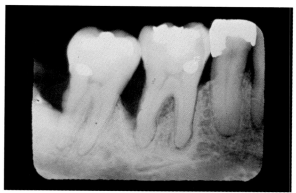

Figure VI-7. This radiograph shows an osseous defect in the furcation area and along the distal root. This is the radiograph of the chronic periodontal abscess shown in Figure VI-5.

STUDY EXERCISES

A periodontal abscess develops in the ____gingival____ ____sulcus____ arising from the microbial flora of the ____sulcus____.

List five common signs and symptoms of a periodontal abscess.
1. _____ deeper pocket _____
2. _____ gingiva red & swollen _____
3. _____ swelling lingual, labial, buccal or palatal gingiva or mucosa _____
4. _____ purulent drainage upon probing _____
5. _____ pain localized to gingiva & alveolus _____

Periodontal abscesses may be acute or chronic. Below, describe the differences in symptoms for these two.

	Chronic	Acute
Onset	slow	rapid
Color change	little or none	red
Swelling	little	much
Radiographic bone loss	may seen like	may not cause overt changes
Severity of pain	less	more

□ Pericoronitis — Pericoronal Abscess

Definition: Pericoronitis is an inflammation of the tissue surrounding the crown of an erupted or partially erupted tooth. A pericoronal abscess occurs when infection localizes in the tissues surrounding an erupting or partially erupting impacted tooth. Most commonly this occurs with mandibular third molars. This condition is really a special type of periodontal abscess.

Pathogenesis

As with periodontal abscesses, this process is initiated when oral flora, food debris, plaque and/or calculus are introduced under the operculum or into the gingival sulcus of a partially erupted tooth. If drainage is restricted, suppuration will accumulate. Further spread of the infection may result in swelling, trismus, dysphagia, and serious complications. The microbial flora around a partially erupted mandibular third molar can be significantly different from the flora found in

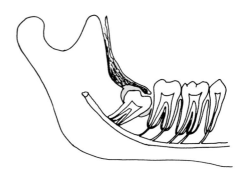

Figure VI-8. Sketch of pericoronitis.

most other parts of the mouth and can contain higher numbers of highly invasive species (e.g. *bacteroides).* There also appears to be a higher concentration of penicillin-resistant microorganisms in this area, thus pericoronal abscesses around third molars **must initially be considered more serious than pericoronal abscesses in other areas of the mouth.**

Another reason pericoronal abscesses occurring in the mandibular third molar region present an increased risk for patients is the proximity to the fascial spaces of the neck. Infections in this area may rapidly spread to the **parapharyngeal** and **pterygomandibular** spaces and can cause respiratory obstruction or mediastinal involvement which may be life threatening.

Signs and Symptoms

The typical signs and symptoms of pericoronitis or pericoronal abscess include the following:
- **Pain** — May range from a dull ache to continuous painful throbbing.
- **Redness** — In acute pericoronitis gingival tissues surrounding the partially erupted tooth may become redder than adjacent tissues, while in chronic pericoronitis color change will be less pronounced.
- **Swelling** — Associated with soft tissues, particularly those surrounding an unerupted tooth, which often proceeds to cellulitis and invasion of other spaces.
- **Trismus** — Inflammation of the masseter and/or medial pterygoid muscles plus regional soft tissue tenderness may severely decrease ability to open mouth.
- **Suppuration** — Pus may frequently be seen exuding from under the pericoronal tissue. Usually this is seen associated with partially erupted mandibular third or second molars.
- **Bad taste** — Suppurative exudate in oral cavity will cause a bad taste in the mouth.
- **Lymphadenitis** — Inflammation and enlargement of regional lymph nodes.
- **Dysphagia** — If infection invades floor of mouth or parapharyngeal areas, difficulties in eating or swallowing can result.
- **Cellulitis** — Cellulitis extending to surrounding areas can rapidly proceed to adjacent fascial spaces.

Pericoronitis may range from a **mild chronic** inflammation of the operculum or pericoronal tissue surrounding the partially erupted impacted mandibular third molar to a **dangerously acute** infection extending to the anterior pillar area, pterygomandibular space, parapharyngeal spaces, submandibular space, buccal space, infratemporal and deep temporal and/or submasseteric space.

NOTE: When describing a patient's condition which involves pericoronitis, you should describe associated tissue involvement and whether or not the problem is chronic or acute.

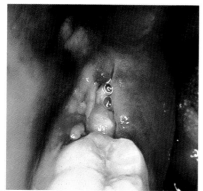

Figure VI-9. A clinical example of a chronic pericoronal abscess.

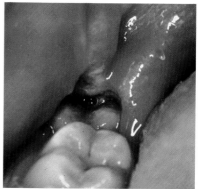

Figure VI-10. A clinical example of an acute pericoronal abscess.

NOTE: When treating acute pericoronitis it is best to control or resolve any soft tissue or fascial space infection prior to surgically removing the partially erupted mandibular third molar. A failure to heed this advice can result in extremely serious postsurgical infections which may be masked by the pain and swelling associated with the surgery.

STUDY EXERCISES

Pericoronal abscesses involving mandibular third molars may be more serious than in other areas of the mouth because they often are caused by ___penicillin___ *-resistant microorganisms or species such as bacteroides which are highly* ___invasive___.

Define:
pericoronitis ___inflammation of coronal portion of tooth___
pericoronal abscess ___infection around surrounding tissues___

Symptoms of pericoronal infection include: ___dull ache → painful throbbing;___
___redness with acute g/t tissue swelling, possible trismus___
___suppuration, bad taste, enlargement of lymph nodes___

☐ Periapical Alveolar Abscess

Definition: A periapical alveolar abscess is an abscess which develops secondarily to pulpal necrosis. Pulpal necrosis may result from thermal, physical, bacterial or chemical trauma to the tooth pulp. There are two general categories for these abscesses.

- **Acute periapical abscesses** usually have a very rapid onset of infection which often spreads rapidly through alveolar bone into surrounding soft tissue and adjacent fascial spaces. Alveolar bone loss is minimal in early stages, and periapical radiographs may show little evidence of pathosis other than a localized destruction of the lamina dura near the exit of the involved root canal.

- **Chronic periapical abscesses** are slower to develop and the infection is usually confined to the periapical region producing a radiolucency in this area.

There can be various types of transformations between these two general categories. For example, a chronic abscess can progress to an acute abscess at any time. An acute abscess can partially resolve, leaving a chronic periapical lesion which can later become acute. Your training in the area of endodontics should provide a discussion of these transformations in much greater detail.

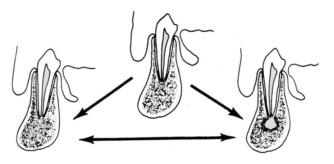

Figure VI-11. Acute periapical abscess and chronic alveolar abscess. Note transformations can occur between these two general classifications.

Signs and Symptoms

The following signs and symptoms may be associated with periapical alveolar abscesses:

- **Pain** — Dull throbbing pain to intense pain.
- **Percussion sensitivity** — Involved tooth may be percussion sensitive.
- **Extrusion of the tooth** — Edema of periodontal ligament may cause tooth to rise in its socket and hyperocclude with the opposing tooth.
- **Mobility** — Affected tooth may become extremely mobile.

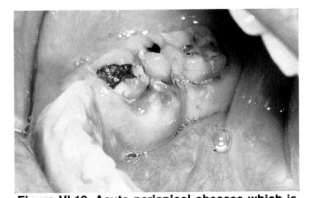

Figure VI-12. Acute periapical abscess which is causing signs of soft tissue inflammation.

- **Swelling** — Soft tissue swelling will be minimal until the abscess erodes through alveolar bone and invades soft tissue.
- **Vitality loss** — Tooth fails to respond to vitality testing.

Radiographic Appearance

Discontinuities or attenuations of the lamina dura, widening of the periodontal ligament space and periapical radiolucencies are usually the first radiographic changes noted following an apical infection secondary to pulpal necrosis. In the early stages of acute apical infections, there may be no radiographic evidence because no substantial alteration in calcific content is visible on the radiograph.

Later (about 8-10 days or longer) enough resorption of bone takes place to become radiographically observable. Less frequently an apical infection may initiate a proliferative reaction of the bone thus causing new bone to be deposited at the apex of the tooth. A condition termed **condensing osteitis** or **sclerosing osteitis** may be seen radiographically as an area of increased radiodensity at or near the apex of the affected tooth.

The apical infection may penetrate entirely through the alveolar bone and invade the soft tissues without greatly increasing the periapical radiolucency.

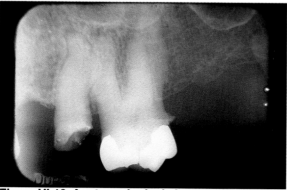

Figure VI-13. Acute periapical abscess. Notice that little change in radiodensity has occurred in trabecular (medullary) bone.

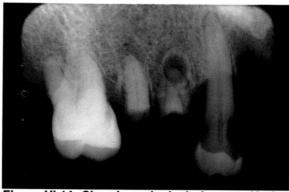

Figure VI-14. Chronic periapical abscess. Notice evidence of bone loss associated with chronic infection.

STUDY EXERCISES

Acute periapical abscesses have a _____*rapid*_____ onset often spreading into surrounding ___*soft*___ ___*tissue*___. Bone loss is ___*small*___ in early stages.

Chronic periapical abscesses develop ___*slowly*___ and are usually confined to ___*periapical*___ regions producing ___*radiolucency*___.

The symptoms often associated with periapical alveolar abscesses include: Involved tooth will test non-___*vital*___ and may have ___*percussion*___ sensitivity and be ___*mobile*___ from the socket. Pain can range from ___*dull*___ ___*throbbing*___ to ___*intense*___. Soft tissue swelling will be present if ___*abscess*___ ___*erodes*___ ___*through*___ ___*bone*___ ___*& into soft tissue*___.

Radiographic signs of periapical abscess may include:
___*widening of PDL*___ in early stages of acute infection
___*bone resorption*___ — 8-10 days later
___*condensing osteitis*___ — less frequently caused by a proliferative reaction.

Will you always find radiographic changes in the presence of a periapical abscess?
___*no*___

☐ Post-surgical (Post-Dental Treatment) Infections

Infections can develop following surgery or other invasive dental procedures. The source of microorganisms for these infections can be from:
- **Normal oral flora** which is displaced into soft tissue or bone during the procedure.
- **An existing abscess** if instruments used for injections or incisions carry the abscess flora into previously uninvolved areas.
- **External sources** if sterile instruments and aseptic techniques are not employed. (This route of infection will not be discussed in detail in this book.)

Post-surgical infections can involve soft tissue, periosteum and even extend to involve hard tissue. These infections include:
- **Post-surgical infections of soft tissue**
- **Subperiosteal infections from retained surgical debris**
- **Expression of periapical suppuration into surround soft tissue**
- **Post-injection infections**

The following discussion is a brief review of post-surgical infections:

Post-Surgical or Post-Dental Treatment Infections
These infections include a variety of soft tissue infections which occur following dental treatment. Included in this group are infections resulting from:
- Contaminated partial thickness flaps
- Curettage of deep periodontal pockets
- Use of contaminated dental instruments
- Puncture wounds
- Endodontic treatment

You should always be alert to the possibility of post-dental treatment infections and advise your patients to contact you immediately if swellings develop or if they experience fever and/or chills within a few days of dental treatment.

Subperiosteal Infections
By definition, subperiosteal infections are a category of infections involving periosteum and will be discussed later.

Expression of periapical suppuration into surrounding soft tissue
Soft tissue infections may result if suppuration from a localized periapical abscess is pumped through the alveolus and periosteum into surrounding soft tissue during extraction movements. Generally these infections will drain through the extraction socket; however, occasionally this drainage path may be closed and the infection then spreads into soft tissue spaces.

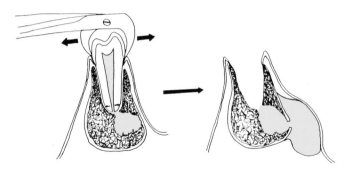

Figure VI-15. Soft tissue infection resulting from suppuration expressed from a localized periapical abscess during extraction.

Post-injection infections
Infection can develop when microorganisms are carried into tissue along with the needle used for injection of local anesthetic or during needle aspiration of lesions. Post-injection infections are illustrated in **Figure VI-16** through **VI-18**. The incidence of these infections can be reduced through adequate preparation of the injection site and taking care **not** to inject anesthetic solutions through areas of infection (either abscess or cellulitis). When aspirating a lesion, the needle should not pass through the lesion into deeper tissues.

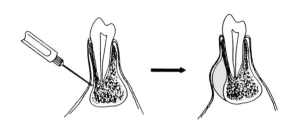

Figure VI-16. Post-injection infection. Suppuration may be subperiosteal or in overlying soft tissue.

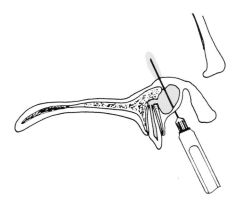

Figure VI-17. Post-injection infection from a seeding of deeper tissues when injecting through an abscessed area. These infections may or may not be subperiosteal.

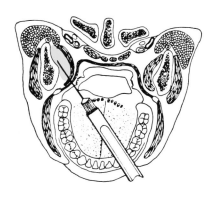

Figure VII-18. Post-injection infection of the pterygomandibular space following inferior alveolar block anesthesia. These infections are usually not subperiosteal. Although these infections rarely occur, they usually are serious and require hospitalization.

Signs and Symptoms

Soft tissue infections resulting from surgery or other invasive dental procedures have similar signs and symptoms in their earlier stages, and can develop into more serious infections if not recognized early. The following signs and symptoms may be seen.

- **Firm, tense, red swelling over abscess site**
- **Tenderness to palpation**
- **Development of facial edema**
- **Increase in body temperature**

Radiographic Appearance

These infections are not usually radiographically apparent in earlier stages, however if chronic infection persists they may extend through periosteum and involve cortical bone, then progress to osteomyelitis of trabecular (medullary) bone.

STUDY EXERCISES

Post-injection infections can result from:

a) post surgical infections of soft tissue

b) retained surgical debris

c) expression of periapical suppuration into surround soft tissue

The occurrence of post-injection infections can be reduced by preparation
of the injection site and by being careful not to place your needle
through an area of infection *either* abscess *or* cellulitis .

☐ Maxillary Sinusitis

Definition: An inflammation or infection of the maxillary sinus involving lining mucosa and periosteum.

Pathogenesis

Infections of the maxillary sinus are not usually of dental origin. The following list represents some dentally related causes of maxillary sinusitis.

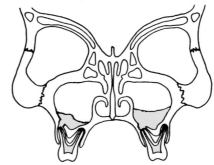

- **Direct spread** of periapical abscess from maxillary posterior teeth which perforates the antral floor to involve the sinus mucosa.
- **Facial fractures** involving the maxillary sinus rarely cause sinusitis except when tooth or bone fragments are dislodged into the sinus or normal drainage is obstructed by the displaced fractured segments.
- **Tooth or root fragments** surgically displaced into the maxillary sinus can cause a chronic sinusitis.
- **Oro-antral openings** can cause an acute or chronic sinusitis producing a purulent discharge via the oro-antral fistula. The chronic discharge can prevent healing of the oro-antral fistula.

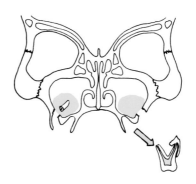

Figure VI-19. The spread of dentally related infections to the maxillary sinus.

Signs and Symptoms
- **Pain** — Throbbing, aching in upper cheek or entire side of the face if the infection process is acute
- **Percussion** — Sensitivity to skeletal jarring, jumping, or head down position
- **Discharge** — Foul-smelling in nasal or pharyngeal cavity
- **Mild systemic symptoms** — If present, fever, chills, sweating
- **Generalized maxillary posterior toothache.**
- **Transillumination** — Failure to illuminate involved sinus by transoral lighting.
- **Radiographic** — Radiopaque antra, mucosal thickening, air-fluid level, or foreign bodies may be seen

Radiographic Appearance

The earliest radiographic changes seen in the maxillary sinus from abscessed maxillary posterior teeth may be a thickening of the antral mucosa overlying the floor of the antrum. The thickening of the antral mucosa (mucositis) may be seen on periapical or panoramic radiographs as a thick, soft tissue density overlying the bony antral floor.

If a periapical infection progresses to invade the entire maxillary antrum, a generalized thickening of the antral mucosa is seen with or without fluid levels of suppurative material. If the apical infection continues, bony destruction of the antral floor may occur. The following radiographic changes may be seen:
- Localized thickening of antral mucosa overlying tooth apex
- Large thickening of antral mucosa overlying the entire antral floor
- Generalized antral mucosal thickening which may entirely fill the sinus
- Observed fluid levels in the sinus
- Bony destruction of antral floor and/or antral walls

NON-DENTAL SOFT TISSUE INFECTIONS

Several non-dental soft tissue infections may present signs and symptoms similar to odontogenic infections. You should be aware of this possibility and include these in your differential diagnosis. By identifying these infections early, you can refer your patients to appropriate specialists. We have provided a brief description of five soft tissue infections which may be mistaken for odontogenic infections. These include **peritonsillar infections, salivary gland infections, superficial skin infections, ear infections,** and **maxillary sinusitis.** When evaluating patients with oral and/or maxillofacial swellings, you should consider these as possible causes, especially if you find no obvious dental source in your clinical examination of the patient.

☐ Peritonsillar Infections

Definition: A localized infection in the connective tissue bed of the faucial tonsil lying between the superior constrictor muscle and the overlying mucous membranes.

Signs and Symptoms

* **Pain** on side of throat radiating to the ear
* **Dysphagia**
* **Speech** changes
* **Fever,** malaise, anorexia
* **Tense** swelling of anterior tonsillar pillar
* **Bulging** of soft palate
* **Fetor oris** once drainage has begun
* **Marked uvular edema**

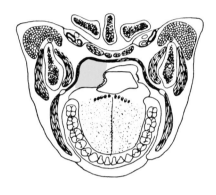

Figure VI-20. Anatomical location of peritonsillar infections.

NOTE: Peritonsillar abscesses should generally be referred for management.

☐ Salivary Gland Infections

Definition: Bacterial or viral infection of any of the salivary glands.

Signs and Symptoms:

* **Swelling** of the gland in either the preauricular area or submandibular space
* **Lymph node** involvement of the preauricular or submandibular nodes
* **Inflammation** of skin overlying the gland
* **Purulence** can often be seen intraorally at the duct opening
* **Tenderness to palpation** in the region of the affected gland
* **Pain** especially diagnostic if occurring at mealtime
* **Fever** is often present

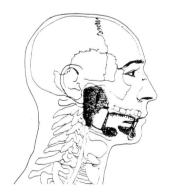

Figure VI-21. Anatomical location of the major salivary glands.

Radiographic Appearance

Salivary gland infections may develop secondarily to **obstruction of the salivary ducts.** Sialoliths may be seen in mandibular occlusal, lateral jaw, or panoramic radiographs. **Sialography** may be necessary to visualize mucous plugs or ductal constriction.

☐ Superficial Skin Infections

The head and neck regions are prone to dermal infections. Infected hair follicles, acne, and actinomyces infections are examples of infections in this area. Occasionally skin infections may produce signs and symptoms similar to those produced by dental infections. Swelling, increased tenderness, increased temperature, pain and edema can result from acute superficial skin infections. Skin infections can progress from a cellulitis to an acute abscess to a chronic abscess.

NOTE: Physicians frequently overlook possible dental etiologies as the cause for superficial skin infections and dentists may prematurely assume a dental origin for superficial skin infections. The incidence of these diagnostic errors can be reduced by performing a thorough dental examination prior to establishing a diagnosis and beginning treatment.

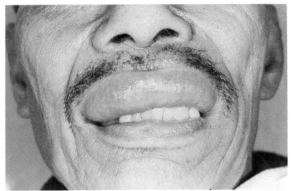

Figure VI-22. Inflammation of this patient's upper lip was caused by an infected hair follicle. No dental etiology was involved.

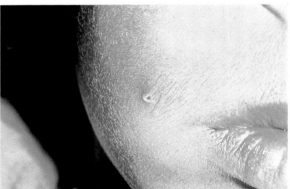

Figure VI-23. The skin lesion in this patient was initially diagnosed as a "pimple" and treated as a superficial skin lesion. Dental examination revealed that this lesion was caused by repeated puncture wounds from an orthodontic headgear wire.

☐ Ear Infections

Ear infections such as **otitis externa, otitis media,** and **mastoiditis** can cause ear pain. In addition, dental infections of the mandibular molar area can **refer pain** to the ear if the pathological process affects the inferior alveolar nerve. **The cause of any ear pain symptoms should be identified as either non-dental or dental and appropriate consultation should be obtained.**

If a patient's symptoms include ear pain an **otoscopic examination** of the ear should be performed. The presence of suppuration, inflammation of the eardrum and bulging of the ear drum are signs of ear infections.

True ear pain can be distinguished from **referred pain** to the ear by applying direct pressure on the external ear or by gently pulling on the pinna of the ear. **If immediate pain is elicited** then the ear pain is most likely associated with an ear infection or other related ear problems. If no immediate pain is elicited by these tests, then the symptom of ear pain is most likely referred pain from a pathological process involving the mandibular molar area and the inferior alveolar nerve.

STUDY EXERCISES

Four potential dentally related causes of maxillary sinusitis include:

1) ___*Direct*___ spread of periapical abscess from _*posterior maxillary*_ ___ teeth which _*perforate antral floor*_

2) Facial fracture with ___*tooth*___ or ___*root*___ *tip* dislodged into the sinus.

3) ___*Tooth*___ or ___*root fragments*___ surgically displaced into the sinus.

4) ___*Antro-Oral*___ openings.

The earliest radiographic changes seen in maxillary sinusitis may be a thickening of the ___*antral*___ ___*mucosa*___. *Other radiographic signs which may occur if the infection becomes more severe include* ___*suppurative fluid*___ *in the sinus and destruction of* ___*antral floor*___.

Signs and symptoms associated with peritonsillar infection include pain located ___*side of throat*___, *swelling of the* ___*anterior tonsillar*___ ___*pillar*___, *bulging of the* ___*soft*___ ___*palate*___, ___*uvular*___ *edema, dysphagia, and often producing the systemic sign of* ___*Dysphagia*___.

A patient presenting with pain and swelling in the pre-auricular area may have a dentally caused buccal space infection or a parotid infection. What signs and symptoms would suggest parotid infection? _*Swelling of gland, purulence from duct, tenderness to palpation, pain, lymph node involvement, fever*_

If a patient presents with swelling of the upper lip yet all the maxillary teeth test vital and there is no periodontal tissue inflammation, what non-dental source would you suspect? _*lacerations or cuts*_

A patient presents to your office complaining of pain that seems to be coming from around his ear. If an ear infection is causing the pain, what might you see in an otoscopic examination? _*Suppuration*_, _*inflammation*_ *or* _*bulging*_ *of the eardrum. How could you determine whether this is true ear pain or referred pain?* _*Pull on ear. If true ear pain, will feel pain immediately*_

Name four (4) non-dental causes of soft tissue infections which should be included in your differential diagnosis of oral and maxillofacial swellings:

1) _*ear infection*_
2) _*Skin*_
3) _*peritonsillar*_
4) _*salivary gland*_

INFECTIONS OF PERIOSTEUM

Infections involving the periosteum may arise from three sources:

- **Extension of hard tissue infections**
- **Extension of soft tissue infections**
- **Direct deposition of microorganisms between the periosteum and cortical bone**

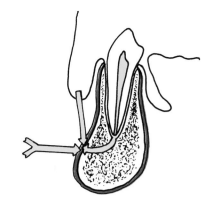

Infections of periosteum can spread into soft tissue causing soft tissue inflammation or abscess if the periosteum is penetrated or into bone causing erosion of cortical bone and osteitis or osteomyelitis.

Figure VI-24. Summary of the origin or pathways by which microorganisms gain access to the potential space between the periosteum and cortical bone.

Infections or inflammation of periosteum can result in two general reactions:

- **Acute subperiosteal abscess formation (post-surgical periosteal abscess)**
- **Chronic periosteal inflammation (periostitis)**

☐ Post-surgical subperiosteal abscess

Subperiosteal infections most frequently result from the entrapment of surgical debris or salivary contamination under periosteal flaps following closure of full-thickness flaps. These infections can also result from the use of non-sterile water during the surgical procedure. If surgical flaps are closed tightly, the microorganisms trapped under the flap can create a subperiosteal abscess. Subperiosteal abscesses present clinically as hard, firm, painful swellings below the periosteum. These infections may penetrate the periosteum and involve the overlying soft tissue and/or extend into the adjacent fascial spaces. These infections may also erode cortical bone and involve medullary bone, thus producing an osteomyelitis or may drain through an extraction socket. Generally, acute abscesses do not result in bone deposition. Radiographic data may provide useful information if foreign objects or bone chips are large.

NOTE: **Copious irrigation with sterile saline and a careful inspection of areas under surgical flaps should be performed just prior to suturing in order to reduce the occurrence of post-surgical subperiosteal infections.**

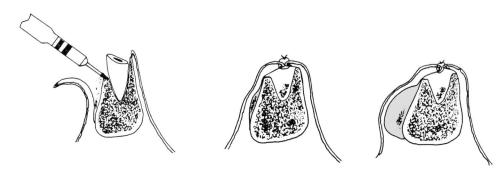

Figure VI-25. Subperiosteal infection resulting from entrapment of surgical debris or salivary contamination.

☐ Periostitis

Definition: Periostitis is an inflammation of the periosteum surrounding bone. Periostitis of the jaws is generally confined to the mandible. Another term for this inflammation is periosteitis.

Pathogenesis

Periostitis usually arises from a **periapical abscess** but can also arise from osteomyelitis. If pressure from intra-bony abscess pushes an infection through cortical bone but fails to penetrate the periosteum, the periosteum may be elevated from underlying bone. Chronic intra-bony infections (either chronic periapical abscesses or osteomyelitis) can result in repeated insults to the periosteum which in turn will form concentric layers of bone thus producing a laminated or "onion-skin" radiographic appearance. This process of sequential bone deposition requires active osteoblastic activity, thus it occurs primarily in young children (1-5 years) and to a lesser extent in adolescents.

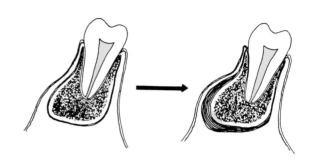

Figure VI-26. Periostitis usually exhibits an "onion-skin" appearance of new bone deposition.

Periostitis has also been termed chronic osteomyelitis with proliferative periostitis, Garre's chronic non-suppurative sclerosing osteitis, or periostitis ossificans.

NOTE: This condition must be distinguished from various neoplastic processes which can also produce firm swellings of the mandible.

Signs and Symptoms

Periostitis is first seen clinically as a **hard, firm swelling** on the medial, lateral, or inferior surfaces of the mandible. A summary of signs and symptoms includes:

- **Pain** — dull, throbbing, continuous.
- **Hard, firm swelling** — generally confined to mandible.
- **Slight increase in WBC** — usually less than increase seen with acute infections.
- **Radiographic signs** — carious teeth or necrotic bone seen in area of swelling, occlusal radiograph showing laminated bone deposition adjacent to soft tissue.

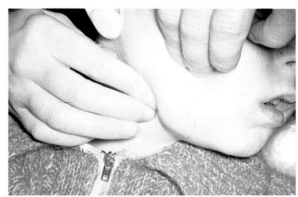

Figure VI-27. A clinical example of periostitis is seen as a firm extraoral swelling near angle of the mandible. Since swelling is confined by the periosteum, no signs of soft tissue inflammation are evident.

Radiographic Appearance

Again, laminated or "onion-skin" radiographic appearance on occlusal radiographs is highly indicative of periostitis. Presence of a periapical radiolucency and absence of sequestrum as seen in periapical views will help distinguish periostitis from osteomyelitis or establish the presence of both osteomyelitis and periostitis.

STUDY EXERCISES

The three potential sources for periosteal infections are extension of infection from _____soft_____ tissue or _____hard_____ tissue and _____deposition_____ of microorganisms between the periosteum and cortical bone.

Periostitis is defined as _____inflamation of periosteum around bone_____ and is generally confined to the _____mandible_____.

Periostitis usually arises from _____periapical_____ _____abscess_____ but can also arise from _____osteomyelitis_____.

List four signs and symptoms usually associated with periostitis:
1) _____hard firm swelling on lat. borders of mandible_____
2) _____slight ↑ WBC_____
3) _____carious teeth + radiographically "onion peel"_____
4) _____dull throbbing pain_____

Radiographically, periostitis often presents with an _____onion_____-_____peel_____ appearance. Periostitis differs from osteomyelitis in not resulting in _____sequestrum_____ or periapical _____radiolucency_____ on radiographic examination.

INFECTIONS INVOLVING HARD TISSUE

Infections involving trabecular (medullary) and cortical bone are referred to as infections of hard tissue. The source of microorganisms which lead to hard tissue infections include:
- Necrotic dental pulps
- Extension of soft tissue or periosteal infections
- Trauma (e.g. fractures, tooth extraction and osseous surgery)
- Hematogenous spread from another area of the body (e.g. tuberculosis)

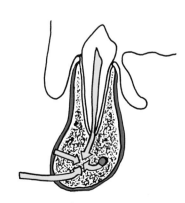

Figure VI-28. Summary of the origin or pathway by which microorganisms gain access to hard tissue.

☐ Acute Alveolar Osteitis — "Dry Socket"

Definition: An inflammatory process involving the alveolar bone of a tooth socket which can develop secondary to tooth extraction.

Pathogenesis

Following the removal of a tooth an inflammatory reaction may initiate the release of tissue activators which transform plasminogen into plasmium with subsequent fibrinogen lysis and loss of the blood clot in the extraction socket. The exposed bony alveolus is thus exposed to oral fluids causing marked pain from stimulation of free nerve endings.

Acute alveolar osteitis is most likely associated with mandibular third molar extractions but may occur with mandibular second molar extractions and to a lesser extent the other mandibular teeth. Rarely does this occur in the maxillary arch.

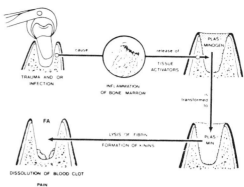

Figure VI-29. Etiology and pathogenesis of fibrinolytic alveolitis (from H. Birn, "Etiology and Pathogenesis of Fibrinolytic Alveolitis," *Int J Oral Surg*, 2:252, 1973, with permission).

Signs and Symptoms

Your patient will present with an extraction socket which has lost its blood clot and is lined with foul-smelling necrotic tissue and complaints of dull aching and/or throbbing pain.

- **Pain** — Dull aching, throbbing
- **Gingival inflammation**
- **Empty alveolar socket**
- **Halitosis**
- **Lymphadenopathy**
- **Minimal systemic symptoms**

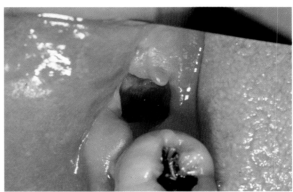

Figure VI-30. Clinical appearance of "dry socket." Notice the absence of organized blood clot in the socket.

Although not a true suppurative infection, a pronounced osteomyelitis of the surrounding alveolar bone marrow can be seen at the histological level.

Radiographic Data

A radiograph of alveolar osteitis will reveal an unremarkable empty socket. Generally there are no radiographic changes in this condition.

STUDY EXERCISES

Acute alveolar osteitis is an ___inflammatory___ process involving the ___alveolar___ bone of a ___tooth___ ___socket___ which can develop secondary to tooth ___extraction___. The disease process is believed to involve the release of ___tissue___ ___activators___ which transform into ___plasminogen___ and the subsequent ___fibrinogen___ lysis and loss of ___blood___ ___clot___. The exposed bone is then ___exposed___ to oral fluids causing ___stimulation___ _____ of free nerve endings. It is most commonly associated with the extraction of ___mandibular___ ___3rd___ ___molars___, however can also occur following extraction of ___other mandibular teeth___. Typical signs and symptoms include:

- ___dull throbbing pain___
- ___empty alveolar socket___
- ___lymphadenopathy___
- ___gingival inflammation___
- ___halitosis___
- ___minimal systemic symptoms___

Radiographs will generally show ___unremarkable empty socket___.

□ Osteomyelitis

Definition: The term osteomyelitis refers to an inflammation of bone. Inflammation can involve the cancellous tissue, bone marrow, cortical bone, and even the periosteum. Osteomyelitis most frequently occurs in the mandible and only rarely in the maxilla. Osteomyelitis can be acute or chronic.

Pathogenesis

Several causes of osteomyelitis have been described. However we will only discuss:
- Acute pyogenic osteomyelitis
- Chronic osteomyelitis

Acute or **chronic osteomyelitis** can develop from the invasion of microorganisms from periapical abscesses, from extension of soft tissue or periosteal infections, from fractures, or from contamination of surgical sites. Inflammation accumulates inside the cancellous bone spaces compromising blood supply and

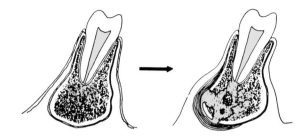

Figure VI-31. Osteomyelitis can initially develop from the contamination of an extration site or progressive invasion of bone following periapical abscess. Notice sequestrum formation and "onion skin" deposition of bone when periosteum is involved.

produces suppuration that leads to death of bone tissue. Continuation of this process eventually leads to **demineralization of bone and radiographic appearance of a lesion in which sequestra are visible.** Sequestra are islands of bone surrounded by areas of demineralization and necrosis. **Paresthesia** may develop if the process involves the mandibular nerve canal. Lower lip paresthesia will occur if infection is distal to the mental foramen. Osteomyelitis can erode the cortical plate of the mandible and allow spread of the infection to the periosteum causing either acute or chronic periostitis. Acute periostitis can spread along the periosteum to the submasseteric space or penetrate the periosteum causing infection of soft tissue and fascial spaces. **Chronic osteomyelitis** with periosteal involvement will frequently produce a characteristic "onion-skin" radiographic appearance (see page 187 for discussion of periostitis).

The reasons why osteomyelitis rarely develops from dentoalveolar or periapical abscesses remain unclear at this time. However, an increased incidence of osteomyelitis is seen in patients with reduced body defenses due to diabetes, syphilis, tuberculosis, extreme malnutrition, or other conditions which impair local blood circulation. **Osteoradionecrosis** is a special form of osteomyelitis which will be discussed in more detail on page 195.

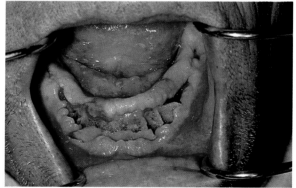

Figure VI-32. A clinical example of osteomyelitis showing exposure of infected bone.

Osteomyelitis resulting from bacterial invasion of bone usually results in the production of pus and extension of the lesion can progress rapidly, hence the term acute pyogenic osteomyelitis. A low-grade, slow-growing osteomyelitis can also result and is termed **chronic osteomyelitis.**

Actinomycotic osteomyelitis is usually a slow-growing condition caused by species of *Actinomyces.* These infections can be difficult to diagnose and treatment often extends over several months.

NOTE: If treatment of a small osteomyelitis infection does not resolve, then referral to a specialist is indicated.

Signs and Symptoms

Typical signs and symptoms of osteomyelitis include:

- **Pain** — severe and deep within bone
- **Paresthesia** — of anterior teeth if anterior to or anterior teeth and lower lip if posterior (distal) to mental foramen
- **Fever** — Usually low-grade fever (approx. 100°F, 37.8°C)
- **Elevated WBC** — greater than 10,000 per mm^3 white blood cell count
- **Radiographic signs** — reduced trabecular definition, radiolucent lesions with indistinct borders, presence of sequestra

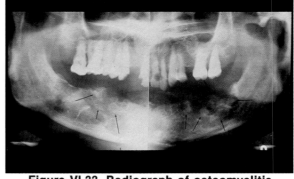

Figure VI-33. Radiograph of osteomyelitis showing areas of sequestrum formation.

- **Sinus tract formation**
- **Exposed bone** — oral mucosa may be destroyed, exposing infected bone
- **Positive culture** — obtained from lesion (it is best to culture bone tissue rather than pus collected at sinus tract stomas)
- **Histological evidence** — bone biopsy will show inflammation, bone resorption and necrosis
- **Increased ESR values**

Radiographic Appearance

Radiographic changes can only be seen when 30-60% of the mineral content of bone has been lost, thus the radiographic signs of osteomyelitis develop over weeks. The following radiographic pattern is usually observed:

- The earliest sign of osteomyelitis is loss of bony trabeculae in the involved area. This may appear as a blurring of the trabeculae.
- Next, irregular bony destruction occurs either isolated or in multiple

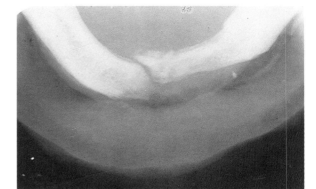

Figure VI-34. Radiograph of advanced osteomyelitis showing advanced destruction of the mandible.

areas separated by what appears to be normal bone. In this stage the bone has a "moth-eaten" appearance.
- Sequestrum formation may be seen in later stages of osteomyelitis. The sequestrum may be quite small (several millimeters) or extensive, involving large segments of the jaws. The sequestra appear as radiopaque islands surrounded by radiolucent bands of soft tissue which separate the dead bone from the vital bone.
- Subperiosteal new bone formation is also seen in osteomyelitis of the jaws. The new bone may appear as laminated or multiple thin layers of new bone. The inferior border of the mandible is a common site for this to be seen, although it also occurs in other areas.
- In children, the loss of the cortex of the bony crypt surrounding unerupted teeth may be radiographic evidence of osteomyelitis.

NOTE: **The treatment of osteomyelitis should either be performed by a specialist or by a general dentist in close consultation with a specialist because extensive osseous surgery and reconstruction may be necessary if conservative treatment is unsuccessful.**

☐ Osteitis

The term **osteitis** refers to inflammation of bone but generally does not result in the death of significant amounts of bone tissue. Osteitis may initially produce demineralization of bone and is often followed by bone deposition (seen as an area of increased radiographic density). Often this response follows resolution of periapical osteitis associated with an acute or chronic periapical abscess.

☐ Osteoradionecrosis

Osteoradionecrosis will be discussed in the next section on **infections of special significance.**

STUDY EXERCISES

_____Osteomyelitis_____ refers to inflammation of trabecular (and/or cortical bone), (does/does not) ____does____ result in the death of significant amounts of bone tissue. Initially the condition may cause ___demineralization___ of bone which is often followed by ___necrosis___ ___sequestra___.

_____Osteomyelitis_____ can be a serious infection of hard tissue and is usually diagnosed by the radiographic presence of sequestra or areas of necrotic bone surrounded by areas of radiolucency. Osteomyelitis can be either ___chronic___ or ___acute___ and in all cases should receive prompt treatment. Acute pyogenic osteomyelitis is caused by ___bacteria___ while a more chronic form is associated with **actinomyces** species.

INFECTIONS OF SPECIAL SIGNIFICANCE

For the purposes of this book we have created a category of **infections of special significance** to emphasize the extreme seriousness of the following infections:
- ☐ Acute cellulitis
- ☐ Ludwig's angina
- ☐ Osteoradionecrosis
- ☐ Cavernous sinus thrombosis

All of these infections are or can lead to life-threatening conditions and require **immediate hospitalization.** Early recognition and referral is essential.

☐ Acute Cellulitis

The term **cellulitis** is used to describe the first stage of inflammation associated with an infection (or other causes of inflammation, e.g. trauma). When an infectious process is involved, cellulitis is characterized by a diffuse (non-confined, non-circumscribed) area of inflammation with increased redness and temperature, capillary dilation and edema, leucocytic infiltration, and rapidly multiplying microorganisms. The area of cellulitis may expand into surrounding tissue or along fascial planes to involve areas away from the primary site of infection.

Once an infectious process results in the formation of a cellulitis, the final outcome of the infection is **always** in question. One cannot predict the **critical turning point** when the patient's host defense mechanisms will **gain control** over the invasive microorganism(s) and **initiate** the process of localization (formation of pus and drainage). In some patients the turning point of localization **fails** to occur before essential body functions are affected and **death results**.

Clinically, the degree of seriousness of a cellulitis ranges from a relatively minor local area of redness (e.g. pimple on the skin) to a massive condition in which death of the patient is imminent. Recognizing the degree of seriousness of a cellulitis is a key factor in planning appropriate management of an infection. Early recognition of a potentially serious cellulitis will enable you to refer your patient to a specialist and/or hospital for immediate and aggressive treatment.

Acute cellulitis is a clinical term commonly used to describe a **rapidly progressing cellulitis involving large anatomical areas (frequently away from the initial site of infection) and producing significant systemic effects.**

Signs and Symptoms

The clinical signs and symptoms of acute cellulitis may include the following:
- **Pain** (can be acute)
- **Redness** — if superficial tissues are involved. May not be seen if deeper tissues are involved
- **Loss of function** — dysphagia, laryngeal edema, ptosis (restricted eye opening)
- **Rapid onset** — 1-2 days
- **Involves fascial spaces or anatomical areas of the head and neck**
- **Fever**
- **Dehydration**
- **Systemic toxicity**
- **Increased pulse rate**
- **Increased respiratory rate**
- **Malaise and weakness**
- **Increased ESR (sed. rate)**
- **Increased WBC count**
- **Increased polys and shift to the left**

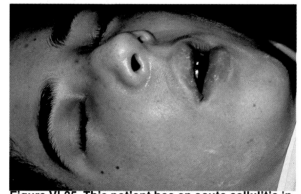

Figure VI-35. This patient has an acute cellulitis involving the buccal space and infraorbital area. Signs of systemic toxicity were also present. She was appropriately referred to an oral and maxillofacial surgeon and immediately hospitalized.

Acute cellulitis may accompany **any** of the soft tissue infections thus far discussed, including those of **both dental and non-dental origins**. The **management** of acute cellulitis must often **take precedence over treatment of the primary cause** of the infection and referral to a specialist and/or hospital is indicated. For this reason, we have placed acute cellulitis in the category of **infections of special significance**.

☐ **Ludwig's Angina**

Definition: An extensive bilateral phlegmonous cellulitis involving the submental, sublingual, and submandibular spaces. The infection may also progress to involve the lateral pharyngeal and retropharyngeal spaces as well as fascial spaces of the neck. (See further discussion on pages 66 to 67.)

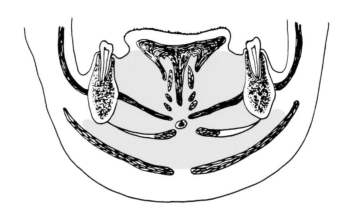

Figure VI-36. Ludwig's angina involves the sublingual, submental and submandibular spaces as shown in yellow in the above illustration.

Signs and Symptoms

Ludwig's angina resulting from dental infections frequently develops within a few days following infection of one of the three fascial spaces. Any of these spaces can also become involved secondarily to infection of other fascial spaces of the head. The following signs and symptoms are associated with the symptom complex known as Ludwig's angina:

- Brawny, indurated swelling of submental, sublingual and submandibular spaces bilaterally
- Elevation of tongue and floor of mouth
- Dysphagia
- Respiratory difficulty
- Speech may be difficult
- Drooling because of painful swallowing
- Systemic toxicity
- Fever, anorexia, malaise

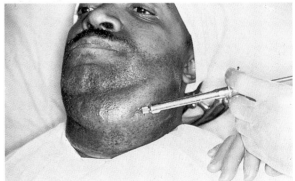

Figure VI-37. Ludwig's angina produces bilateral swelling of the submandibular, submental, and sublingual spaces.

Management

Management of a patient with Ludwig's will involve extraoral incision and drainage and requires close supervision to monitor for airway obstruction. Patients with Ludwig's angina should be treated by an oral and maxillofacial surgeon or other hospital practitioner experienced in management of Ludwig's. **It is essential that you refer these patients immediately for treatment** as this condition, if untreated, can progress rapidly to respiratory obstruction and death.

☐ Osteoradionecrosis

Definition: Osteoradionecrosis is a disease process which involves a pyogenic infection of previously irradiated bone.

Pathogenesis

Bone exposed to high doses of radiation will show a decreased ability to manage local infections. This is because of the injurious effect of radiation upon the individual cells as well as regional microcirculation. The radiotherapy causes a progressive diminution fibrosis of the vascularity of the bone at an arteriolar level (obliterative endarteritis). Irradiated bone is extremely susceptible to ischemic death and infection.

Three predisposing conditions which most usually will be present in order for osteoradionecrosis to occur include:

- **Previous direct irradiation of the maxilla/mandible.** Generally local irradiation in excess of **4,000 rads** is sufficient to predispose a patient to osteoradionecrosis. It is important to know the exact location of any radiation therapy.
- **Trauma to soft tissue or bone.** Frequently routine dental procedures and minor tooth extractions are enough trauma to allow an ingress of oral microorganisms into the bone and initiate osteoradionecrosis.
- **Surgical intervention** following radiotherapy may cause an acute pyogenic osteomyelitis in the avascular bone which may result in progressive massive destruction of the jaws. The high risk of osteoradionecrosis from surgical intervention following radiotherapy necessitates the careful evaluation of the oral status prior to radiation treatments. Teeth in the line of the radiation should be removed before radiation if there is any question of their long-term prognosis. If there is any question about the patient's ability and willingness to perform meticulous oral hygiene, you may want to perform extractions and denture construction prior to radiation treatment.

Signs and Symptoms

The signs and symptoms of osteoradionecrosis are similar to those of osteomyelitis. The key to diagnosis is a previous history of radiation therapy of the jaws or head region.

Management

Any patient with a history of radiation to the jaw area must be closely followed if not totally managed by one specially trained in the management of post-irradiated patients. Any surgical needs

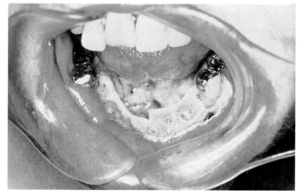

Figure VI-38. A clinical example of osteoradionecrosis.

should be carefully reviewed and referred to a specialist. The example of osteoradionecrosis shown in **Figure VI-38** above was initiated by the extraction of periodontally compromised anterior teeth by a general dentist for a patient who received radiation therapy 12 years prior.

☐ Cavernous Sinus Thrombosis

Definition: A condition in which a thrombosis (blood clot) is formed in the cavernous sinus of the brain.

Pathogenesis

Thrombus (blood clot) formation in blood vessels is promoted by several factors including: **stasis** (stoppage of blood flow), **increased platelet count, shock,** and **inflammation** of vessel walls in the midface region. The angular, ophthalmic, and pterygoid plexus veins connect with both the cavernous sinus and facial vein (which flows into the external jugular vein). Usually, blood in these veins flows into the external jugular vein; however, these vessels **lack valves** to prevent retrograde blood flow into the cavernous sinus. Infections of the **midface region** and **infratemporal space** (pterygoid plexus) initiate an inflammatory response result-

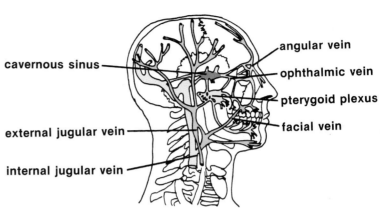

Figure VI-39. Venous system of the head. Cavernous sinus is shown in red; yellow indicates the major veins which communicate with the cavernous sinus.

ing in an increase in extravascular fluid pressure (edema and abscess formation). Increased pressure can **reverse the direction of venous blood flow** causing stasis in the cavernous sinus or transport of microorganisms to the cavernous sinus. **Both consequences of retrograde blood flow can initiate thrombus formation.**

Signs and Symptoms

Headache, irritability, drowsiness, vomiting, and neck stiffness are signs of intracranial spread. Edema of both the upper and lower eyelids indicates impending cavernous sinus thrombosis. There is a high fever with sweats and a rapid pulse. The abducens nerve is paralyzed early in the condition, but soon an ophthalmoplegia develops. The signs and symptoms that can be indicative of cavernous sinus thrombosis include:

- **Pyrexia — fluctuating**
- **Edema of eyelids**
- **Exophthalmos**
- **Pulsating exophthalmos**
- **Abducens nerve paralysis**
- **Ophthalmoplegia**
- **Edematous conjunctivae**

- **Papilledema and retinal hemorrhages**
- **C.N.S. signs of meningeal irritation**
- **Lacrimation**
- **Positive blood cultures**
- **Dilated pupils and photophobia**
- **Systemic toxicity**

Odontogenic Origin

Cavernous sinus thrombosis can result from dental **infections of the midface region** and **periorbital area** (from maxillary anterior teeth) or from **infections of the infratemporal space** (from maxillary posterior teeth or extension of pterygomandibular space infections from maxillary or mandibular second or third molars). The midface region (nose, base of the upper lip, and infraorbital area) is often called the "**danger triangle.**" **Needle track contamination** of the infratemporal (pterygoid plexus) and pterygomandibular spaces can occur especially if poor aseptic technique is used.

NOTE: Cavernous sinus thrombosis is an extremely serious complication which can develop from infections of the jaws. Patients require immediate hospitalization with intravenous antibiotics and anti-coagulants.

POST-TEST — UNIT VI

- Answer each of the following questions.
- Check your answers with the correct responses on page 202.
- If all questions are answered correctly, proceed to Unit VII, page 203.
- If you do not answer all questions correctly, read and study the content of this unit.

QUESTIONS

1. Which of the following clinical signs and symptoms of maxillofacial swelling are considered swellings of non-microbial origin? *(circle correct answer(s))*
   - (a) Swelling in the area of the angle of the mandible within 24 hours following removal of an impacted mandibular third molar
   - (b) Growth of tissue around the border of a loose-fitting denture
   - (c) Swelling of the eyes of an allergic patient after exposure to a specific allergen
   - (d) Swelling of the palate which is of normal color when all maxillary teeth are vital and no sinus infection is present
   - e. Swelling of the submental space which developed 24 hours after endodontic treatment of an abscessed mandibular central incisor

2. Which of the following signs and/or symptoms are associated with neoplastic swellings?
   - a. shock
   - (b) normal vital signs
   - (c) hard, firm and indurated lesion
   - d. fractured teeth
   - (e) non-tender, enlarged lymph nodes

3. Which of the following statements describes the pathways for the spread of infection between soft tissue, periosteum, and hard tissue?
   - a. soft tissue infection —→ periosteum —→ hard tissue
   - b. hard tissue —→ periosteum —→ soft tissue
   - c. soft tissue —→ hard tissue (no periosteal involvement) —→ soft tissue —→ periosteum —→ hard tissue
   - d. hard tissue —→ soft tissue (no periosteal involvement)
   - (e) all of the above pathways can occur

4. Match the numbers corresponding to the routes of microbial invasion with the names of the infections given.
   - a. _1_ pericoronitis
   - b. _2_ periapical abscess
   - c. _3_ tuberculosis of the mandible
   - d. _1_ periodontal abscess
   - e. _4_ osteoradionecrosis
   - f. _5_ post-injection infection

   1. **growth in enclosed pouch**
   2. **invasion of dental pulp**
   3. **hematogenous spread**
   4. **breakdown of tissue defenses**
   5. **introduction of oral flora into deeper tissues**

5. Select the term on the right which matches the following statements:
   - a. _2_ firm, brawny, painful swelling with pus histologically present but not confined to a clinically distinct area
   - b. _3_ a diffuse inflammation of soft tissue which is free to spread to adjacent tissues
   - c. _4_ an opening in skin or mucosa through which pus may drain
   - d. _1_ presence of pus in a clinically distinct area

   1. **abscess**
   2. **infiltrate**
   3. **cellulitis**
   4. **fistula**

6. Name three (3) ways microorganisms can gain access to the potential space between periosteum and cortical bone.
   a. _needle track_
   b. _soft tissue extension_
   c. _hard tissue extension_

7. Fill in the missing words:
   Inflammation of periosteum causes dilation of blood vessels and a) _edema_ to accumulate between periosteum and cortical bone. As pressure increases, the periosteum is b) _suspended_ from cortical bone, which in turn activates c) _osteoblast_ to form new d) _bone_ along the inner side of the elevated periosteum. This can produce a radiographic appearance termed e) " _onion_ _peel_ " if the process is associated with f) _chronic_ inflammation.

8. We have established a category of "infections related to dental treatment. These infections can be classified as:
   a. odontogenic
   b. non-odontogenic
   c. either odontogenic or non-odontogenic

9. Match the numbered terms at the right with the following signs and symptoms.
   a. _2_ inflammatory response in bone which is similar to cellulitis
   b. _3_ death of bone with formation of sequestrum in a patient with no history of radiation therapy
   c. _1_ inflammation of the cortical bone lining a tooth socket following extraction
   d. _X 2_ inflammation of bone at the apex of a tooth in which an infection penetrates cortical bone and periosteum without marked alteration in the radiodensity of trabecular bone
   e. _4_ formation of sequestrum in the mandible of a patient who has received greater than 7,000 rads of x-ray irradiation

   1. alveolar osteitis
   2. osteitis
   3. osteomyelitis
   4. osteoradionecrosis

10. Match the following numbered terms with the statements below: 1) odontogenic infections. 2) non-odontogenic infections
    a. _1_ carious invasion of dental pulp followed by a soft tissue infection
    b. _1_ growth of microorganisms in the sulcus between soft tissue and the crown of a partially erupted tooth
    c. _2_ abscess of the tonsils
    d. _1_ infection involving the lining of the maxillary sinus with all teeth vital and no chronic periodontal abscess present
    e. _2_ infected hair follicle of the chin which is causing pain in mandibular anterior teeth
    f. _1_ bulging of the attached gingiva or alveolar mucosa caused by growth of an abscess in the periodontal pocket
    g. _2_ subperiosteal abscess resulting from entrapment of contaminated surgical debris under a full-thickness flap

11. Match the names of the soft tissue infections on the right with each of the following statements.
 a. ___2___ associated with partially erupted teeth
 b. ___3___ associated with pulpal necrosis
 c. ___4___ associated with infection of partial thickness flaps
 d. ___1___ associated with deep periodontal pockets and associated bone loss in furcation area
 e. ___3___ associated with loss of tooth vitality
 f. ___4___ associated with soft tissue infection which develops secondarily to extraction of a tooth which has a chronic periapical abscess
 g. ___5___ associated with an infection which develops 2-4 days following injection of local anesthetic.

 1. **periodontal abscess**
 2. **pericoronitis-pericoronal abscess**
 3. **dento-alveolar abscess**
 4. **post-surgical infection**
 5. **post-injection infection**

12. Match the name of the condition with each of the following statements:
 a. ___3___ results from loss of a normal blood clot from an extraction socket and inflammation of nerve endings
 b. ___2___ can lead to periostitis and deposition of new bone in an "onion-skin" appearance
 c. ___2___ can denude bone
 d. ___2___ may require surgical removal of sequestra and reconstructive surgery in non-irradiated patients
 e. ___2___ may cause paresthesia if nerve canals are involved
 f. ___3___ halitosis, dull pain and history of recent third molar extraction are present
 g. _1 2_ may cause demineralization of bone without sequestra and upon resolution, may have an area of increased radiodensity.

 1. **osteitis**
 2. **osteomyelitis**
 3. **acute alveolar osteitis**

13. Match the names of the conditions involving periosteum on the right with each of the following statements:
 a. ___1___ deposition of new bone giving "onion-skin" appearance on radiographs (chronic inflammation)
 b. ___1___ implies inflammation and edema of periosteum
 c. _1 2_ implies presence of pus between periosteum and cortical bone
 d. _3 2_ generally results from inadequate irrigation of full thickness flaps
 e. _2 3_ can result from injection of microorganisms between periosteum and cortical bone

 1. **periostitis**
 2. **subperiosteal abscess**
 3. **post-injection, subperiosteal abscess**

14. Which of the following sign and symptom complex names are classified in this book as infections of special significance?
 a. acute alveolar osteitis
 b. acute dento-alveolar abscess
 c. Ludwig's angina
 d. acute cellulitis
 e. acute pericoronitis
 f. osteoradionecrosis
 g. acute periodontal abscess
 h. cavernous sinus thrombosis

15. Match the sign and symptom complexes for non-dentally related infections on the right with the correct statements below (choices may be made more than once).

a. _3_ pus visible at duct opening

b. _2_ can produce dysphagia, speech changes and uvular edema

c. _3_ pain increases at mealtime

d. _3 3_ preauricular swelling

e. _1_ may cause pain in teeth

f. _4_ immediate pain elicited by pulling on pinna

g. _1_ pain in vital maxillary posterior teeth

1. **non-dental maxillary sinusitis**
2. **peritonsillar abscess**
3. **salivary gland infection**
4. **ear infection**
5. **superficial skin infection**
6. **superficial mucosal infection**

For each of the clinical conditions described in Questions 16-20,
   a. Give the **name** applied to this collection of signs and symptoms.
   b. Briefly **describe** the pathological process for this condition.

16. **Case description:** This 23-year-old male complains of acute pain in the area behind his right mandibular molar teeth. He says this condition has occurred before, but was not as serious as it is now. He reports no trismus, but does have some pain on swallowing. Vital signs are normal except for a slight rise in temperature.

a. **Name:** _Pericoronitis_   b. **Pathogenesis:** _____
periodontal pockets creating a nedus for food
& bacteria to collect. Causing inflammation

17. **Case description:** This 55-year-old female previously had all of her teeth removed before receiving 8,000 rads of radiation to her lower jaw area during therapy for a sublingual squamous cell carcinoma. She has worn a lower denture for 6 years, but has had trouble with small "denture sores" for some time. Presently she complains of dull, constant pain under her denture. Clinical examination of her present condition revealed exposed necrotic bone in the anterior region of the mandible. Radiographs reveal presence of sequestrae in the anterior area of the mandible.

a. **Name:** _Osteoradionecrosis_   b. **Pathogenesis:** _____
Radiation decrease patient ability to fight infection
hence trauma & infections go unchecked & cause
necrosis of bone.

18. **Case description:** *This 30-year-old female has a 9 mm periodontal pocket on the buccal side of her right maxillary second premolar. Vital signs are normal. All teeth are vital, and she has no history of trauma in this area. Probing of the pocket produced profuse bleeding and pus.*

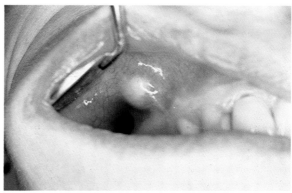

a. **Name:** *Acute Periodontal Abcess*   b. **Pathogenesis:** *Large pocket created by bacteria causing inflammation forming an abscess*

19. **Case description:** *This 26-year-old female had been to an emergency dental clinic five days ago where the dentist repaired broken fillings in her mandibular right 2nd premolar and first molar with zinc oxide cement. Since that time, swelling of the lingual tissue, buccal vestibule, and buccal fascial space have developed. Both the second premolar and molar are now non-vital, sensitive to palpation, percussion, and are extremely mobile. She has some pain on swallowing and the facial swelling is also painful. Periapical radiographs show extensive coronal caries in these two teeth, but only slight disruption of the lamina dura and enlargement of the periodontal ligament space near the apex of the premolar and distal root of the first molar.*

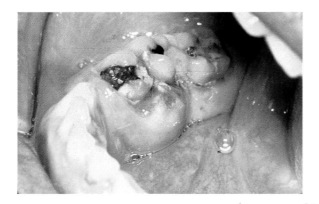 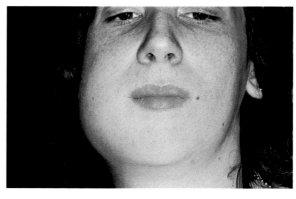

a. **Name:** *Acute Periapical Alveolar Abcess*   b. **Pathogenesis:** *Infection originated in pulp & worked itself through bone to soft tissues*

POST-TEST ANSWERS

1. a, b, c, d

2. b, c, e

3. e

4. a = 1, b = 2, c = 3, d = 1, e = 4, f = 5

5. a = 2, b = 3, c = 4, d = 1

6. Any three (3) of the following routes may be given, and any order is acceptable.
  - *extension of a soft tissue infection*
  - *extension from hard tissue through cortical bone*
  - *direct deposition of microorganisms below full thickness flaps*
  - *direct deposition of microorganisms along a needle track*

7. a. edema (pus is not correct)   d. bone
  b. elevated or detached   e. "onion-skin"
  c. osteoblasts   f. chronic

8. c

9. a = 2, b = 3, c = 1, d = 2, e = 4

10. a = 1, b = 1, c = 2, d = 2, e = 2, f = 1, g = 2

11. a = 2, b = 3, c = 4, d = 1, e = 3, f = 4, g = 5

12. a = 3, b = 2, c = 2, d = 2, e = 2, f = 3, g = 1

13. a = 1, b = 1, c = 2, d = 2, e = 3

14. c, d, f, h

15. a = 3, b = 2, c = 3, d = 3, 4, e = 1, f = 4, g = 1

*16. a. **Name:** Pericoronitis (pericoronal abscess).*
    *b. **Pathogenesis:** This condition is initiated by microbial growth in the space surrounding the crown of a partially erupted tooth (usually partially impacted mandibular third molars). Regional inflammation (acute or chronic) can result. If microorganisms invade the tissue, this infection may spread to adjacent facial spaces or the bloodstream (see page 176-177 for more details).*

*17. a. **Name:** Osteoradionecrosis.*
    *b. **Pathogenesis:** Previous irradiation of the oral region reduces the defense mechanisms of local tissues (both soft tissue and bone) to microbial invasion, thus allowing an infection to involve adjacent areas (see page 195 for more details).*

*18. a. **Name:** Acute periodontal abscess.*
    *b. **Pathogenesis:** Growth of microorganisms in deep periodontal pockets can result in the invasion of mucosal soft tissues. In this instance, microorganisms from the deep buccal sulcus have invaded the soft tissue of the maxillary buccal vestibule and the infection has become localized in this location. These infections may, however, spread to adjacent fascial spaces and/or enter the bloodstream and cause systemic involvement (see pages 174-175 for additional details).*

*19. a. **Name:** Acute periapical alveolar abscess.*
    *b. **Pathogenesis:** Infections originating in a dental pulp can exit the tooth through a root canal (usually the periapical canal(s)), rapidly penetrate trabecular (medullary) and cortical bone, periosteum and involve surrounding soft tissues (see pages 178-179 for additional details). In this case, the infection has produced swelling of both buccal and lingual soft tissues and has also spread to involve the buccal fascial space.*

UNIT VII
DIAGNOSTIC DECISIONS

OVERVIEW AND OBJECTIVES

The purpose of this unit is to review the process for diagnosing the cause and degree of seriousness for oral and maxillofacial infections. We first present a review of terminology, then review the relationships between an initial and definitive diagnosis. A **checklist for diagnostic decisions** is presented to assist you with the diagnostic process. The **first step** in diagnosis is to **summarize relevant patient problems. Next,** initial determination is made as to the microbial or non-microbial origin of the underlying pathological process followed by a refinement of causes until the etiology of the microbial problem is identified and a determination is made as to whether the problem is chronic, acute, or dangerously acute. An evaluation of **modifying factors** will allow you to generalize the overall seriousness of the infection. An **initial diagnosis** of the problem and degree of risk can then be made. You can then decide to treat the problem yourself, refer, and/or obtain additional data. The process for obtaining a **definitive diagnosis** is discussed including evaluation of laboratory and clinical data and you can again decide to treat, refer, and/or obtain additional data. Following completion of this unit you will:

1. Describe why the establishment of a diagnosis (either initial or definitive) is an essential step in the overall management of infections including five (5) ways the diagnostic process can be of assistance in data organization, identification of etiology, and planning management.

2. Describe the importance of an **initial** and **definitive** diagnosis in the management of oral infections.

3. Describe why the process to obtain a definitive diagnosis should be initiated simultaneously with development of an initial diagnosis when managing moderate to serious infections.

4. Given a complete description of patient data or a list of problems for an oral and/or maxillofacial swelling, correctly follow the decision process to obtain an **initial diagnosis** of the problem. Included in this objective process is your ability to **defend your choice at each branch** by summarizing the signs and symptoms which are consistent with your choice. In addition, you should also be able to list those signs or symptoms which are not consistent with your choice and state what should be done for these.

5. Given a description of initial patient data, determine the effect of a **patient's overall health**; the **anatomical location** of the problem; and the **microbial factors** on the **overall risk** or seriousness of the infection.

6. For any given infection, state the etiology and modifying factors.

7. Given a description of laboratory, clinical, radiographic, and historical data for an oral infection, **obtain a definitive diagnosis** for the problem.

8. Describe how your **course of action** may be changed as a result of obtaining a definitive diagnosis for an oral and/or maxillofacial infection.

Unit VII
DIAGNOSTIC DECISIONS

INTRODUCTION

A **diagnosis** is a systematic process for determining the nature of a disease process. The following terminology is often used when referring to a diagnosis or the diagnostic process:

- **Clinical diagnosis** — A diagnosis based upon the clinical signs and symptoms of a disease.
- **Confirming Diagnosis** — A definitive diagnosis made after the disease has been resolved through initial treatment.
- **Definitive Diagnosis** — A diagnosis based upon direct clinical data and supporting laboratory and/or radiographic data.
- **Differential Diagnosis** — A diagnosis made by distinguishing between two or more diseases with similar signs and symptoms.
- **Initial Diagnosis** — A diagnosis based upon data derived from the initial clinical and radiographic examination of the patient.
- **Laboratory Diagnosis** — A diagnosis established through chemical, microscopic, microbiologic, or histologic study of blood, tissue, secretions or discharges obtained from a disease.
- **Physical Diagnosis** — A diagnosis based upon data obtained from patient examination using physical measures such as palpation, percussion, auscultation, and inspection.

INITIAL AND DEFINITIVE DIAGNOSIS

The development of a **diagnosis** (either initial or definitive) is an essential step in the overall management of any oral and/or maxillofacial swelling. Through the process of diagnosis you will collect and organize relevant historical, clinical, radiographic and laboratory data in order to:

- develop a list of problems related to the swelling
- identify the etiology or cause of the swelling
- identify the presence of modifying factors which can affect the management of the problems
- develop an initial diagnosis as a basis for initial management (treatment) decisions
- develop a definitive diagnosis as a basis for definitive management (treatment) decisions

The initial diagnosis is a diagnosis based upon your patient's chief complaint, historical data, initial clinical evaluation, initial radiographic data, and initial laboratory data. It is your best **first assessment** of the cause of a patient's problem and forms the basis for initial treatment decisions and/or your decision to refer. An initial diagnosis is not usually derived from laboratory data, additional radiographic data, or any other data that would require significant time to obtain. At this stage your **goal is to treat the most immediate problems** with treatment methods which will **most likely** control the problems. Your initial diagnosis is only as good as the data initially obtained. Occasionally, oral and maxillofacial infections will not respond favorably to treatment which is based upon your initial diagnosis and you must review your diagnostic process and possibly collect additional data. In other instances, you will know that additional diagnostic data will be necessary but you **must institute treatment before this information can be obtained**.

The **definitive diagnosis** is a more refined diagnosis derived from analysis of your initial clinical data, any additional data (laboratory, radiographic), and frequently includes analysis of the results of initial treatment. While initial diagnosis and treatment is based on speculations as to the causative microorganisms and/or effects on the host, definitive diagnosis is based on specific data (e.g. species identification, antibiotic susceptibility).

While the **initial** and **definitive diagnoses** can be linked processes, in clinical practice often they are not. If you **do not obtain** specimens for laboratory analysis during inital data collection then you must collect specimens at a later date and **postpone definitive diagnosis and treatment** until laboratory analysis can be completed. Thus, in order to reach a definitive diagnosis you must begin the diagnostic process again and wait 2-14 days for culture and antibiotic susceptibility (C & S) results before beginning definitive treatment. If, however, you collect specimens for laboratory analysis as part of your initial data collection process, the results will then be available when needed and a **smooth transition can be made from initial to definitive treatment.**

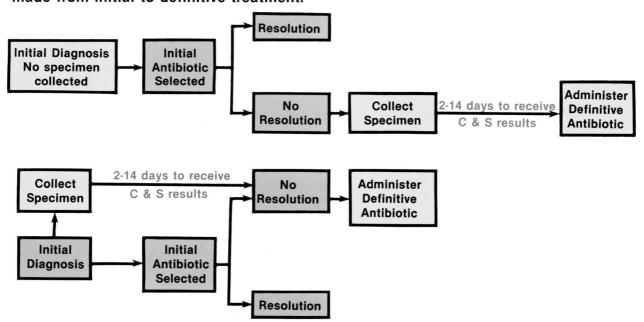

Figure VII-1. Obtaining specimens for laboratory study during initial data collection will enable you to proceed with definitive diagnosis and treatment if initial treatment is unsuccessful.

NOTE: With acute infections, failure to obtain a specimen for microbiological analysis during your initial data collection process can result in a 2- to 14-day delay in administration of definitive treatment (definitive antibiotic) when initial treatment fails to resolve the infection. This time period is also the time period during which patients with acute infections are in the most danger.

DIAGNOSTIC DECISIONS

Once you have collected historical, clinical, radiographic, and laboratory data you are ready to begin the diagnostic process. To assist you in diagnosing the cause of an oral and/or maxillofacial swelling we have developed the **diagnostic decisions checklist.**

DIAGNOSTIC DECISIONS

SUMMARY OF PATIENT'S PROBLEMS

1. _____   6. _____   11. _____
2. _____   7. _____   12. _____
3. _____   8. _____   13. _____
4. _____   9. _____   14. _____
5. _____   10. _____   15. _____

PROCESS FOR INITIAL DIAGNOSIS

Problem is . . . . ☐ Microbial   ☐ Non-Microbial   ☐ Unknown_____

Source of Infection is . . ☐ Odontogenic   ☐ Non-odontogenic   ☐ From Dental Tx   ☐ Unknown _____

Soft Tissue (dentally related)	Periosteum	Special sigificance	Soft tissue (non-dental)
☐ Periodontal Abscess	☐ Subperiosteal abscess	☐ Acute cellulitis	☐ Maxillary sinusitis
☐ Pericoronal Abscess	☐ Post-Injection	☐ Ludwig's angina	☐ Peritonsillar abscess
☐ Dento-Alveolar Abscess	☐ Periostitis	☐ Osteo-	☐ Salivary gland infection
☐ Post-surgical Infection	**Hard Tissue**	radionecrosis	☐ Ear infection
☐ Post-injection Infection	☐ Acute alveolar osteitis	☐ Cavernous sinus	☐ Superficial skin infection
☐ Maxillary Sinusitis	(dry socket)	thrombosis	☐ Superficial mucosal infection
☐ Other _____	☐ Osteitis		☐ Other _____
_____	☐ Osteomyelitis		
	☐ Osteoradionecrosis		

Progress of Infection is . ☐ Chronic (slow)   ☐ Acute (rapid)   ☐ Dangerously Acute (fulminating) _____

EVALUATION OF MODIFYING FACTORS

Patient's Health	Anatomical Factors	Microbial Factors	
☐ Serious medical risk	☐ High risk space(s)	☐ Acute cellulitis	☐ Culture indicated but
☐ Moderate medical risk	☐ Multiple spaces (bi)	☐ Systemic toxicity	not taken
☐ Low medical risk	☐ Involves adjacent areas	☐ Extreme swelling	☐ No Gram stain
☐ No medical risk	but controllable	☑ Fever	☐ Culture taken
Why? _____	☐ Confined to alveolar ridge	☐ Chronic infection	☐ Gram stain obtained
_____	Where?_____	☐ Recent antibiotic	☐ Culture not indicated
	_____	☐ Poor O.H./perio disease	Other _____

INITIAL DIAGNOSIS: _____

_____

_____

INITIAL COURSE OF ACTION

☐ Treat in office   ☐ Refer to a specialist   ☐ Hospitalize. Who/Where? _____

☐ Need additional data. What data? _____

PROCESS FOR DEFINITIVE DIAGNOSIS

Summary of Laboratory Data

MICROBIOLOGY LAB	HEMATOLOGY LAB	HISTOPATHOLOGY LAB
☐ Single species ☐ Mixed ☐ None	☐ WBC count _____	Tissue specimen analysis _____
Predominant species: _____	☐ WBC Differential:	_____
_____	Polys ___% Eosinophils ___%	_____
☐ Aerobic ☐ Anaerobic	Lymphocytes___% Basophils ___%	_____
Antibiotic Sensitivity:	Monocytes ___% Immature? ___	_____
1st choice _____	ESR_____mm/hr	_____
2nd choice _____	Blood Culture _____	_____
3rd choice _____	_____	_____

DEFINITIVE DIAGNOSIS

☐ Agrees/Consistent with initial diagnosis

☐ Differs from initial diagnosis _____

_____

DEFINITIVE COURSE OF ACTION

☐ Treat in office   ☐ Refer to a specialist   ☐ Hospitalize. Who/Where? _____

☐ Need additional data. What data? _____

NOTE: **The diagnostic decisions checklist was designed to lead you to a DIAGNOSIS of dentally related swellings and to lead you to a DIFFERENTIAL DIAGNOSIS of non-dentally related swellings. You should seek additional references for assistance in diagnosing non-dentally related swellings or REFER patients with these problems to a specialist.**

STUDY EXERCISES

Developing a diagnosis is an essential step in the overall management of any oral and/or maxillofacial swelling. This process will guide you in:
- *developing a ___list___ of problems associated with a patient's problem.*
- *identifying the ___etiology___ or ___cause___ of the problem.*
- *identifying the presence of ___modifying___ ___factors___ which can influence your management decisions.*
- *developing an ___initial___ diagnosis as a basis for ___initial___ treatment.*
- *developing a ___definitive___ diagnosis as a basis for ___definitive___ treatment.*

Your goal for developing an initial diagnosis is to gather enough data to begin appropriate ___treatment___ or refer your patient to a specialist. Generally you (will/will not) ___will not___ have information as to the identity of the causative ___causes___ (s) and your selection of treatment methods will be based upon general ___treatment___ methods that will most likely control the problem.

A definitive diagnosis is obtained at a ___later___ time once laboratory results have been ___obtained___ and the results of initial ___treatment___, and additional ___data___ have been assessed.

With acute infections, ___failure___ to obtain a specimen for microbiological analysis during your ___initial___ data collection process can result in a ___2___ to ___14___ day ___delay___ in obtaining a ___definitive___ diagnosis and selecting a definitive ___tx plan___ if initial treatment methods are unsuccessful. This time delay is also the time period when patients with serious infections are in the most ___danger___.

Summarizing Patient Problems

The **initial** step in diagnosing the cause of an oral and/or maxillofacial swelling is to summarize all of your patient's problems that relate to the pathological process including relevant **historical data, clinical signs and symptoms, anatomical location and involved tissues, radiographic data** and **any available laboratory data.** This initial **problem list** is essential for establishing whether your patient has an infection or whether a non-microbial cause is involved. In addition, this problem list will often enable you to determine whether an infection is **odontogenic** (related to teeth or tooth structure), **dentally related** (infection related to previous dental treatment), or is **non-odontogenic** (does not originate from teeth or tooth-related structures). The summary of patient problems should also enable you to identify the specific etiology of the problem and factors which would influence the overall degree of seriousness of the problem. **If insufficient data has been collected to make these decisions, then additional data should be collected.** We have provided the following space on the **diagnostic decisions checklist** for recording patient problems useful in your diagnostic decisions.

Determining the Etiology

Determining the cause of oral and/or maxillofacial swellings with initial data only can be somewhat confusing and you may prematurely arrive at an initial diagnosis which later proves incorrect. The following section will provide you with a systematic method for determining the cause or etiology of oral and/or maxillofacial swellings from the list of problems. Whether or not the diagnosis is an **initial diagnosis** or **definitive diagnosis** will depend upon the completeness of available data. **Figure VII-2** summarizes the decision process used to establish an initial diagnosis which can be refined to a definitive diagnosis if necessary.

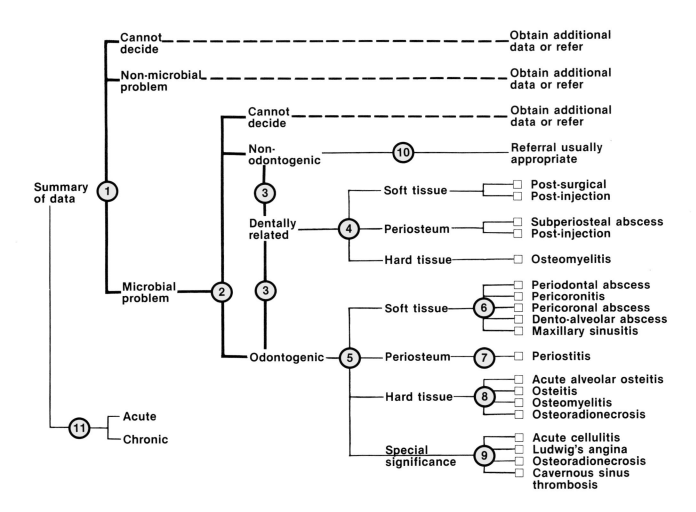

Figure VII-2. Summary of the decision process for establishing a diagnosis for oral and/or maxillofacial swellings. The numbered and circled decision points in the diagram are explained in the text.

NOTE: The criteria provided here are intended as GENERAL GUIDELINES and MAY NOT APPLY in all clinical situations. Extensive training and clinical experience is required in order to diagnose the cause of many oral and/or maxillofacial swellings. The danger associated with this approach is that it may oversimplify the diagnostic process and misdirect your treatment. If you feel the least bit uncomfortable with your diagnosis you should refer the case to a specialist.

① Is the origin of the problem microbial or non-microbial?

After summarizing all available data, your first step in the process of obtaining an initial diagnosis is **to determine if the swelling (problem) is of microbial origin.** A summary of signs and symptoms for non-microbial and microbial problems is provided in **Figure VII-3.**
- If **ALL** signs and symptoms fall into one category then your decision is obvious.
- If **some** are signs and symptoms of both categories then you must either obtain more data or refer your patient to a specialist.

NOTE: Never overlook the possibility that a non-microbial problem has become secondarily infected and that both categories are present. For example:
- Fractures can be contaminated with oral flora and thus allow soft tissue and/or hard tissue infections to develop.
- Neoplastic lesions may become secondarily infected by oral flora.

SIGNS AND SYMPTOMS OF NON-MICROBIAL AND MICROBIAL ORAL AND/OR MAXILLOFACIAL SWELLINGS

SWELLINGS OF NON-MICROBIAL ORIGIN

Trauma	Neoplastic Swellings	Developmental Swellings
• History of recent trauma • Bruising, ecchymosis, hematoma • Swelling tender to palpation • Fractured teeth, bone • Active bleeding • Malocclusion • Absence of transmitted mobility • Loss of function of mandible • Paresthesia • Shock • Little change in vital signs • Other major trauma	• Slower growing • Absence of inflammation (unless secondary infection) • Hard, firm, indurated • Minimal edema • Normal vital signs • Paresthesia (intrabony) • Ulcers or open lesions with minimal inflammation • Non-tender enlarged lymph nodes (may have slight tenderness)	• Congenital abnormalities • Process associated with growth & maturation • No signs of inflammation • No changes in vital signs **Autoimmune Diseases** • Allergic related angioedema • Usually no changes in vital signs except tachycardia with allergic reactions

SWELLINGS OF MICROBIAL ORIGIN

• Signs of inflammation • History of toothache, caries, periodontal disease • Partially erupted teeth • Hyperocclusion (isolated teeth) • Changes in vital signs (increased temperature) • Trismus	• Dysphagia • Systemic toxicity • Toxic shock syndrome • Aspiration of pus • Fluctuance in swelling • Isolation of microbes in sufficient numbers • Tender enlarged lymph nodes	• Radiographic lesions associated with teeth or tooth-related structures • Respiratory obstruction • History of needle puncture • Recent dental treatment • Pain • Tenderness to palpation

Figure VII-3. Major signs and symptoms or problems associated with non-infectious and infectious swellings of the head and neck.

After making this decision, you should check the appropriate box on the diagnostic decisions checklist indicating you **initially** believe a patient's problem to be of microbial or non-microbial origin. **If you believe both etiologies are present check both.** In this situation **additional data** may be needed or **refer** your patient to a specialist. If the cause is still **unknown**, again either **obtain more data** or **refer** your patient to a specialist. Remember, this first decision is based upon your initial data only and that re-evaluation of your first choice may be necessary once additional laboratory and/or clinical data is obtained.

② **Is the microbial problem (infection) of odontogenic or non-odontogenic origin?**

Assuming a microbial origin for a problem, the next step is to decide whether or not the problem is related to teeth or tooth-related structures. If you **erroneously** conclude an infection to be of odontogenic origin you may be led into unnecessary dental treatment (e.g. endodontic treatment, tooth extraction, or other surgery) while leaving the true source of the infection to progress untreated.

An intermediate category of **infections resulting from dental treatment** lies between the truly odontogenic and truly non-odontogenic infections. These will be discussed in ③.

NOTE: Generally the treatment of non-odontogenic infections is beyond the scope of general dentistry and most non-odontogenic infections should be referred to the appropriate specialist.

SIGNS AND SYMPTOMS OF ODONTOGENIC AND NON-ODONTOGENIC SWELLINGS

NON-ODONTOGENIC	ODONTOGENIC
• Infection NOT related to teeth or tooth-supporting structures	• Infection related to teeth or tooth-supporting structures
• Vital teeth (no pathology associated with endodontically treated teeth)	• May have non-vital teeth, periodontal disease or large carious lesions
• Radiographic signs not directly associated with teeth	• Radiographic signs associated with tooth or tooth-related structures
• Culture obtained from soft tissue without signs of tooth involvement	• Culture obtained from teeth or tooth-related structures
• Evidence of involvement of salivary glands, eyes, ears	• Maxillary sinusitis associated with problems with maxillary posterior teeth
• Maxillary sinusitis without tooth-related signs and symptoms	• History of recent dental treatment or surgery
• Dermatologic problems	• Evidence of dentally related trauma

Figure VII-4. Summary of signs and symptoms and/or problems associated with non-odontogenic and odontogenic oral and/or maxillofacial infections.

③ **Is the infection related to dental treatment?**

As briefly mentioned above, infections may develop as a result of dental treatment. While these infections do not fit the strict definition of odontogenic infections, they are associated with treatment of odontogenic problems and are thus considered dentally related **iatrogenic infections**. Iatrogenic infections are technically of non-odontogenic origin. Thus we have provided two routes of the diagnostic decision tree leading to infections resulting from dental treatment (see **Figure VII-2**).

SOME EXAMPLES OF INFECTIONS RESULTING FROM DENTAL TREATMENT

POST-SURGICAL INFECTIONS	**ACCIDENTAL INTRODUCTION OF MICROBES INTO TISSUE WHEN PERFORMING OTHER DENTAL TREATMENT**
• Soft tissue infections	
• Maxillary sinus infections from oro-antral openings or displaced root tips	• Dento-alveolar abscess following endodontic treatment
• Subperiosteal abscesses from surgical debris	• Infections which develop following subgingival procedures (e.g. curettage, tissue packing for impressions, etc.)
• Osteomyelitis, osteitis	
• Suture tract infections (suture abscess)	
POST-INJECTION INFECTIONS	
• Subperiosteal infections	**INFECTIONS FOLLOWING USE OF UNSTERILE INSTRUMENTS OR POOR ASEPTIC TECHNIQUE**
• Soft tissue infections	
• Fascial space infections	

NOTE: This list was not intended to be all inclusive.

Figure VII-5. Some examples of iatrogenic infections which may result from dental treatment.

④   **What is the etiology of the infection related to dental treatment?**

NOTE: **Dentists must be able to identify and appropriately manage infections which may result from their treatment of a patient's dental problems.**

Signs and Symptoms

The signs and symptoms of infections related to dental treatment can vary with the location of the problem and, in most cases, are similar to odontogenic infections of the areas involved. The key to diagnosing dental treatment infections includes:

- A recent history of intra-oral surgery (e.g. tooth extractions, endodontic or periodontic surgery, etc.).
- A recent history of other dental procedures (e.g. anesthetic injection, aspiration of lesions, endodontic treatment, subgingival procedures, etc.).

SIGNS AND SYMPTOMS OF INFECTIONS RELATED TO DENTAL TREATMENT

MAXILLARY SINUS	POST INJECTION	POST SURGICAL	OTHER
• History of maxillary posterior tooth extraction with oro-antral communication • Radiographic evidence of maxillary root tip located in the sinus	• Recent history of local anesthetic injection or attempts to culture from a swelling • Soft tissue infection adjacent to oral cavity with no apparent odontogenic cause	• Recent history of surgical flap reflection • Soft tissue infection in surgical area	• Soft tissue infection following other dental procedures such as tissue packing, sulcular curettage, or impression procedures • Endodontic therapy

Figure VII-6. Summary of the signs and symptoms or problems associated with the various types of dentally related non-odontogenic infections.

Following your diagnostic decisions for ② and ③ you should record your decision on the checklist. If source is unknown, collect more data or refer to a specialist.

STUDY EXERCISES

Based on data from the following summary of patient problems, complete the first two steps of the diagnostic process and explain the basis for your choices.

Case #1

SUMMARY OF PATIENT'S PROBLEMS
1. *Hist. of toothache mand. (R) c.I.*
2. *Poor nutrition*
3. *Excessive alcohol consumption*
* 4. *Penicillin Allergy*
5. *Lives alone in 1 Room hotel*
6. *Temp = 102°F*
7. *Fluctuant (R) Submental swelling*
8. *Red & Tender (R) Submandib. area*
9. *Radiolucency Apex mand (R) c.I.*
10. *Dysphagia*
11. *Dyspepsia*
12. *WBC = 18,000*
13. *Pus aspirated*
14. *Gram stain 4+ cocci*
15. *No c&s data*

PROCESS FOR INITIAL DIAGNOSIS
Problem is .... ☒ Microbial   ☐ Non-Microbial   ☐ Unknown_____
Source of Infection is .. ☒ Odontogenic   ☐ Non-odontogenic   ☐ From Dental Tx   ☐ Unknown _____
What data supports this choice? _____history of toothache___ + gram stain___

Case #2

SUMMARY OF PATIENT'S PROBLEMS
1. *Swelling in Submandib. area*
2. *Normal temperature of skin*
3. *No dysphagia*
4. *No redness*
5. *Temp = 97.2°F*
6. *indurated swelling - non fluct.*
7. *Dyspepsia*
8. *oral exam - Normal*
9. *Enlarged lymph nodes Area #3*
10. *WBC = 6,800*
11. *Recent weight loss*
12. *Radiographs - Neg.*
13. *Aspiration - Neg.*
14. *cachetic appearance*
15.

PROCESS FOR INITIAL DIAGNOSIS
Problem is .... ☐ Microbial   ☒ Non-Microbial   ☐ Unknown_____
Source of Infection is .. ☐ Odontogenic   ☒ Non-odontogenic   ☐ From Dental Tx   ☐ Unknown _____
What data supports this choice? ___WBC, temp, atp. weight___

Discussion of Cases

Case #1

PROCESS FOR INITIAL DIAGNOSIS
    Problem is .... ☑ Microbial   ☐ Non-Microbial   ☐ Unknown_____
    Source of Infection is .. ☑ Odontogenic   ☐ Non-odontogenic   ☐ From Dental Tx   ☐ Unknown _____

This case clearly falls into a microbial infection because of Temp. = 102°F, fluctuant swelling, redness, tender, W.B.C. = 18,000, suppuration present with positive Gram stain for bacteria. In addition, the evidence strongly suggests an association between the mandibular left central incisor and the submental swelling, radiolucency, history of toothache in the mandibular left central incisor.

Case #2

PROCESS FOR INITIAL DIAGNOSIS
    Problem is .... ☐ Microbial   ☑ Non-Microbial   ☑ Unknown_____
    Source of Infection is .. ☐ Odontogenic   ☑ Non-odontogenic   ☐ From Dental Tx   ☑ Unknown _____

There is no evidence to suggest a microbial etiology for the submandibular swelling. In addition, there is no evidence for odontogenic cause of swelling, i.e. normal oral exam, no radiographic evidence, normal W.B.C., neg. aspiration. The clinician, however, should be suspecting a neoplastic condition or possible salivary gland pathology.

⑤   What is the general classification of the odontogenic infection?

As discussed in Unit VI, the commonly seen odontogenic infections are classified into the categories of **soft tissue, periosteum, hard tissue,** and problems of **special significance.** The signs and symptoms or problems used for this classification are summarized in **Figure VII-7.**

**SIGNS AND SYMPTOMS USED
TO CATEGORIZE TISSUES INVOLVED**

SOFT TISSUE	PERIOSTEUM	HARD TISSUE	SPECIAL SIGNIFICANCE
• Soft tissue inflammation	• Dull pain	• Radiographic changes	• See Ludwig's angina
• Trismus	• Firm, indurated swelling	• Exposed bone	• See acute cellulitis
• Cellulitis	• Subperiosteal bone formation	• Dull pain	• See osteoradio-necrosis
• Redness	• Subperiosteal radiolucent space	• Sequestra formation	• See cavernous sinus thrombosis
• Increased temperature		• Bone loss	
• Swelling		• Pathologic fracture	

Figure VII-7. Summary of signs and symptoms or problems
used to categorize various tissues involved.

Once an odontogenic infection is placed into the general classification, you must then determine the specific etiology of the infection. Decision points ⑥, ⑦, and ⑧ provide criteria for making these decisions.

NOTE: It is possible to have signs and symptoms of soft tissue, periosteum, hard tissue and special infections present simultaneously. Your diagnosis must reflect multiple involvement and your management of the infection should involve the management of all associated signs and symptoms.

STUDY EXERCISE

How would the following summary of patient's problems (signs and symptoms) be categorized? Support your answer by writing the problem number in the supporting evidence section.

SUMMARY OF PATIENT'S PROBLEMS

1. Toothache - max ⓡ 2nd premolar
2. on tetracycline for acne
3. toxic appearance
4. Dehydration
5. Temp = 102° F
6. Fluctuant ⓛ Buccal space swelling
7. moderate trismus
8. Radiolucency Apex max ⓡ 2nd p.m.
9. WBC = 14,000 w/ shift to left.
10. fluid in ⓡ max sin. antrum
11. Dull Pain ⓡ post max area
12. Gram stain = ++++ cocci
13. subperiosteal bone formation
14. max ⓡ 2nd p.m. Non-vital
15. _____

Problem is:
- ☒ Microbial
- ☐ Non-microbial
- ☐ Both
- ☐ Unknown

Supporting evidence:
Lab results - Gram Stain
Temp

Source is:
- ☒ Odontogenic
- ☐ Non-odontogenic
- ☐ Related to dental treatment
- ☐ Unknown

Supporting evidence:
Toothache

Infection involves:
- ☒ Soft tissue
- ☒ Periosteum
- ☐ Hard tissue
- ☐ "Special"

Supporting evidence:
trismus , ⓑ space swelling
Subperiosteal bone formation

ANSWER

Problem is:
- ✔ Microbial
- ☐ Non-microbial
- ☐ Both
- ☐ Unknown

Supporting evidence:
Temp. = 102° F
WBC = 14,000
Gram stain Positive for bacteria
Fluctuance , Toxic appearance

Source is:
- ✔ Odontogenic
- ☐ Non-odontogenic
- ☐ Related to dental treatment
- ☐ Unknown

Supporting evidence:
toothache and non-vital max ⓡ 2nd p.m.
Buccal swelling & Radiolucency @ apex max ⓡ 2nd p.m.

Infection involves:
- ✔ Soft tissue
- ✔ Periosteum
- ☐ Hard tissue
- ☐ "Special"

Supporting evidence:
Soft tissue swelling - buccal space
Subperiosteal bone formation
No evidence of bone changes in maxillary bone

⑥ What is the etiology of odontogenic soft tissue infections?

The etiologies for soft tissue infections are summarized from the diagnostic checklist form as shown by the insert to the right.

Soft Tissue (dentally related)
☐ Periodontal Abscess
☐ Pericoronal Abscess
☐ Dento-Alveolar Abscess
☐ Post-surgical Infection
☐ Post-injection Infection
☐ Maxillary Sinusitis
☐ Other _____
_____

NOTE: We have also included the dentally related non-odontogenic soft tissue infections in this list. Diagnostic criteria have already been given for the dentally related non-odontogenic etiologies and will not be repeated here.

SIGNS AND SYMPTOMS OF
ODONTOGENIC SOFT TISSUE INFECTIONS

PERIODONTAL ABSCESS	PERICORONITIS	PERIAPICAL ABSCESS
• Deep pockets • Gingivae red and swollen • Pus on pocket probing • Pain localized to gingiva • Swelling usually localized to alveolar ridge or vestibule • Radiographs may or may not show bony defects	• Presence of partially erupted tooth (usually mandibular third molar) • Redness of pericoronal tissue • Swelling of anterior pillar or fascial space involvement • Suppuration may exude from around the tooth • Fetor oris • Dysphagia • Trismus • Bone loss due to chronic infection	• Continuous pain • Pain to heat and cold • Percussion sensitivity • Increased mobility • Pain on palpation • Extrusion of tooth from socket • Purulence in the sulcus with a narrow deep defect • Non-vital tooth or root of a multirooted tooth • Bone loss around root apex • Loss of PDL and lamina dura continuity • Condensing osteitis near root apex • Intraoral or extraoral sinus tract stoma • Deep sinus tract probing in periodontal ligament space

Figure VII-8. Summary of signs and symptoms or problems associated with odontogenic soft tissue infections.

⑦ What is the etiology of periosteal infections?

Infections involving the periosteum can originate from soft tissue or hard tissue infections or from entrapment of surgical debris under full-thickness flaps and subperiosteal injections.

Periosteum
☐ Subperiosteal abscess
☐ Post-Injection
☐ Periostitis

- **Subperiosteal abscesses** usually have a history of full-thickness flap surgery but can also have a history of subperiosteal injections. Pus can frequently be aspirated from these infections.
- **Post-injection** infections of the periosteum have a histoy of subperiosteal injections.
- **Periostitis** usually involves "onion skin" deposition of bone. A history of chronic bone infection is usually associated. Usually pus cannot be aspirated from these lesions.

⑧   What is the etiology of odontogenic hard tissue infections?

Hard tissue odontogenic infections are classified as shown in the insert to the right. **Figure VII-9** summarizes the signs and symptoms or problems associated with the types of hard tissue infections.

Hard Tissue
☐ Acute alveolar osteitis (dry socket)
☐ Osteitis
☐ Osteomyelitis
☐ Osteoradionecrosis

SIGNS AND SYMPTOMS OF HARD TISSUE INFECTIONS

ACUTE ALVEOLAR OSTEITIS
- **Recent history of tooth extraction (especially mandibular third molars)**
- **Dull aching pain**
- **Halitosis**
- **Lymphadenopathy**
- **Gingival inflammation**

OSTEOMYELITIS
- **Dull pain in jaws**
- **Fever**
- **Swelling**
- **Paresthesia**
- **Sinus tract formation**
- **Increased ESR values**
- **Increased WBC counts**
- **Exposed bone**
- **Radiolucencies in bone with indistinct borders**
- **Blurred trabeculae**
- **Sequestrum formation**
- **May show onion skin if associated with periostitis**

OSTEITIS
- **Inflammation of bone**
- **Pain**
- **May cause radiolucency from bone resorption followed by bone deposition (condensing osteitis)**
- **Lacks sequestrum formation**

OSTEORADIONECROSIS
- **Same signs and symptoms as osteomyelitis; distinguishing factor is a history of radiation therapy**

Figure VII-9. Summary of signs and symptoms or problems asociated with hard tissue infections.

NOTE: Osteomyelitis may also arise from non-dental causes. Thus, if no dental causes can be found, you will check NON-ODONTOGENIC in the above box and OSTEO-MYELITIS in this section and refer your patient to a specialist.

⑨   Is the infection of special significance?

Infections of special significance are those with potentially very serious outcomes if not diagnosed and treated immediately. Infections in this category are summarized on the checklist as shown to the right.

We have discussed the signs and symptoms of each of these infections in detail earlier in this book.

Special sigificance
☐ Acute cellulitis
☐ Ludwig's angina
☐ Osteo-radionecrosis
☐ Cavernous sinus thrombosis

NOTE: These infections (with the exception of osteoradionecrosis) can develop from both odontogenic and non-odontogenic sources. All of these require immediate hospitalization.

⑩   What is the origin of non-odontogenic infections?

If an infection cannot be linked to a dental origin, then you should **look** for a **non-dental origin** or **refer** your patient to a specialist. Most frequently, dentists will decide that an infection is not of dental origin following review of historical and clinical data in which:

- Normal vital teeth are present
- There is absence of periodontal or pericoronal disease
- No recent history of dental treatment is given
- Presence of other facial infections (acne, lacerations, etc.) is seen

Soft tissue (non-dental)
☐ Maxillary sinusitis
☐ Peritonsillar abscess
☐ Salivary gland infection
☐ Ear infection
☐ Superficial skin infection
☐ Superficial mucosal infection
☐ Other _____

⑪ Is the problem acute or chronic?

It is important to know whether the problem is **acute** or **chronic. Generally this can be determined through historical data and by clinical and radiographic examination. Figure VII-10** summarizes the typical signs and symptoms associated with acute and chronic infections. You should determine whether the infection is acute or chronic and record this assessment in the space provided.

SIGNS AND SYMPTOMS
OF ACUTE AND CHRONIC INFECTIONS

ACUTE
- **Rapid onset (a few days)**
- **Red color**
- **Cellulitis present (lacks localization)**
- **Lack signs of bone resorption**
- **Acute pain**

CHRONIC
- **Long term (can be present for weeks to months)**
- **May have developed from acute infection**
- **Purple in color**
- **May be fluctuant**
- **May have drainage site**
- **May show signs of bone resorption or deposition**
- **Less acute pain**

Figure VII-10. Summary of typical signs and symptoms of acute and chronic infections.

SUMMARY

We have presented you with a diagnostic system for identifying the etiology of odontogenic and non-odontogenic infections. We have also provided you with a method for classifying non-odontogenic infections and non-infectious swellings into general categories allowing you to formulate a differential diagnosis and seek appropriate referral for problems beyond the level of your training.

The **Diagnostic Decisions Checklist** was developed in order to help you summarize your decisions. You should complete the following study exercises in order to see how this approach can be directly applied to clinical situations.

DIAGNOSTIC DECISIONS

SUMMARY OF PATIENT'S PROBLEMS

1. _____ 6. _____ 11. _____
2. _____ 7. _____ 12. _____
3. _____ 8. _____ 13. _____
4. _____ 9. _____ 14. _____
5. _____ 10. _____ 15. _____

PROCESS FOR INITIAL DIAGNOSIS

Problem is . . . . ☐ Microbial   ☐ Non-Microbial   ☐ Unknown_____
Source of Infection is . . ☐ Odontogenic   ☐ Non-odontogenic   ☐ From Dental Tx   ☐ Unknown _____

Soft Tissue (dentally related)
☐ Periodontal Abscess
☐ Pericoronal Abscess
☐ Dento-Alveolar Abscess
☐ Post-surgical Infection
☐ Post-injection Infection
☐ Maxillary Sinusitis
☐ Other _____
_____

Periosteum
☐ Subperiosteal abscess
☐ Post-Injection
☐ Periostitis
Hard Tissue
☐ Acute alveolar osteitis
   (dry socket)
☐ Osteitis
☐ Osteomyelitis
☑ Osteoradionecrosis

Special sigificance
☑ Acute cellulitis
☑ Ludwig's angina
☑ Osteo-
   radionecrosis
☑ Cavernous sinus
   thrombosis

Soft tissue (non-dental)
☐ Maxillary sinusitis
☐ Peritonsillar abscess
☐ Salivary gland infection
☐ Ear infection
☐ Superficial skin infection
☐ Superficial mucosal infection
☐ Other _____

Progress of Infection is . ☐ Chronic (slow)   ☐ Acute (rapid)   ☐ Dangerously Acute (fulminating) _____

EVALUATION OF MODIFYING FACTORS

Patient's Health
☑ Serious medical risk
☑ Moderate medical risk
☑ Low medical risk
☑ No medical risk
Why? _____
_____

Anatomical Factors
☑ High risk space(s)
☑ Multiple spaces (bi)
☑ Involves adjacent areas
   but controllable
☑ Confined to alveolar ridge
Where? _____

Microbial Factors
☑ Acute cellulitis
☑ Systemic toxicity
☑ Extreme swelling
☑ Fever
☑ Chronic infection
☑ Recent antibiotic
☑ Poor O.H./perio disease

☐ Culture indicated but
   not taken
☐ No Gram stain
☐ Culture taken
☐ Gram stain obtained
☐ Culture not indicated
Other _____

STUDY EXERCISES

Given data and/or a problem list for each of the following oral and/or maxillofacial swellings, complete the following checklist for each case and state your reasoning.

Case #1. *A 29-year-old male presented for routine operative dentistry for placement of a small occlusal amalgam restoration in his maxillary right first molar following a local anesthetic injection in the right pterygomaxillary area. Approximately 10 days following this treatment, tenderness over the right temporal region and a moderate trismus was present. Following vital signs were obtained: Pulse 72, Respiration 19, Blood pressure 120/70, Temperature 100.1°F. The patient felt lethargic and was not eating well. Radiographic evidence of the teeth and jaws were normal as well as the oral examination. Oral penicillin given to the patient for 5 days decreased the swelling which began to return after discontinuing the penicillin. Laboratory values showed: W.B.C. — 9,000. The swelling increased in the temporal region as well as the trismus and tenderness in the pterygomandibular space, infratemporal and deep temporal spaces. Aspiration failed to obtain suppuration, but some saline and hematogenous material was sent for culture and sensitivity.*

SUMMARY OF PATIENT'S PROBLEMS

1. *tenderness over (R) temporal*
2. *trismus*
3. *fever*
4. *lethargic*
5. *tenderness*
6. _____
7. _____
8. _____
9. _____
10. _____
11. _____
12. _____
13. _____
14. _____
15. _____

PROCESS FOR INITIAL DIAGNOSIS

Problem is .... ☒ Microbial   ☐ Non-Microbial   ☐ Unknown _____

Source of Infection is .. ☐ Odontogenic   ☐ Non-odontogenic   ☒ From Dental Tx   ☐ Unknown _____

Soft Tissue (dentally related)	Periosteum	Special sigificance	Soft tissue (non-dental)
☐ Periodontal Abscess	☐ Subperiosteal abscess	☐ Acute cellulitis	☐ Maxillary sinusitis
☐ Pericoronal Abscess	☒ Post-Injection	☐ Ludwig's angina	☐ Peritonsillar abscess
☐ Dento-Alveolar Abscess	☐ Periostitis	☐ Osteo-radionecrosis	☐ Salivary gland infection
☐ Post-surgical Infection	**Hard Tissue**		☐ Ear infection
☒ Post-injection Infection	☐ Acute alveolar osteitis	☐ Cavernous sinus thrombosis	☐ Superficial skin infection
☐ Maxillary Sinusitis	(dry socket)		☐ Superficial mucosal infection
☐ Other _____	☐ Osteitis		☐ Other _____
_____	☐ Osteomyelitis		
	☐ Osteoradionecrosis		

Progress of Infection is . ☐ Chronic (slow)   ☐ Acute (rapid)   ☒ Dangerously Acute (fulminating) _____

What data indicates the swelling is or is not of microbial origin?

fever

oral pen. giving some relief

What data indicates the presence of odontogenic, non-odontogenic, or dental treatment related infection?

hx of dental tx

What is the data supporting your specific diagnosis of etiology?

hx of injection

Case #2. A 24-year-old male student presents to your office with an obvious, painful swelling over the right canine fossa area. His maxillary right canine was tender to percussion and had a radiolucent lesion at the apex. Intraorally a fluctuant swelling was present that yielded 3 cc of purulent exudate on aspiration. Stat Gram stain revealed 4+ gram positive cocci, 2+ gram negative rods. No other abnormalities or physical findings were available.

SUMMARY OF PATIENT'S PROBLEMS

1. _Swelling_
2. _canine tender to percussion_
3. _radiolucent lesion @ apex_
4. _purulent exudate_
5. _4+ gram positive cocci_

6. _____
7. _____
8. _____
9. _____
10. _____

11. _____
12. _____
13. _____
14. _____
15. _____

PROCESS FOR INITIAL DIAGNOSIS

Problem is .... ☒ Microbial   ☐ Non-Microbial   ☐ Unknown_____

Source of Infection is .. ☒ Odontogenic   ☐ Non-odontogenic   ☐ From Dental Tx   ☐ Unknown _____

Soft Tissue (dentally related)	**Periosteum**	**Special sigificance**	**Soft tissue (non-dental)**
☐ Periodontal Abscess	☐ Subperiosteal abscess	☒ Acute cellulitis	☐ Maxillary sinusitis
☐ Pericoronal Abscess	☐ Post-Injection	☒ Ludwig's angina	☐ Peritonsillar abscess
☒ Dento-Alveolar Abscess	☐ Periostitis	☒ Osteo-	☐ Salivary gland infection
☐ Post-surgical Infection	**Hard Tissue**	radionecrosis	☐ Ear infection
☐ Post-injection Infection	☐ Acute alveolar osteitis	☒ Cavernous sinus	☐ Superficial skin infection
☐ Maxillary Sinusitis	(dry socket)	thrombosis	☐ Superficial mucosal infection
☐ Other _____	☐ Osteitis		☐ Other _____
_____	☐ Osteomyelitis		
	☒ Osteoradionecrosis		

Progress of Infection is . ☒ Chronic (slow)   ☒ Acute (rapid)   ☒ Dangerously Acute (fulminating) _____

What data indicates the swelling is or is not of microbial origin?

purulent exudate   _gram (-) rods_
swelling
gram + cocci

What data indicates the presence of odontogenic, non-odontogenic, or dental treatment related infection?

radiolucent lesion at apex
canine tender to percussion

What is the data supporting your specific diagnosis of etiology?

Per Apical radiolucency along
with sensitivity on the
canine suggest acute
periapical periodontitis

Discussion of Cases

Case #1

SUMMARY OF PATIENT'S PROBLEMS

1. tenderness: deep temporal,
2. pterygomandibular, infra temp.
3. on (R)
4. moderate trismus
5. Fever - 100.1°F
6. Lethargic, loss of appetite
7. Previous antibiotic (Pen)
8. improved but condition
9. reappeared when pen discon.
10. No T.O S§S other than
11. Pterygomand involvement.
12. WBC = 9,000
13. _____
14. _____
15. _____

PROCESS FOR INITIAL DIAGNOSIS

Problem is . . . . ☑ Microbial   ☐ Non-Microbial   ☐ Unknown _____

Source of Infection is . . ☐ Odontogenic   ☐ Non-odontogenic   ☑ From Dental Tx   ☐ Unknown _____

Soft Tissue (dentally related)	Periosteum	Special sigificance	Soft tissue (non-dental)
☐ Periodontal Abscess	☐ Subperiosteal abscess	☐ Acute cellulitis	☐ Maxillary sinusitis
☐ Pericoronal Abscess	☐ Post-Injection	☐ Ludwig's angina	☐ Peritonsillar abscess
☐ Dento-Alveolar Abscess	☐ Periostitis	☐ Osteo-	☐ Salivary gland infection
☐ Post-surgical Infection	**Hard Tissue**	radionecrosis	☐ Ear infection
☑ Post-injection Infection	☐ Acute alveolar osteitis	☐ Cavernous sinus	☐ Superficial skin infection
☐ Maxillary Sinusitis	(dry socket)	thrombosis	☐ Superficial mucosal infection
☐ Other _____	☐ Osteitis		☐ Other _____
_____	☐ Osteomyelitis		
	☐ Osteoradionecrosis		

Progress of Infection is . ☑ Chronic (slow)☑ Acute (rapid)   ☐ Dangerously Acute (fulminating) _____

What data indicates the swelling is or is not of microbial origin?

Elevated temp. 100.1°F low grade   Positive responce to penicillin
Tender swelling
WBC = 9,000

What data indicates the presence of odontogenic, non-odontogenic, or dental treatment related infection?

This infection is most likely related   of odontogenic infection were found
to dental treatment but is not   during oral examination or on radiographs.
odontogenic in origin because no s§s

What is the data supporting your specific diagnosis of etiology?

Recent history of local anesthetic   genic source evident, s§s support infection
injection into the involved area, No odonto-   and no non-odontogenic source is evident.

suspect low-grade infection - possibly Actino.

See page 220 for discussion of **Case #2.**

Case #2

SUMMARY OF PATIENT'S PROBLEMS

1. *Pain & swelling ® canine fossa*
2. *Fluctuance*
3. *Max ® canine Percussion Sens.*
4. *Radiographic lesion apex Max*
5. *® canine*
6. _____
7. _____
8. _____
9. _____
10. _____
11. _____
12. _____
13. _____
14. _____
15. _____

PROCESS FOR INITIAL DIAGNOSIS

Problem is . . . . ☑ Microbial ☐ Non-Microbial ☐ Unknown_____

Source of Infection is . . ☑ Odontogenic ☐ Non-odontogenic ☐ From Dental Tx ☐ Unknown _____

Soft Tissue (dentally related)	Periosteum	Special sigificance	Soft tissue (non-dental)
☐ Periodontal Abscess	☐ Subperiosteal abscess	☐ Acute cellulitis	☐ Maxillary sinusitis
☐ Pericoronal Abscess	☐ Post-Injection	☐ Ludwig's angina	☐ Peritonsillar abscess
☑ Dento-Alveolar Abscess	☐ Periostitis	☐ Osteo-	☐ Salivary gland infection
☐ Post-surgical Infection	**Hard Tissue**	radionecrosis	☐ Ear infection
☐ Post-injection Infection	☐ Acute alveolar osteitis	☐ Cavernous sinus	☐ Superficial skin infection
☐ Maxillary Sinusitis	(dry socket)	thrombosis	☐ Superficial mucosal infection
☐ Other _____	☐ Osteitis		☐ Other _____
_____	☐ Osteomyelitis		
	☐ Osteoradionecrosis		

Progress of Infection is . ☐ Chronic (slow) ☑ Acute (rapid) ☐ Dangerously Acute (fulminating) _____

What data indicates the swelling is or is not of microbial origin?

Gram stain Positive for bacteria *Radiographic lesion at apex - Max ® canine*
Percussion sensitive Max ® canine
Fluctuance in swelling

What data indicates the presence of odontogenic, non-odontogenic, or dental treatment related infection?

tooth related signs & symptoms - Max ® canine
Percussion sensitivity
Radiolucency at root apex

What is the data supporting your specific diagnosis of etiology?

Dento-alveolar abscess associated w/ Max ® canine with spread to infra- orbital area (canine fossa)

EVALUATION OF MODIFYING FACTORS

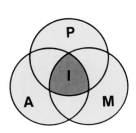

Once the cause of an infection is identified you should then evaluate your data to identify any **modifying factors** which could increase the degree of seriousness of the infection. A seemingly minor infection may become a life-threatening problem if your **patient's body resistance** is compromised, the infection is **located in a critical anatomical area**, or if the **microorganism(s) is(are) extremely aggressive**. We have provided the following space on the diagnostic decisions checklist for you to evaluate and summarize the **degree of risk** in each of these three areas.

EVALUATION OF MODIFYING FACTORS

Patient's Health	Anatomical Factors	Microbial Factors	
☐ Serious medical risk	☐ High risk space(s)	☐ Acute cellulitis	☐ Culture indicated but
☐ Moderate medical risk	☐ Multiple spaces (bi)	☐ Systemic toxicity	not taken
☐ Low medical risk	☐ Involves adjacent areas	☐ Extreme swelling	☐ No Gram stain
☐ No medical risk	but controllable	☑ Fever	☐ Culture taken
Why? _____	☐ Confined to alveolar ridge	☐ Chronic infection	☐ Gram stain obtained
_____	Where?_____	☐ Recent antibiotic	☐ Culture not indicated
		☐ Poor O.H./perio disease	Other

Decreased Patient Resistance

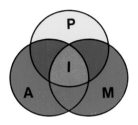 Factors which can reduce a patient's normal body resistance and/or prolong the resolution of an otherwise minor infection should be identified during the data collection and diagnosis stages of infection management strategy. This process will form the basis for defining management objectives directed toward reducing the effects of these factors during treatment. Early identification of these factors can also help you determine the need for referral.

Major factors that can affect a patient's resistance to infection include:
- **Systemic disease processes**
- **Medications**
- **Allergies**
- **Previous radiation therapy**
- **Age**
- **Nutritional status**
- **Alcohol consumption**
- **Psychological condition**
- **Family and social environment**
- **Presence of any serious signs**
- **Predisposing factors**

A review of these factors is presented in Unit I, pages 21 to 26.

The following categories are used to evaluate your patient's medical risk and/or other factors which could contribute to a decrease in a patient's body resistance.

☐ **Serious medical risk or problem**

Serious medical problem(s) or other serious predisposing factor(s) is(are) present. Management of oral infections in seriously compromised patients should be referred to a specialist and/or hospital. When managing these patients, serious complications can develop rapidly and have fatal consequences, i.e. severe uncontrolled diabetes mellitis.

☐ **Moderate Medical Risk**

A moderate decrease in a patient's body resistance due to a controlled medical problem or moderate predisposing condition may be managed by general practitioners in conjunction with appropriate consultation with the patient's physician or other specialists. These patients require close monitoring both during treatment and for at least two to three weeks after treatment. These patients should be immediately referred to a specialist if problems develop. Patients in this medical risk category can be a major area of concern for general dental practitioners. If you are unsure of your abilities to control moderate risk patients, then refer these patients to a specialist trained to handle these problems. An example of moderate medical risk might be a patient who is a controlled insulin dependent diabetic.

☐ **Low medical risk**

Often a patient will have minor medical problems or other minor factors which could compromise their resistance to infection. While close monitoring is essential, a practitioner should not hesitate to initiate appropriate treatment; however, a referral should be made if complications develop. An example of a low medical risk might be a patient with a mild asthmatic condition requiring antihistamines.

☐ **No medical risk**

If no medical risk is identified, then proceed with treatment. However, if complications develop, referral should be considered.

Following a review of factors which can decrease a patient's body resistance to infection, you should make a judgment as to the **overall degree of seriousness** and **check** the appropriate box on the checklist. Briefly describing the reasons for your rating will help you keep these factors in mind when considering management objectives.

STUDY EXERCISES

Briefly explain the criteria for evaluation of the modifying factors affecting a patient's health:

☐ Serious medical risk *uncontrolled medical problems*
☐ Moderate medical risk *Controlled medical problem*
☐ Low medical risk *minor medical problems*
☐ No medical risk *No medical risks present*

NOTE: *If you cannot decide in which medical risk category a patient's illness should be classified, it is better to place it into a more serious risk than a less serious category.*

Anatomical Factors

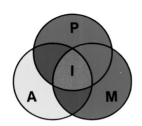

The anatomical location of an infection is a **critical factor** contributing to the overall seriousness of an infection. The anatomical location of infections may result in problems such as trismus, dysphagia, and/or respiratory restriction or allow rapid progression of an infection to the cavernous sinus, fascial planes of the neck and mediastinum. Conversely, infections may be confined to easily controlled areas. Between these extremes are infections which may respond to conservative treatment or may rapidly progress into critical areas.

After you have identified areas of anatomical involvement you should again **rate the overall degree of risk associated with the anatomical location of an infection.**

☐ **Infections of high risk spaces or areas**

Infections of the following spaces **must be considered extremely dangerous** because of their anatomical location and high potential for creating life-threatening conditions or because the treatment methods to control them are usually beyond the training of general practitioners. A general practitioner should **refer any of these space infections to a specialist or hospitalize the patient immediately.**

☐ **Parapharyngeal space**   ☐ **Pterygomandibular space**
☐ **Fascial planes of the neck**   ☐ **Parotid space**
☐ **Temporal spaces**   ☐ **Multiple fascial space infection**
☐ **Periorbital space**

☐ **Multiple Space Infections**

If an infection involves multiple fascial spaces (**especially if any of the above critical spaces are also involved**) the infection may rapidly progress to a critical condition. Multiple space involvement may be **unilateral** or **bilateral.** It is erroneous to consider multiple **unilateral** space infections involving any of the high risk spaces as less serious than bilateral space infections. Respiratory obstruction **can result from unilateral internal swellings** of the lateral pharyngeal space in conjunction with swellings of the submandibular, sublingual, submental and/or fascial planes of the neck.

The frequently recognized multiple fascial space infection is Ludwig's angina. This name implies involvement of the submandibular, sublingual, and submental spaces. It is unfortunate that other infections involving multiple spaces do not have a name that **creates concern** in the minds of clinicians in a way similar to the term Ludwig's angina.

☐ **Infections of fascial spaces adjacent to alveolar ridges (moderate to serious risk)**

Infections which have spread to the following anatomical areas must be regarded as anatomically more serious than infections localized to the alveolar ridges and palate. These infections can cause facial swelling, lingual swelling, trismus, and some dysphagia. They can also be more painful. Infections of these spaces can range from **moderate to severe.**

- ☐ **Base of the upper lip**
- ☐ **Mentalis space**
- ☐ **Submental space**
- ☐ **Sublingual space**
- ☐ **Peritonsillar area**

- ☐ **Submandibular space**
- ☐ **Buccal space**
- ☐ **Submasseteric space**
- ☐ **Infraorbital space**
- ☐ **Soft palate**

While infections of these anatomical areas are usually controlled by conservative treatment methods including intraoral incision and drainage, **they have significant potential for spread to more serious anatomical areas if initial treatment methods are unsuccessful.** These infections may or may not be referred to a specialist depending upon other factors, such as the patient's general health and characteristics of the microorganisms. You should obtain a specimen for Gram stain, culture and antibiotic sensitivity testing from infections of these spaces or refer the patient to a specialist to perform these procedures. **The progress of these infections must be monitored daily and quickly referred to a specialist if not controlled within 24 to 48 hours.**

☐ **Infections confined to the alveolar ridges (low risk areas)**

Infections confined to the alveolar ridges, palate or buccal vestibules do not generally pose serious anatomical problems for your patients. If these infections **do not** progress beyond these areas, conservative treatment methods such as **irrigation, curettage, endodontic treatment, tooth extraction** and possibly **intraoral incision and drainage** will usually resolve the problem. The following anatomical areas are usually classified as **low risk areas:**

- ☐ **Maxillary Alveolar Ridge**
- ☐ **Mandibular Alveolar Ridge**

- ☐ **Hard Palate**
- ☐ **Facial Vestibules**

To assist you in determining the degree of risk associated with the anatomical location of an infection, page two of the checklist uses the same color coding as shown below.

SUMMARY OF INVOLVED ANATOMICAL AREAS

Involves dento-alveolar ridges
- ☐ Maxillary ridge. Where? _____
- ☐ Mandibular ridge. Where? _____

Mandible & Below	Cheek & Lateral Face	Pharyngeal Spaces	Mid-face Region
☐ 1 Facial vestibule of mandible	☐ 7 Buccal vestibule of maxilla	☐ 13 Pterygomandibular	☐ 17 Palatal
☐ 2 Body of mandible	☐ 8 Buccal space	☐ 14 Parapharyngeal	☑ 18 Infraorbital
☐ 3 Mentalis space	☐ 9 Submasseteric space	– Lateral pharyngeal	☐ 19 Periorbital
☐ 4 Submental space	☐ 10 Deep Temporal space	– Retropharyngeal	☑ 20 Base of upper lip
☐ 5 Sublingual space	☐ 10 Superficial Temporal	☐ 15 Peritonsillar	☐ 21 Maxillary sinus
☐ 6 Submandibular space	☐ 11 Infratemporal		
	☐ 12 Parotid space	☐ 16 Cervical Spaces	

STUDY EXERCISES

*Briefly describe the significance of the ratings used to describe the degree of risk associated with the **anatomical factors** and name two (2) fascial spaces or areas in each category.*

- ☐ *High risk spaces* ~~should be referred~~   parapharyngeal,   periorbital
- ☐ *Multiple spaces* ~~may progress to high risk~~   soft palate,   submental
- ☐ *Involves adjacent areas but controllable*
  ~~conservative~~   buccal,   submandibular
- ☐ *Confined to alveolar ridge* ~~low risk~~   hard palate,   facial vestibules

Microbial factors

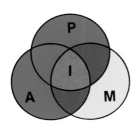

The characteristics of the microorganism involved in an infection can have significant impact upon the course of the infection and your selection of treatment methods. In your **initial diagnosis** you will usually have little information as to the identity and characteristics of the microorganism (unless a Gram stain is performed). However, an evaluation of the clinical course of the infection can allow you to assess the risk associated with microbial factors. While considerable overlap (green) exists between the anatomical location of the infection and the effects of the infection upon host defense mechanisms, the following factors are strongly influenced by the characteristics of the microorganisms involved with an infection. You will notice that **the overall risks are increased if basic information is not initially obtained. Failure to obtain basic information during initial data collection can delay definitive treatment if initial treatment proves ineffective.**

☐ **Acute cellulitis**

Acute cellulitis with a rapid clinical outset and/or progress suggests that the microorganism(s) is(are) highly invasive or that large numbers of microorganisms are present. Prompt, aggressive, and effective management is essential. Referral to a specialist and/or hospital is indicated.

☐ **Systemic toxicity**

Systemic toxicity is a sign that indicates an infection has spread into the bloodstream and is having effects beyond the local area of infection. Referral is indicated.

☐ **Extreme swelling**

Extreme swelling may be indicative of either large numbers of microorganisms or that the microorganism(s) has(have) evoked an exaggerated inflammatory response. Extreme swelling can severely restrict anatomic functions (swallowing, respiration, trismus, or even eye function) or may increase the rate of spread to adjacent areas (fascial spaces or cavernous sinus).

☑ **Fever**

Fever is usually indicative of bacteremia and is caused by circulation of the pyrogens produced by the host leucocytes.

☐ **Chronic infection**

A chronic infection which has not resolved after initial therapy may require extensie or prolonged treatment. Bacterial infections (such as *staphylococcus*), *actinomyces*, fungal infections or osteomyelitis may require several weeks of antimicrobial medications and/or surgical intervention. These infections may best be managed by a specialist.

☐ **Recent antibiotic therapy**

A history of recent antibiotic therapy (especially tetracycline and penicillin, but other antibiotics as well) may have altered the normal oral flora and selected for flora that are resistant to these antibiotics. Penicillin should not be used in initial treatment of patients who have recently taken this antibiotic for other reasons.

☐ **Poor oral hygiene or periodontal disease**

Poor oral hygiene and presence of active periodontal disease increases the numbers of microorganisms present in the oral cavity and also favors an increase in anaerobic species. These factors can increase the risk for an infection over a similar infection in a clean and healthy mouth.

☐ **Culture indicated but not taken**

If an infection has spread into the fascial spaces of the head and neck, a specimen should be obtained for laboratory analysis during initial data collection. This initiates action by the laboratory which will provide species identification, antibiotic sensitivity, etc. **If a specimen collection is indicated but not initially collected, you should consider the risks associated with microbial factors to be increased.** If you initially attempt to obtain a specimen for culturing but are unsuccessful, then try again at the earliest opportunity (e.g. next day) or refer your patient to a specialist.

☐ **Gram stain indicated but not obtained**

Again, if a Gram stain is indicated but not obtained, then the infection should be considered more serious. The importance of the Gram stain to the overall management of oral infections has been discussed on page 137. If Gram stain information is not available you cannot establish the presence of microorganisms, identify the morphological characteristics of species involved, select proper antibiotic therapy, nor verify future laboratory data (did the lab lose some species?). The risks for treating oral infections are thus increased if a Gram stain is indicated but not obtained.

☐ **Culture taken**

If culturing is indicated and a specimen is collected (and sent for microbiological analysis), then the results will be available if changes in initial treatment are needed. Initiating this information chain will reduce the time required to obtain a definitive diagnosis, thus reducing the risks associated with microbial factors.

☐ **STAT Gram stain obtained**

Obtaining Gram stain results will enable you to be more accurate in selection of antibiotics and planning other treatment.

☐ **Culture not indicated**

If culturing is not essential because the infection is confined to alveolar ridges and can probably be controlled by conservative treatment, then this would be a favorable factor.

STUDY EXERCISES
Briefly explain why the following microbial factors have been color coded as indicated:
☐ *Acute cellulitis* rapid onset & progression, microbes highly invasive
☐ *Systemic toxicity* infection in bloodstream
☐ *Extreme swelling* large numbers of organisms may restrict anatomy
☑ *Fever* indicates bacteremia
☐ *Chronic infection* may require long term tx
☐ *Recent antibiotic therapy* may select for flora resistance
☐ *Poor O.H./Perio disease* indicates number of bacteria
☐ *Culture indicated but not taken* increases microbial factors
☐ *No Gram stain* identification of microbes questionable

In this section we have provided categories of risk for **patient health, anatomical location** and **microbial factors.** However, the overlap between these areas is considerable. If **any red** box is checked (**serious** risk factor) then the case should be referred to a specialist for management. If a **yellow box** (moderate risk factor) is checked in **all** categories then the overall risk may be increased to the level of requiring referral. If **two** or more **yellow** boxes are checked, then you should seriously consider referral.

NOTE: Evaluation of modifying factors and the influence of these factors on your decision to treat or refer a patient will depend upon your level of training and clinical experience in treating patients with moderate infections.

INITIAL DIAGNOSIS

Once you have **summarized a patient's problems, made an initial diagnosis** of the cause of an infection, and **identified modifying factors** that can influence the degree of seriousness, you should concisely describe this information in the space provided on the checklist.

INITIAL DIAGNOSIS: _____

_____

_____

INITIAL COURSE OF ACTION

Once your initial diagnosis has been established you must decide whether **you will treat** the infection in your office, **refer** your patient **to a specialist**, or **refer** your patient for immediate **hospitalization**. Your decision should be based upon your evaluation of both the seriousness of the infection and your experience in managing infections. This decision is a value judgment and specific criteria cannot be provided. However, you should not be reluctant to refer patients to a specialist at this stage.

NOTE: It is better to refer a patient at this early stage than risk further deterioration of your patient's condition.

If you feel additional data is needed for a more thorough diagnosis or if **no specimen** can be obtained for a Gram stain or for culture and antibiotic susceptibility testing, then you should indicate the need for specimen collection at the earliest opportunity.

NOTE: You should always keep in mind that an initial diagnosis is usually based on incomplete information as to the causative microorganisms and the overall health of your patient.

You should summarize your initial course of action on the checklist in the space provided.

INITIAL COURSE OF ACTION

☐ Treat in office   ☐ Refer to a specialist   ☐ Hospitalize. Who/Where? _____

☐ Need additional data. What data? _____

DEFINITIVE DIAGNOSIS

Once you have received the results from laboratory studies and any additional data you may have obtained following your initial diagnosis a definitive diagnosis can usually be made.

NOTE: Because of the variable times required to perform laboratory tests and some variation in time required to obtain material for microbiological studies, you may frequently refine your definitive diagnosis over a 2- to 14-day period. Occasionally additional data will be required, thus further delaying your definitive diagnosis.

The following process should enable you to efficiently proceed with a definitive diagnosis and effective management of the problem.

- ## Summary of results from laboratory studies

Results of laboratory studies are summarized in this portion of the checklist.

Summary of Laboratory Data

MICROBIOLOGY LAB	HEMATOLOGY LAB	HISTOPATHOLOGY LAB
☐ Single species ☐ Mixed ☐ None	☐ WBC count _____	Tissue specimen analysis _____
Predominant species: _____	☐ WBC Differential:	_____
_____	Polys ___% Eosinophils ___%	_____
	Lymphocytes ___% Basophils ___%	_____
☐ Aerobic ☐ Anaerobic	Monocytes ___% Immature? ___	_____
Antibiotic Sensitivity:	ESR_____mm/hr	_____
1st choice _____	Blood Culture _____	_____
2nd choice _____	_____	_____
3rd choice _____	_____	_____

The purpose of laboratory data is to provide additional information in the areas of host reactions to the problem and more complete information about the identity and characteristics of any causative microorganisms. The significance of these data has been described in Unit V — Laboratory Data (pages 124-164) and will not be reviewed here.

SUMMARY OF DEFINITIVE DIAGNOSIS

This portion of the checklist requires you to make a judgment as to whether laboratory data support your initial diagnosis or whether your initial diagnosis needs modification. At this time you should re-define your diagnosis if indicated.

DEFINITIVE DIAGNOSIS

☐ Agrees/Consistent with initial diagnosis
☐ Differs from initial diagnosis _____

DEFINITIVE COURSE OF ACTION

The checklist then asks you to re-examine your initial course of action and to re-evaluate whether or not your patient should be referred for treatment. At this time you should also identify any additional data that are necessary to more thoroughly understand the underlying factors associated with your patient's problem.

DEFINITIVE COURSE OF ACTION

☐ Treat in office   ☐ Refer to a specialist   ☐ Hospitalize. Who/Where? _____
☐ Need additional data. What data? _____

SUMMARY OF DIAGNOSTIC DECISION PROCESS

In this unit we have presented a process for identifying patient problems, developing an initial diagnosis, and identifying modifying factors which will influence your treatment or referral decisions. In addition we have provided a mechanism for refining your initial diagnosis to reach a definitive diagnosis through laboratory data, and again to evaluate your decision to treat or refer your patient.

NOTE: While this may seem to be a laborious process, the stakes are high and attention to detail is extremely important. There are few areas in the field of dentistry which parallel the importance of accurate diagnosis and effective management of oral and/or maxillofacial infections.

POST-TEST — UNIT VII

- *Answer each of the following questions.*
- *Check your answers with the correct responses on page 234.*
- *If all questions are answered correctly, proceed to Unit VIII, page 239.*
- *If you do not answer all questions correctly, re-read and re-study the contents of this unit.*

QUESTIONS:

1. *Which of the following statements is/are* **true** *regarding the value of the diagnostic process in the overall management of oral and/or maxillofacial swellings?*
   - a. *It will help you to formulate a list of problems related to the swelling.*
   - b. *It may enable you identify the etiology or cause of the swelling.*
   - c. *It will enable you to identify the presence of modifying factors which can affect the management of the problems.*
   - d. *It allows you to develop a basis for initial management (treatment) decisions.*
   - e. *It allows you to develop a basis for definitive management (treatment) decisions.*

2. *An* **initial** *diagnosis will allow you to:*
   - a. *Make an initial decision to treat or refer the patient.*
   - b. *Begin initial treatment before all data are received.*
   - c. *Allow you to choose an antibiotic that has been shown effective against the involved microorganism(s).*

3. *When diagnosing an oral infection, which of the following statements is/are* **true** *regarding a* **definitive** *diagnosis?*
   - a. *Identification of the involved microorganism(s) is required.*
   - b. *The time required by a microbiology laboratory to identify the organisms and perform antibiotic susceptibility testing can range from 2-14 days.*
   - c. *When managing minor infections, it is important to begin the definitive diagnosis process before beginning initial treatment.*
   - d. *When managing moderate to serious infections it is important to begin the definitive diagnosis process prior to beginning initial treatment.*

4. **Case Description:** *A toxic-looking 62-year-old male with a red, painful swelling of the left submandibular region presents to your office. The swelling began 4 days previously and has steadily increased in size. The patient complains of pain, inability to open his mouth, and pain on swallowing.*

   Past Medical History: *Mild, chronic, obstructive pulmonary disease. Myocardial infarction 3 years ago, currently with occasional angina pectoris. Medications: Diuretics (hydrochlorthiazide), Nitroglycerin as required.*

   Clinical Data: *A large, tender, red, fluctuant swelling fills the left submandibular space. Moderate trismus and moderate dysphagia are present.*

   Vital Signs: *Temp. 101.2°F; P — 72; R — 17; B.P. 135/90.*

   Radiographic Data: *A poor-quality panoramic film revealed a 1 cm radiolucent lesion at the apex of the mandibular left first molar.*

   Laboratory Data: *W.B.C. = 13,000/mm^3 with shift to the left. E.S.R. = 50 mm/hr. Stat Gram stain of suppuration obtained from an extraoral aspirate of the fluctuance revealed 4+ Gram negative rods.*

4. a. Summarize the patient's problems.

SUMMARY OF PATIENT'S PROBLEMS

1. _swelling_   6. _suppuration_   11. _____
2. _pain_   7. _____   12. _____
3. _trismus_   8. _____   13. _____
4. _dysphagia_   9. _____   14. _____
5. _indurated tissue_ 10. _____   15. _____

4. b. Indicate your initial diagnosis. _Acute periapical periodontitis_

PROCESS FOR INITIAL DIAGNOSIS
Problem is . . . . ☒ Microbial   ☐ Non-Microbial   ☐ Unknown_____
Source of Infection is . . ☒ Odontogenic   ☐ Non-odontogenic   ☐ From Dental Tx   ☐ Unknown _____

Supporting data:

malodorous lesion   _____   _____
+ gram (-) rods   _____   _____

4. c. Determine the etiology and progress of the infection.

Soft Tissue (dentally related)
☐ Periodontal Abscess
☐ Pericoronal Abscess
☒ Dento-Alveolar Abscess
☐ Post-surgical Infection
☐ Post-injection Infection
☐ Maxillary Sinusitis
☐ Other _____
_____

Periosteum
☐ Subperiosteal abscess
☐ Post-Injection
☐ Periostitis
Hard Tissue
☐ Acute alveolar osteitis (dry socket)
☐ Osteitis
☐ Osteomyelitis
☐ Osteoradionecrosis

Special sigificance
☒ Acute cellulitis
☐ Ludwig's angina
☐ Osteo-radionecrosis
☐ Cavernous sinus thrombosis

Soft tissue (non-dental)
☐ Maxillary sinusitis
☐ Peritonsillar abscess
☐ Salivary gland infection
☐ Ear infection
☐ Superficial skin infection
☐ Superficial mucosal infection
☐ Other _____

Progress of Infection is . ☐ Chronic (slow)   ☒ Acute (rapid)   ☐ Dangerously Acute (fulminating) _____

Supporting data:

indurant tissue   _____   _____
swelling   _____   _____

4. d. Identify and evaluate modifying factors.

EVALUATION OF MODIFYING FACTORS

Patient's Health
☒ Serious medical risk
☒ Moderate medical risk
☐ Low medical risk
☐ No medical risk
Why? _not_
Hygiene
_____

Anatomical Factors
☐ High risk space(s)
☒ Multiple spaces (bi)
☒ Involves adjacent areas but controllable
☐ Confined to alveolar ridge
Where? _parapharyngeal_
submandibular

Microbial Factors
☒ Acute cellulitis
☒ Systemic toxicity
☒ Extreme swelling
☒ Fever
☐ Chronic infection
☐ Recent antibiotic
☐ Poor O.H./perio disease

☐ Culture indicated but not taken
☐ No Gram stain
☐ Culture taken
☒ Gram stain obtained
☐ Culture not indicated
Other _____

INITIAL DIAGNOSIS: _____
Acute periapical periodontitis

4. e. State and justify your initial course of action.

INITIAL COURSE OF ACTION
☐ Treat in office   ☐ Refer to a specialist   ☒ Hospitalize. Who/Where? _____
☐ Need additional data. What data? _____

Why? _Events of spreading_
_____
_____

5. **Case Description:** *A healthy 16-year-old female presents to your office for the surgical removal of her four partially erupted, impacted third molars. The surgery was uneventful; however, on the fourth post-operative day, an increase in the swelling of the right cheek area was noted by the patient and she returned to your office.*

Past Medical History: *Non-contributory.*

Clinical Data: *No serious general signs were present. A red, firm swelling which was tender to palpation over the right buccal space was noted. No fluctuance was noted at this time. There was one tender right submandibular lymph node.*

Vital Signs: *Temp. 101.1°F; P — 72; R — 17; B.P. 115/70.*

Radiographic Data: *Non-contributory except recent extraction sites of four third molars.*

Laboratory Data: *No blood tests were performed. An extraoral aspiration failed to obtain material for Stat Gram stain. The patient was placed on oral penicillin, 500 mg every 6 hours, and told to relax at home and to take plenty of fluids.*

a. *Complete the checklist below for this case.*

DIAGNOSTIC DECISIONS

SUMMARY OF PATIENT'S PROBLEMS

1. _Swelling_
2. _Tender lymph node_
3. _____
4. _____
5. _____
6. _____
7. _____
8. _____
9. _____
10. _____
11. _____
12. _____
13. _____
14. _____
15. _____

PROCESS FOR INITIAL DIAGNOSIS

Problem is .... ☒ Microbial   ☐ Non-Microbial   ☐ Unknown_____

Source of Infection is .. ☐ Odontogenic   ☐ Non-odontogenic   ☒ From Dental Tx   ☐ Unknown _____

Soft Tissue (dentally related)	Periosteum	Special sigificance	Soft tissue (non-dental)
☐ Periodontal Abscess	☐ Subperiosteal abscess	☐ Acute cellulitis	☐ Maxillary sinusitis
☐ Pericoronal Abscess	☐ Post-Injection	☐ Ludwig's angina	☐ Peritonsillar abscess
☐ Dento-Alveolar Abscess	☐ Periostitis	☐ Osteo-	☐ Salivary gland infection
☒ Post-surgical Infection	**Hard Tissue**	radionecrosis	☐ Ear infection
☐ Post-injection Infection	☐ Acute alveolar osteitis	☐ Cavernous sinus	☐ Superficial skin infection
☐ Maxillary Sinusitis	(dry socket)	thrombosis	☐ Superficial mucosal infection
☐ Other _____	☐ Osteitis		☐ Other _____
_____	☐ Osteomyelitis		
	☐ Osteoradionecrosis		

Progress of Infection is . ☐ Chronic (slow)   ☒ Acute (rapid)   ☐ Dangerously Acute (fulminating) _____

EVALUATION OF MODIFYING FACTORS

Patient's Health	Anatomical Factors	Microbial Factors	
☐ Serious medical risk	☐ High risk space(s)	☐ Acute cellulitis	☒ Culture indicated but
☐ Moderate medical risk	☐ Multiple spaces (bi)	☐ Systemic toxicity	not taken
☐ Low medical risk	☒ Involves adjacent areas	☐ Extreme swelling	☒ No Gram stain
☒ No medical risk	but controllable	☒ Fever	☐ Culture taken
Why? _____	☐ Confined to alveolar ridge	☐ Chronic infection	☐ Gram stain obtained
_____	Where? _R buccal_	☐ Recent antibiotic	☒ Culture not indicated
	_____	☐ Poor O.H./perio disease	Other _____

INITIAL DIAGNOSIS: _post oper infection_
_____
_____

INITIAL COURSE OF ACTION

☒ Treat in office   ☐ Refer to a specialist   ☐ Hospitalize. Who/Where? _____
☐ Need additional data. What data? _culture & sensitivity test_

b. **Clinical Course:** *Two days later the patient felt better and the right buccal space swelling was fluctuant. An extraoral aspiration obtained 6 cc of yellow suppuration. The culture and sensitivity revealed: Sensitivity to penicillin, ampicillin and erythromycin. Single species; 4 + streptococcus species.*

Complete the portion of the checklist below.

PROCESS FOR DEFINITIVE DIAGNOSIS
Summary of Laboratory Data

MICROBIOLOGY LAB	HEMATOLOGY LAB	HISTOPATHOLOGY LAB
☑ Single species ☐ Mixed ☐ None	☐ WBC count _____	Tissue specimen analysis ____
Predominant species: _____	☐ WBC Differential:	_____
4+ strep	Polys ____% Eosinophils ____%	_____
_____	Lymphocytes____% Basophils ____%	_____
☐ Aerobic ☐ Anaerobic	Monocytes ____% Immature? ____	_____
Antibiotic Sensitivity:	ESR_____mm/hr	_____
1st choice_____	Blood Culture _____	_____
2nd choice _____	_____	_____
3rd choice_____	_____	_____

DEFINITIVE DIAGNOSIS
☑ Agrees/Consistent with initial diagnosis
☐ Differs from initial diagnosis _____

DEFINITIVE COURSE OF ACTION
☑ Treat in office   ☐ Refer to a specialist   ☐ Hospitalize. Who/Where? _____
☐ Need additional data. What data? _____

6. **Case Description:** *A 21-year-old male college student presented to the emergency dental clinic during final exam week complaining of pain and swelling around his partially erupted, impacted mandibular left third molar. He reported that the pain had been increasing steadily for the past three days along with increasing difficulty in opening his mouth. He had not been able to eat solid food and had been taking fluids by mouth only intermittently.*

Past Medical History: *Asthma as a child, but without recent exacerbations of any significance. Allergic reaction to oral penicillin — severe skin rash.*

Clinical Data: *A red, diffuse swelling was observed intraorally over and around the mandibular left third molar. Moderate trismus and slight dysphagia were observed clinically. A panoramic radiograph revealed a partial bony impacted lower left third molar.*

Vital Signs: *Temp. 100.6°F; R — 17; P — 68; B.P. 120/70 without significant orthostatic drop.*

Radiographic Data: *Periapical radiographs could not be obtained due to the restriction in mouth opening.*

Laboratory data: *A cotton swab was used to obtain a specimen of intraoral suppuration obtained from the gingival margin of the lower left third molar. The swab was sent to the microbiology lab for Stat Gram stain, culture and antibiotic susceptibility tests.*

STAT Gram Stain Results

☐ Single specie   ☑ Mixed   ☐ No microbes present
☐ Gram (+) cocci *+++*   ☐ Gram (−) cocci *++*
☐ Gram (+) rods   *++*   ☐ Gram (−) rods *+++*
☐ Other _____

a. *Complete this portion of the checklist.*

SUMMARY OF PATIENT'S PROBLEMS

1. *pain*   6. _____   11. _____
2. *swelling*   7. _____   12. _____
3. *trismus*   8. _____   13. _____
4. *pen allergy*   9. _____   14. _____
5. _____   10. _____ 15. _____

PROCESS FOR INITIAL DIAGNOSIS

Problem is . . . . ☑ Microbial   ☐ Non-Microbial   ☐ Unknown_____
Source of Infection is . . ☑ Odontogenic   ☐ Non-odontogenic   ☐ From Dental Tx   ☐ Unknown_____

Soft Tissue (dentally related)	Periosteum	Special sigificance	Soft tissue (non-dental)
☐ Periodontal Abscess	☐ Subperiosteal abscess	☐ Acute cellulitis	☐ Maxillary sinusitis
☑ Pericoronal Abscess	☐ Post-Injection	☐ Ludwig's angina	☐ Peritonsillar abscess
☐ Dento-Alveolar Abscess	☐ Periostitis	☐ Osteo-	☐ Salivary gland infection
☐ Post-surgical Infection	**Hard Tissue**	radionecrosis	☐ Ear infection
☐ Post-injection Infection	☐ Acute alveolar osteitis	☐ Cavernous sinus	☐ Superficial skin infection
☐ Maxillary Sinusitis	(dry socket)	thrombosis	☐ Superficial mucosal infection
☐ Other _____	☐ Osteitis		☐ Other _____
_____	☐ Osteomyelitis		
	☑ Osteoradionecrosis		

Progress of Infection is . ☐ Chronic (slow)   ☑ Acute (rapid)   ☐ Dangerously Acute (fulminating) _____

EVALUATION OF MODIFYING FACTORS

Patient's Health	Anatomical Factors	Microbial Factors	
☐ Serious medical risk	☐ High risk space(s)	☐ Acute cellulitis	☐ Culture indicated but
☐ Moderate medical risk	☐ Multiple spaces (bi)	☐ Systemic toxicity	not taken
☐ Low medical risk	☑ Involves adjacent areas	☑ Extreme swelling	☐ No Gram stain
☑ No medical risk	but controllable	☑ Fever	☑ Culture taken
Why? _____	☐ Confined to alveolar ridge	☐ Chronic infection	☑ Gram stain obtained
_____	Where?_____	☐ Recent antibiotic	☐ Culture not indicated
		☑ Poor O.H./perio disease	Other _____

INITIAL DIAGNOSIS: *pericoronitis* _____
_____

INITIAL COURSE OF ACTION

☑ Treat in office   ☐ Refer to a specialist   ☐ Hospitalize. Who/Where? _____
☐ Need additional data. What data? _____

Treatment: *This patient was given a prescription for 28 erythromycin tablets (250-mg) and instructed to take one tablet every 6 hours. In addition, he was instructed to take one 30 mg codeine tablet and 2 aspirin (650 mg) every 3 hours to control his pain. He was instructed in the use of a plastic syringe to irrigate the pericoronal area in the area of the involved third molar and told to use intraoral hot saline rinses hourly. He was reappointed to return to the clinic in 4 days.*

The patient returned two days later and apologized for returning earlier than recommended. His condition has now beome much worse. Trismus has increased to the degree that mouth opening is all but restricted. Pain on swallowing has greatly increased and his roommate says he has been up all night and has not eaten any food or consumed any water for the last 36 hours and, because of these problems, he has not been able to take the antibiotic and pain medication as you prescribed. His temperature has increased to 103.4°F, respiration rate has increased to 20, and he must lean forward with his nose elevated in order to breathe. Pulse rate has increased to 82.

Extraoral Examination: *Red, firm, non-fluctuant swelling on the left side of head over area of the submasseteric space, submandibular space and lateral side of the neck. The left jugulo omohyoid lymph nodes are tender and enlarged.*

Intraoral Examination: *Could not perform complete intraoral examination due to trismus. However, a fluctuant swelling of the posterior mandibular left buccal vestibule could be seen without opening the jaws.*

Radiographic Data: *No new radiographs were obtained.*

Laboratory Data: *A specimen was obtained from the fluctuant vestibular swelling and submitted for Stat Gram stain followed by culture and antibiotic susceptibility testing. The results are shown to the right. The lab was con-*

STAT Gram Stain Results

☑ Single specie ☐ Mixed ☐ No microbes present
☑ Gram (+) cocci   + ☐ Gram (−) cocci 0
☐ Gram (+) rods   0 ☐ Gram (−) rods 0
☐ Other ++++ WBC

*tacted for results from the earlier specimen and it reported "normal oral flora" with **strepto-coccus** as the predominant species and **staphylococcus epidermidis** also present. Antibiotic susceptibility tests are not as yet available.*

b. How would you now evaluate this patient's condition? You can re-use the initial portion of the checklist because you do not have a definitive diagnosis at this time.

SUMMARY OF PATIENT'S PROBLEMS

1. pain
2. trismus
3. temperature
4. resp↑
5. breathing problem
6. node involvement
7. ___
8. ___
9. ___
10. ___
11. ___
12. ___
13. ___
14. ___
15. ___

PROCESS FOR INITIAL DIAGNOSIS

Problem is . . . . ☒ Microbial ☐ Non-Microbial ☐ Unknown____
Source of Infection is .. ☒ Odontogenic ☐ Non-odontogenic ☐ From Dental Tx ☐ Unknown ____

Soft Tissue (dentally related)	Periosteum	Special sigificance	Soft tissue (non-dental)
☐ Periodontal Abscess	☐ Subperiosteal abscess	☒ Acute cellulitis	☐ Maxillary sinusitis
☒ Pericoronal Abscess	☐ Post-Injection	☐ Ludwig's angina	☐ Peritonsillar abscess
☐ Dento-Alveolar Abscess	☐ Periostitis	☐ Osteo-	☐ Salivary gland infection
☐ Post-surgical Infection	**Hard Tissue**	radionecrosis	☐ Ear infection
☐ Post-injection Infection	☐ Acute alveolar osteitis	☐ Cavernous sinus	☐ Superficial skin infection
☐ Maxillary Sinusitis	(dry socket)	thrombosis	☐ Superficial mucosal infection
☐ Other ____	☐ Osteitis		☐ Other ____
	☐ Osteomyelitis		
	☒ Osteoradionecrosis		

Progress of Infection is . ☒ Chronic (slow) ☐ Acute (rapid) ☒ Dangerously Acute (fulminating) ____

EVALUATION OF MODIFYING FACTORS

Patient's Health	Anatomical Factors	Microbial Factors	
☒ Serious medical risk	☒ High risk space(s)	☒ Acute cellulitis	☐ Culture indicated but
☐ Moderate medical risk	☒ Multiple spaces (bi)	☒ Systemic toxicity	not taken
☒ Low medical risk	☐ Involves adjacent areas	☒ Extreme swelling	☐ No Gram stain
☐ No medical risk	but controllable	☒ Fever	☒ Culture taken
Why?____	☐ Confined to alveolar ridge	☐ Chronic infection	☒ Gram stain obtained
____	Where?____	☐ Recent antibiotic	☐ Culture not indicated
		☐ Poor O.H./perio disease	Other ____

INITIAL DIAGNOSIS: ____ Exacerbation of condition: Spreading to adj area ____

c. What errors in data collection and/or diagnosis could have contributed the deterioration of this patient's condition? ____ underestimated danger - cotton swab ____ method sample poor

POST-TEST ANSWERS

1. a, b, c, d, e
2. a and b only
3. a, b, d only
4. a.

SUMMARY OF PATIENT'S PROBLEMS

1. *toxic looking 63 y.o.*
2. *progressive submand. swelling*
3. *pain, trismus, dysphagia*
4. *C.O.P.D. – mild*
5. *M.I. – 3 years ago*
6. *Meds- diuretics, Nitroglycerin*
7. *V.S. – fever 101.2° F*
8. *L submand. space swelling*
9. *red, tender, fluctuant*
10. *radiolucency apex L.L. first molar*
11. *WBC – 13,000*
12. *E.S.R. – 60 mm/hr.*
13. *needle aspirate culture*
14. *4+ Gram (–) rods*
15. _____

4. b.

PROCESS FOR INITIAL DIAGNOSIS

Problem is . . . . ☑ Microbial   ☐ Non-Microbial   ☐ Unknown_____
Source of Infection is . . ☑ Odontogenic   ☐ Non-odontogenic   ☐ From Dental Tx   ☐ Unknown _____

Supporting data:

inflammation signs: redness, swelling, pain
systemic toxicity, fever

loss of function: trismus, dysphagia
fluctuant swelling

bacteria in aspirate

4. c.

Soft Tissue (dentally related)	Periosteum	Special sigificance	Soft tissue (non-dental)
☐ Periodontal Abscess	☐ Subperiosteal abscess	☑ Acute cellulitis	☐ Maxillary sinusitis
☐ Pericoronal Abscess	☐ Post-Injection	☐ Ludwig's angina	☐ Peritonsillar abscess
☑ Dento-Alveolar Abscess	☐ Periostitis	☐ Osteo-radionecrosis	☐ Salivary gland infection
☐ Post-surgical Infection	**Hard Tissue**	☐ Cavernous sinus thrombosis	☐ Ear infection
☐ Post-injection Infection	☐ Acute alveolar osteitis (dry socket)		☐ Superficial skin infection
☐ Maxillary Sinusitis	☐ Osteitis		☐ Superficial mucosal infection
☐ Other _____	☐ Osteomyelitis		☐ Other _____
_____	☐ Osteoradionecrosis		

Progress of Infection is . ☐ Chronic (slow) ☑ Acute (rapid)   ☐ Dangerously Acute (fulminating) _____

Supporting data:

apical radiolucency of mandibular Ⓛ 1st molar

swelling in submandibular space

4. d.

EVALUATION OF MODIFYING FACTORS

Patient's Health	Anatomical Factors	Microbial Factors	
☑ Serious medical risk	☐ High risk space(s)	☑ Acute cellulitis	☐ Culture indicated but not taken
☐ Moderate medical risk	☐ Multiple spaces (bi)	☑ Systemic toxicity	☐ No Gram stain
☐ Low medical risk	☑ Involves adjacent areas but controllable	☐ Extreme swelling	☐ Culture taken
☐ No medical risk		☑ Fever	☑ Gram stain obtained
Why? _____	☐ Confined to alveolar ridge	☐ Chronic infection	☐ Culture not indicated
_____	Where?_____	☐ Recent antibiotic	Other _____
		☐ Poor O.H./perio disease	

INITIAL DIAGNOSIS: *Left submandibular space infection secondary to dento-alveolar (periapical) infection of the mandibular Ⓛ 1st molar*

4. e.

INITIAL COURSE OF ACTION

☐ Treat in office   ☑ Refer to a specialist   ☑ Hospitalize. Who/Where? *Refer & hospitalize NOW!*
☑ Need additional data. What data? *need culture and sensitivity tests*

This patient has several critical factors which should be managed in a hospital facility: acute cellulitis, serious medical risks, signs of systemic toxicity. In addition, culture and antibiotic suceptibility tests must be initiated immediately to obtain a definitive diagnosis.

5. a.

DIAGNOSTIC DECISIONS

SUMMARY OF PATIENT'S PROBLEMS

1. surgical removal, 4 3rd molars
2. swelling ® cheek 4 days postop
3. temp 101.1°F
4. meds - 500 mg pen. q6h
5. no aspirate obtained
6. swelling over buccal space
7. is red, firm, nonfluctuant
8. tender ® submand node
9. _____
10. _____
11. _____
12. _____
13. _____
14. _____
15. _____

PROCESS FOR INITIAL DIAGNOSIS

Problem is . . . . ☑ Microbial   ☐ Non-Microbial   ☐ Unknown _____

Source of Infection is . . ☑ Odontogenic   ☐ Non-odontogenic   ☐ From Dental Tx   ☐ Unknown _____

Soft Tissue (dentally related)	Periosteum	Special sigificance	Soft tissue (non-dental)
☐ Periodontal Abscess	☐ Subperiosteal abscess	☐ Acute cellulitis	☐ Maxillary sinusitis
☐ Pericoronal Abscess	☐ Post-Injection	☐ Ludwig's angina	☐ Peritonsillar abscess
☐ Dento-Alveolar Abscess	☐ Periostitis	☐ Osteo-	☐ Salivary gland infection
☑ Post-surgical Infection	**Hard Tissue**	radionecrosis	☐ Ear infection
☐ Post-injection Infection	☐ Acute alveolar osteitis	☐ Cavernous sinus	☐ Superficial skin infection
☐ Maxillary Sinusitis	(dry socket)	thrombosis	☐ Superficial mucosal infection
☐ Other _____	☐ Osteitis		☐ Other _____
_____	☐ Osteomyelitis		
	☐ Osteoradionecrosis		

Progress of Infection is . ☐ Chronic (slow)   ☐ Acute (rapid)   ☐ Dangerously Acute (fulminating) _____

EVALUATION OF MODIFYING FACTORS

Patient's Health	Anatomical Factors	Microbial Factors	
☐ Serious medical risk	☐ High risk space(s)	☐ Acute cellulitis	☑ Culture indicated but
☐ Moderate medical risk	☐ Multiple spaces (bi)	☐ Systemic toxicity	not taken
☐ Low medical risk	☑ Involves adjacent areas	☐ Extreme swelling	☑ No Gram stain
☑ No medical risk	but controllable	☑ Fever	☐ Culture taken
Why? _____	☐ Confined to alveolar ridge	☐ Chronic infection	☐ Gram stain obtained
P.M.H. - negative	Where? ® buccal space	☐ Recent antibiotic	☐ Culture not indicated
		☐ Poor O.H./perio disease	Other _____

INITIAL DIAGNOSIS: postoperative ® buccal space infection. Most likely resident oral flora which may be sensitive to penicillin

INITIAL COURSE OF ACTION

☑ Treat in office   ☐ Refer to a specialist   ☐ Hospitalize. Who/Where? _____
☑ Need additional data. What data? Culture and sensitivity testing

5. b.

DEFINITIVE DIAGNOSIS

☑ Agrees/Consistent with initial diagnosis
☐ Differs from initial diagnosis _____

DEFINITIVE COURSE OF ACTION

☑ Treat in office   ☐ Refer to a specialist   ☐ Hospitalize. Who/Where? _____
☐ Need additional data. What data? _____

6. a.

DIAGNOSTIC DECISIONS

SUMMARY OF PATIENT'S PROBLEMS

1. pain
2. moderate trismus
3. slight dysphagia
4. swelling around mand. 3rd molar
5. decreased oral intake
6. penicillin allergy
7. asthma - childhood
8. fever - 100.6° F
9. red, diffuse, tender swelling
10. partially impacted 3rd molar
11. _____
12. _____
13. _____
14. _____
15. _____

PROCESS FOR INITIAL DIAGNOSIS

Problem is . . . . ☑ Microbial ☐ Non-Microbial ☐ Unknown_____

Source of Infection is . . ☑ Odontogenic ☐ Non-odontogenic ☐ From Dental Tx ☐ Unknown_____

Soft Tissue (dentally related)	Periosteum	Special sigificance	Soft tissue (non-dental)
☐ Periodontal Abscess	☐ Subperiosteal abscess	☑ Acute cellulitis	☐ Maxillary sinusitis
☑ Pericoronal Abscess	☐ Post-Injection	☑ Ludwig's angina	☐ Peritonsillar abscess
☐ Dento-Alveolar Abscess	☐ Periostitis	☑ Osteo-	☐ Salivary gland infection
☐ Post-surgical Infection	**Hard Tissue**	radionecrosis	☐ Ear infection
☐ Post-injection Infection	☐ Acute alveolar osteitis	☑ Cavernous sinus	☐ Superficial skin infection
☐ Maxillary Sinusitis	(dry socket)	thrombosis	☐ Superficial mucosal infection
☐ Other _____	☐ Osteitis		☐ Other _____
	☐ Osteomyelitis		
	☐ Osteoradionecrosis		

Progress of Infection is . ☐ Chronic (slow) ☑ Acute (rapid) ☐ Dangerously Acute (fulminating) _____

EVALUATION OF MODIFYING FACTORS

Patient's Health	Anatomical Factors	Microbial Factors	
☐ Serious medical risk	☐ High risk space(s)	☐ Acute cellulitis *see note below* ☒	☐ Culture indicated but
☑ Moderate medical risk	☐ Multiple spaces (bi)	☐ Systemic toxicity	not taken
☐ Low medical risk	☑ Involves adjacent areas	☐ Extreme swelling ☒	☐ No Gram stain
☐ No medical risk	but controllable	☑ Fever *invalid technique*	☑ Culture taken
Why? ↓ food & fluid intake	☐ Confined to alveolar ridge	☐ Chronic infection	☐ Gram stain obtained
penicillin allergy	Where? possibly pterygomand.	☐ Recent antibiotic	☐ Culture not indicated
asthma history	lat. pharyngeal, submasseteric	☐ Poor O.H./perio disease	Other swab used

INITIAL DIAGNOSIS: acute pericoronal abscess of mandibular (L) 3rd molar with possible spread into pterygomandibular, lateral pharyngeal and/or submasseteric space

DEFINITIVE COURSE OF ACTION

☐ Treat in office   ☑ Refer to a specialist   ☐ Hospitalize. Who/Where? _____

☑ Need additional data. What data? Culture and sensitivity

NOTE: While an attempt was made to culture material from this infection, the use of cotton swabs was inappropriate and provided irrelevant data. The cotton swab would probably have been contaminated with oral flora and thus the results would not detect the true identity of the microorganisms responsible for the infection. Since the swelling was not localized or fluctuant at the initial appointment, culturing at that time was premature. Culturing should have been postponed until needle aspirate technique could be used.

6. b.

DIAGNOSTIC DECISIONS

SUMMARY OF PATIENT'S PROBLEMS
1. *severe trismus & dysphagia*
2. *no food or liquid intake 36 hrs*
3. *temp ↑ 103.4F pulse ↑ 82*
4. *resp. rate ↑ 20*
5. *unable to take oral meds*
6. *Swelling: red, firm, nonfluctuant*
7. *involved spaces: Ⓛ submandibular,*
8. *submasseteric, lateral neck*
9. *node involvement: tender, enlarged*
10. *L juguloomohyoid*
11. *fluctuance in Ⓛ buccal*
12. *vestibule*
13. *respiratory difficulty*
14. ___
15. ___

PROCESS FOR INITIAL DIAGNOSIS
Problem is ....☑ Microbial ☐ Non-Microbial ☐ Unknown___
Source of Infection is ..☑ Odontogenic ☐ Non-odontogenic ☐ From Dental Tx ☐ Unknown ___

Soft Tissue (dentally related)
☐ Periodontal Abscess
☑ Pericoronal Abscess
☐ Dento-Alveolar Abscess
☐ Post-surgical Infection
☐ Post-injection Infection
☐ Maxillary Sinusitis
☐ Other ___
___

Periosteum
☐ Subperiosteal abscess
☐ Post-Injection
☐ Periostitis
Hard Tissue
☐ Acute alveolar osteitis (dry socket)
☐ Osteitis
☐ Osteomyelitis
☐ Osteoradionecrosis

Special sigificance
☑ Acute cellulitis
☐ Ludwig's angina
☐ Osteo-radionecrosis
☐ Cavernous sinus thrombosis

Soft tissue (non-dental)
☐ Maxillary sinusitis
☐ Peritonsillar abscess
☐ Salivary gland infection
☐ Ear infection
☐ Superficial skin infection
☐ Superficial mucosal infection
☐ Other ___

Progress of Infection is . ☐ Chronic (slow) ☐ Acute (rapid) ☑ Dangerously Acute (fulminating) ___

EVALUATION OF MODIFYING FACTORS

Patient's Health
☑ Serious medical risk
☐ Moderate medical risk
☐ Low medical risk
☐ No medical risk
Why? *↓ eating and fluid intake respiratory difficulty*

Anatomical Factors
☑ High risk space(s)
☐ Multiple spaces (bi)
☐ Involves adjacent areas but controllable
☐ Confined to alveolar ridge
Where? *lateral neck*

Microbial Factors
☑ Acute cellulitis
☑ Systemic toxicity
☑ Extreme swelling
☑ Fever
☐ Chronic infection
☐ Recent antibiotic
☐ Poor O.H./perio disease

☐ Culture indicated but not taken
☐ No Gram stain
☑ Culture taken
☑ Gram stain obtained
☐ Culture not indicated
Other ___

INITIAL DIAGNOSIS: *acute cellulitis involving multiple spaces and spreading into cervical spaces. Serious general signs of toxicity and respiratory difficulty are present. Source of infection - pericoronal abscess. Medical risk increased due to dehydration*

INITIAL COURSE OF ACTION
☐ Treat in office ☑ Refer to a specialist ☑ Hospitalize. Who/Where? ___
☑ Need additional data. What data? *culture and sensitivity testing*

6. c.

The errors or inadequacies in data collection and/or diagnosis include:
1. *The potential seriousness of this problem was initially underestimated based on the nutritional status, clinical signs and symptoms, and anatomical areas involved.*
2. *Use of a cotton swab to collect the initial specimen was inappropriate and wasted both time and the patient's money.*
3. *Use of 250 mg of erythromycin was insufficient (this will be discussed in the next unit).*
4. *No mention of curettage around the partially erupted tooth was made (this will be discussed in the next unit).*
5. *The four-day follow-up schedule was much too long, thus not permitting the clinician to detect the worsening of the condition at an early stage (this will be discussed in the next unit).*

Overall, this patient should have been referred to a specialist when first seen because of dehydration and lack of nutritional intake, the anatomical areas involved, the probable inability to take antibiotics orally due to trismus and dysphagia. The diagnosis of acute pericoronitis is correct, however, if no mention was made of the seriousness of the modifying factors in the diagnosis, the true seriousness of the problem would not have been reflected.

TREATMENT

The next two units of this book focus on the treatment of odontogenic and dentally related oral and/or maxillofacial infections. In the **treatment phase** of infection management the information obtained during **data collection** and **diagnosis** is utilized to select appropriate treatment methods and the results of these treatment methods are **monitored** to permit rational alterations in treatment when needed. The need for referral to a specialist and/or hospital should be evaluated at each phase.

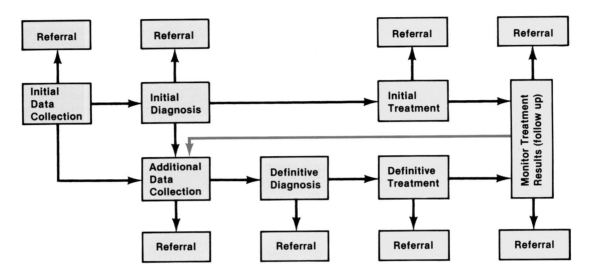

Unit VIII — Management of Odontogenic and Dentally Related Infections — This unit reviews the process of defining management objectives and choosing treatment methods appropriate to manage the degree of severity of patient problems. Emphasis is placed on the spectrum of treatment options ranging from procedures that can be performed by the patient or in the setting of a general dentist's office to those requiring hospitalization. This unit also reviews the concepts involved in monitoring the results of treatment. A summary of infection management is provided at the end of this unit.

NOTE: **The effective and efficient management of oral infections requires both theoretical knowledge and clinical experience. Selection of treatment options should be carefully planned in relationship to the overall condition of each individual patient. Use of treatment methods which are not justified by supporting data can lead to unnecessary treatment and expense to your patient and, in addition, may actually confuse the clinical picture and thus compromise and/or delay appropriate treatment.**

Unit IX — Checklist for Diagnosing and Managing Oral and/or Maxillofacial Swellings — This short unit collects all of the checklists utilized in this book together in a form that can be used in the clinical management of patients.

UNIT VIII
MANAGEMENT OF ODONTOGENIC AND DENTALLY RELATED INFECTIONS

OVERVIEW & OBJECTIVES

The purpose of this unit is to summarize the management options for treating patients with dentally related oral and/or maxillofacial infections. In this unit we will present an overall philosophy for treating infections. Management objectives are defined from the areas of **improving patient health, anatomical factors,** and **microbial characteristics. Initial** treatment methods are selected as a result of your initial diagnosis and often changed to **definitive** methods once a definitive diagnosis is obtained. **Monitoring the results of treatment** is an essential component in the overall management of infections and prompt appropriate referral to a specialist or hospital is stressed for infections whose management requirements are beyond usual training of general dentists. Following completion of this unit you will:

1. Describe the overall philosophy for the management of dentally related oral and/or maxillofacial infections.
2. Diagram the three (3) general areas that must be considered when formulating management objectives **and** the effects each area can have on the other two components.
3. Diagram the treatment options that are directed toward treatment of each area of the overlapping circle diagram.
4. Describe the relationship between initial and definitive treatment in terms of:
     a. availability of data   b. knowledge of cause   c. specificity of treatment
5. Given a diagnosis of any critical conditions, describe the proper management procedures.
6. Name seven (7) **management objectives** which must be considered in the area of **improving a patient's resistance.**
7. Name and describe each of the **specific treatment options** for each of the seven (7) management objectives for improving patient resistance.
8. Name three (3) management objectives directed toward **reducing the numbers of microorganisms** present in an oral infection.
9. Name three (3) treatment methods used to obtain **drainage** of an infected area **without the use of incision and drainage** and describe the limitations of these methods.
10. Name two (2) approaches to **incision** and **drainage** and describe why the external methods should usually be performed by a specialist.
11. Describe the technique for intraoral incision and drainage.
12. Describe which intraoral anatomical areas should be incised and drained by a specialist and which areas are usually within the training of general dentists.
13. Describe the indications and contraindications for the use of antibiotic therapy.
14. Given Gram stain results and/or a microbiologist's report, select the antibiotic of choice for the management of oral infections.
15. Describe the three (3) management objectives which should be considered in the area of **improving anatomical factors.**
16. Describe the similarities and differences between initial and definitive treatment in terms of timing and techniques used.
17. Given a complete description of data and diagnostic decisions for a patient with an oral infection, identify and describe the appropriate management objectives, treatment methods and monitoring strategy and/or referral decisions which should be planned for the management of the infection.

UNIT VIII
MANAGEMENT OF ODONTOGENIC AND DENTALLY RELATED INFECTIONS

INTRODUCTION

Management of oral and/or maxillofacial infections should not be taken lightly. Even now, in spite of modern medical skills and the latest anti-microbial drugs, dentally related infections occasionally lead to the death of patients. Seemingly simple infections can rapidly progress to complex problems. Therefore, when managing patients with infections, you should direct your treatment toward **all** aspects of improving patient health.

NOTE: Your goal in managing any infection is to restore the health of your patient as rapidly as possible with a minimum of lasting consequences.

We have emphasized earlier the importance of collecting sufficient data to derive an accurate list of patient problems and an accurate diagnosis of the etiology of any oral and/or maxillofacial swelling. We have also stressed the need to identify other factors related to the patient's overall health. In Unit VIII we developed the concept of overlapping circles to illustrate the various components which must be considered in diagnosing the cause of an infection and evaluating the overall seriousness of the problem. In this unit we will present a summary of specific treatment methods or management strategies that can be used to improve your patient's problems. **Figure VIII-1** summarizes the three major areas of concern.

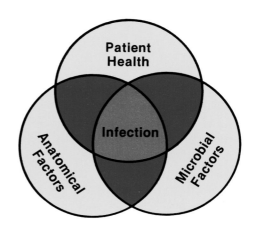

Figure VIII-1. Summary of major areas that must be considered when diagnosing and treating oral and/or maxillofacial infections.

Defining Management Objectives

Prior to initiating any treatment procedures you should identify any specific patient problems that may require management and thus define a list of **management objectives.** Defining this list will then enable you to select treatment methods on a basis of defined need instead of randomly initiating treatment with little knowledge of the desired outcome or reason for the treatment.

Through definition of treatment objectives you can then initiate **specific treatment methods or procedures** and then observe the effects of treatment as related to the objectives of treatment. If the specific treatment does not accomplish the treatment objectives then alternative treatment methods can be initiated and patient progress monitored.

From analysis of **patient resistance, anatomical factors** and **causative microorganisms,** treatment objectives can be divided into the following general categories:
- **improving your patient's overall body resistance** (including management of medical problems)
- **decreasing problems associated with the anatomical location of the problem**
- **eliminating the causative microorganisms**

Each of these general objectives can be divided into specific objectives. **Figure VIII-2** below provides a summary of the relationship between patient problems, management objectives and the various treatment methods used to manage problems associated with infections.

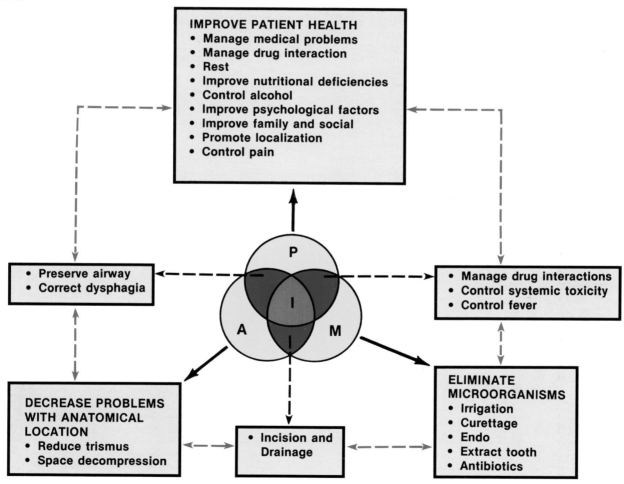

Figure VIII-2. Summary of management objectives and treatment methods used for oral and/or maxillofacial infections. The solid black arrows in this diagram point to the management objectives used for improving patient health (P), decreasing problems with anatomical location (A), and eliminating the causative microorganisms (M). The black dashed arrows point to the management objectives for managing problems which result from the overlap of the three major components of the infection. The blue dashed arrows emphasize the overlapping effects of treatment methods (e.g. incision and drainage can reduce both anatomical and microbial factors).

The checklist on the next page summarizes the general and specific management objectives and the treatment methods commonly used to manage oral and/or maxillofacial infections. You will notice that this section of the form is divided into **initial treatment** and **definitive treatment**. You should check the boxes to the left to define your objectives and then select the treatment method to meet the objective.

MANAGEMENT SUMMARY

MANAGEMENT OF CRITICAL CONDITIONS

Yes	No	Condition Present	Describe Condition	Refer	Hospitalize
☑	☐	Abnormally high fever	_____	☐	☐
☐	☐	Respiratory problems...................	_____	☐	☐
☐	☐	CNS involvement	_____	☐	☐
☐	☐	Systemic toxicity	_____	☐	☐
☐	☐	Dehydration (moderate to severe)	_____	☐	☐
☐	☐	Inadequate nutrition (moderate to severe) ..	_____	☐	☐
☐	☐	Spread to critical areas	_____	☐	☐
☐	☐	Medically compromised patient...........	_____	☐	☐
☐	☐	High potential for alcohol or drug withdrawal	_____	☐	☐

INITIAL TREATMENT (based on initial diagnosis)

Improving body resistance

Yes No

☐ ☐ Manage systemic medical problems. How? _____ ☐ ☐

☐ ☐ Manage possible drug interaction problems. How? _____ ☐ ☐

☐ ☐ Obtain adequate rest .... ☐ Limit activities ☐ Home or bed rest _____ ☐ ☐

☐ ☐ Improve nutritional deficiencies

   ☐ Improve caloric and protein intake. How? _____ ☐ ☐

   ☐ Improve fluid intake. How? _____ ☐ ☐

   ☐ Improve vitamin/mineral intake. How? _____ ☐ ☐

☐ ☐ Control alcohol consumption How? _____ ☐ ☐

☐ ☐ Manage drug addiction problem How? _____ ☐ ☐

☐ ☐ Improve psychological factors How? _____ ☐ ☐

☐ ☐ Improve family & social factors How? _____ ☐ ☐

☐ ☐ Promote localization — Heat ☐ Intraoral ☐ Extraoral How _____ ☐ ☐

☐ ☐ Control pain ☐ Analgesic_____ Dose_____ Route_____ ☐ ☐

   ☐ Sedative dressing _____ ☐

Elimination of causative microorganisms

☐ ☐ Drainage

   ☐ Irrigation with water or saline _____

   ☐ Curettage around the following teeth _____

   ☐ Endodontic treatment of the following teeth _____ ☐

   ☐ Extraction of the following teeth _____ ☐ ☐

☐ ☐ Incise and Drain ..... Location _____ ☐ ☐

   ☒ Intraoral .... Where? _____ ☐ ☐

   ☒ Extraoral .... Where? _____ ☐ ☐

☐ ☐ Remove sequestrum.. Where? _____ ☐ ☐

☐ ☐ Antibiotic therapy_____ Dose_____ Duration_____ ☐ ☐

Improving Anatomical Factors

☐ ☐ Relieve trismus ...... How? _____ ☐ ☐

☐ ☐ Preserving airway .... How? _____ ☐ ☐

☐ ☐ Space decompression How? _____ ☐

DEFINITIVE TREATMENT

☐ No change from initial therapy required

☐ Changes from initial therapy required (describe) _____ ☐ ☐

   ☐ ☐ Manage critical systemic conditions _____ ☐ ☐

   ☐ ☐ Improving body resistance_____ ☐ ☐

      ☐ Change pain medication_____ ☐ ☐

      ☐ Other _____

   ☐ ☐ Elimination of microorganism(s) _____ ☐ ☐

      ☐ Change antibiotic(s) to _____ dose _____ duration _____ ☐ ☐

      _____ dose _____ duration _____

      ☐ Other _____

   ☐ ☐ Manage anatomical factors _____ ☐ ☐

      ☐ Obtain additional drainage _____ ☐ ☐

      ☐ Other _____

Comments_____

MONITORING TREATMENT RESULTS

	Patient Appt.	Seen	Clinical Course of Infection Worse	Same	Better	Resolved	Referred Specialist	Hospital	Comments
Day 0		☒	☐	☐	☐	☐	☐	☐	_____
Day 1	☐	☐	☐	☐	☐	☐	☐	☐	_____
Day 2 ..	☐	☐	☐	☐	☐	☐	☐	☐	_____
Day 3	☐	☐	☐	☐	☐	☐	☐	☐	_____
Day 4 ..	☐	☐	☐	☐	☐	☐	☐	☐	_____
Day 5	☐	☐	☐	☐	☐	☐	☐	☐	_____
Day 6 ..	☐	☐	☐	☐	☐	☐	☐	☐	_____
Day 7	☐	☐	☐	☐	☐	☐	☐	☐	_____
Day 10 ..	☐	☐	☐	☐	☐	☐	☐	☐	_____
Day 14	☐	☐	☐	☐	☐	☐	☐	☐	_____
Long term ..	☐	☐	☐	☐	☐	☐	☐	☐	_____

As you can see, this checklist emphasizes treatment objectives, treatment methods and referral decisions as well as a course of action for monitoring the progress of treatment. It organizes this approach by first listing conditions **requiring immediate referral or hospitalization** then proceeding with **initial** and **definitive management objectives** and **selection of treatment options.** We will discuss each of the following areas of the checklist.

- **Management of critical conditions**
- **Initial management objectives and treatment methods** (based upon initial data)
   Improving patient resistance
   Elimination of causative microorganisms
   Managing problems associated with anatomical factors
- **Definitive treatment methods** (based upon definitive data)
- **Monitoring treatment results**

MANAGEMENT OF CRITICAL CONDITIONS

The first step in the management of any infectious process involves the management of any critical or life-threatening conditions or problems. A thorough review of your data and diagnostic problem list should enable you to detect any of the following problems and seek appropriate referral **immediately.** If no critical conditions are present at this time, you should also indicate this on the management checklist.

MANAGEMENT OF CRITICAL CONDITIONS

Yes	No	Condition Present	Describe Condition	Refer	Hospitalize
☐	☐	Abnormally high fever	_____	☐	☐
☐	☐	Respiratory problems.....................	_____	☐	☐
☐	☐	CNS involvement	_____	☐	☐
☐	☐	Systemic toxicity	_____	☐	☐
☐	☐	Dehydration (moderate to severe)	_____	☐	☐
☐	☐	Inadequate nutrition (moderate to severe) ..	_____	☐	☐
☐	☐	Spread to critical areas	_____	☐	☐
☐	☐	Medically compromised patient	_____	☐	☐
☐	☐	High potential for alcohol or drug withdrawal	_____	☐	☐

NOTE: The treatment of the initial source of an infection must be regarded as SECONDARY to the management of any critical or life-threatening condition.

*Assuming that all other signs and symptoms are within the scope of a general practitioner's ability to manage, which of the following signs and symptoms or patient problems would indicate: **NO** = no critical condition present at this time; **R** = immediate referral to a specialist; and **H** = hospitalization is essential at this time?*

Signs & Symptoms or Problem	NO	R	H	Why?
1. Vital Signs: T = 41°C, BP = 130/82/80, Pulse = 98, Resp. = 22	☑	☐	☒	*only temp up*
2. Vital Signs: T = 38°C, BP = 140/83/83, Pulse = 82, Resp. = 18	☑	☐	☐	
3. Difficulty in swallowing to the degree that food and water cannot be taken in.	☐	☐	☒	*dysplacation of swallowt*
4. Dental infection involving base of upper lip, infraorbital and periorbital areas.	☐	☐	☒	*progressive infecti*
5. Patient must lean forward and stick out her chin to breath.	☐	☐	☒	*''*
6. Patient's eyes appear to bulge, and are very lethargic.			☒	*''*
7. Patient complains of pain in his neck.	☐	☑	☐	*''*
8. Patient is diabetic and cannot be trusted to take insulin injections regularly.	☐	☑	☐	

ANSWERS

1. *H, V.S. show patient in extreme danger.*
2. *NO, V.S. alone do not indicate presence of critical condition.*
3. *H, Aphagia — needs I.V. fluids and nutrients.*
4. *H, Critical anatomic areas — high risk of cavernous sinus thrombosis.*

5. *H, Indicates partial respiratory obstruction. Total obstruction could occur at any time.*
6. *H, CNS involvement likely.*
7. *R and/or H, Spread to cervical spaces indicates expert supervision essential.*
8. *R and/or H. Patient must receive insulin on regular basis under supervision.*

INITIAL MANAGEMENT OBJECTIVES

Treatment of any oral and/or maxillofacial infection should begin immediately following initial data collection, initial diagnosis, and formulation of initial management objectives.

The distinction between **initial** and **definitive treatment** is similar to the distinction between initial and definitive diagnosis. **Initial treatment is based upon your initial clinical findings and initial diagnosis.** An initial diagnosis frequently lacks laboratory information concerning the characteristics of the involved microorganisms, may lack information from other laboratory tests and may lack additional radiographic data. Despite the limitations of initial diagnosis, you must promptly formulate initial management objectives and begin initial treatment while awaiting additional data. Initial treatment is based upon **generally applied** treatment methods which have been proven successful in the management of a wide range of infections. However this approach is not always successful.

Definitive treatment is based upon your definitive diagnosis and employs **specific treatment methods.** Definitive treatment is initiated after you have obtained laboratory results, obtained additional radiographic data and have observed the clinical results of initial treatment methods.

Identification of initial management objectives for **improving patient resistance, eliminating the causative microorganism(s)** and **improving anatomical factors** are shown with boxes on the left side of the checklist below. You should **check the appropriate management objectives** under the "**Yes/No**" columns, thus indicating a need for action in each area **before** selecting the **specific treatment method.**

INITIAL TREATMENT (based on initial diagnosis)
Improving body resistance

Yes	No		Refer	Hospitalize
☐	☐	Manage systemic medical problems. How? _____	☐	☐
☐	☐	Manage possible drug interaction problems. How? _____	☐	☐
☐	☐	Obtain adequate rest .... ☐ Limit activities ☐ Home or bed rest _____	☐	☐
☐	☐	Improve nutritional deficiencies		
		☐ Improve caloric and protein intake. How? _____	☐	☐
		☐ Improve fluid intake. How? _____	☐	☐
		☐ Improve vitamin/mineral intake. How? _____	☐	☐
☐	☐	Control alcohol consumption How? _____	☐	☐
☐	☐	Manage drug addiction problem How? _____	☐	☐
☐	☐	Improve psychological factors How? _____	☐	☐
☐	☐	Improve family & social factors How? _____	☐	☐
☐	☐	Promote localization — Heat ☐ Intraoral ☐ Extraoral How _____	☐	☐
☐	☐	Control pain ☐ Analgesic_____ Dose_____ Route_____	☐	☐
		☐ Sedative dressing _____	☐	☐

Elimination of causative microorganisms

Yes	No		Refer	Hospitalize
☐	☐	Drainage		
		☐ Irrigation with water or saline _____		
		☐ Curettage around the following teeth _____		
		☐ Endodontic treatment of the following teeth _____	☐	
		☐ Extraction of the following teeth _____	☐	☐
☐	☐	Incise and Drain ..... Location _____	☐	☐
		☑ Intraoral .... Where? _____	☐	☐
		☑ Extraoral .... Where? _____	☐	☐
☐	☐	Remove sequestrum.. Where? _____	☐	☐
☐	☐	Antibiotic therapy_____ Dose_____ Duration_____	☐	☐

Improving Anatomical Factors

Yes	No		Refer	Hospitalize
☐	☐	Relieve trismus ...... How? _____	☐	☐
☐	☐	Preserving airway .... How? _____	☐	☐
☐	☐	Space decompression How? _____	☐	☐

STUDY EXERCISES

Initial management objectives are management objectives developed from ___initial___ data. Initial management objectives serve as guidelines for selecting ___initial___ treatment ___methods___. The three general areas that should be evaluated include:

- ___improving body resistance___
- ___causative microorganisms___
- ___improving anatomical factors___
- ___assessing need to refer___

If your initial data and initial diagnosis indicates the need to manage a particular problem, then you should check the ___yes___ box on the checklist. If not, you should check ___no___ box on the checklist. Once an initial management objective has been identified you should then select a treatment ___method___ to manage the problem.

INITIAL TREATMENT METHODS

In the next section of this unit we will discuss the various treatment methods that can be used to satisfy each of the management objectives in the areas of:

- **Improving body resistance**
- **Eliminating the causative microorganism**
- **Improving anatomical factors**

This list is first intended to guide your **initial treatment decisions.** It can also be used later to plan **definitive treatment** if any changes are necessary. You will notice that the right-hand column of the checklist, shown on page 244, indicates need for referral and/or hospitalization. Occasionally, the treatment methods required to satisfy a specific management objective involve techniques usually beyond the scope of general dentistry or placing the patient in a controlled environment.

Improving Body Resistance

Your **first step** in the treatment of an infection is to identify the presence of problems or conditions which could contribute to a decrease in your patient's natural defense mechanisms. Your next step is to choose appropriate treatment methods to correct the problems. Under the category of **improving patient's body resistance**, we will discuss treatment options for the following problems.

Improving body resistance

Yes No
- ☐ ☐ Manage systemic medical problems. How? _____ ☐ ☐
- ☐ ☐ Manage possible drug interaction problems. How? _____ ☐ ☐
- ☐ ☐ Obtain adequate rest .... ☐ Limit activities ☐ Home or bed rest _____ ☐ ☐
- ☐ ☐ Improve nutritional deficiencies
  - ☐ Improve caloric and protein intake. How? _____ ☐ ☐
  - ☐ Improve fluid intake.   How? _____ ☐ ☐
  - ☐ Improve vitamin/mineral intake. How? _____ ☐ ☐
- ☐ ☐ Control alcohol consumption   How? _____ ☐ ☐
- ☐ ☐ Manage drug addiction problem   How? _____ ☐ ☐
- ☐ ☐ Improve psychological factors   How? _____ ☐ ☐
- ☐ ☐ Improve family & social factors How? _____ ☐ ☐
- ☐ ☐ Promote localization − Heat ☐ Intraoral ☐ Extraoral How _____ ☐ ☐
- ☐ ☐ Control pain   ☐ Analgesic_____ Dose_____ Route_____ ☐ ☐
                      ☐ Sedative dressing _____ ☐ ☐

Yes No
☐ ☐ Manage Systemic Medical Problems

You should assess your patient's medical history and seek appropriate counsel for managing any medical problems. Briefly describe your planned management in the space provided. Notice that management of some conditions may require referral or even hospitalization of your patient. A complete discussion of the interaction between infections and systemic medical disorders is beyond the scope of this book.

☐ ☐ Manage Possible Drug Interaction Problems

A careful analysis of all drugs or medications your patient may be taking could reveal underlying medical or psychological problems or potential problems in the management of an infection. A discussion of drug interaction problems is beyond the scope of this book.

☐ ☐ Obtain Adequate Rest

Rest is an often underrated but important factor in raising a patient's body resistance to infection. **The amount of rest required must be proportional to the degree of seriousness of the infection and the general health of the patient.**

Treatment Options

The treatment options for obtaining adequate patient rest include:
- **Advise patient to limit strenuous activities.** You would use this option for healthy patients with relatively minor infections. Frequently very active patients will not follow this advice and more controlled measures are necessary.
- **Advise patient to stay home.** Convalescence at home with or without bed rest.
- **Admit patient to hospital.** If infection involves high-risk fascial spaces or has spread bilaterally in the neck area; if patient has signs and symptoms of systemic toxicity, and/or if patient **will not** or **cannot obtain adequate rest** at home (because of psychological, family or social factors), admission to a hospital is indicated.

☐ ☐ **Improving Nutritional Deficiencies**

You should take measures to improve any nutritional deficiencies. Patients with oral swelling and pain are frequently dysphagic or even aphagic and have dangerously low rates of fluid intake. Adequate caloric, protein, fluid, and vitamin and mineral intake must be established. Again, treatment options can range from **advice** to **hospitalization.**

If a patient is on a special diet for any systemic disorder you must consult with his physician before altering his dietary intake. The patient must be advised of the importance of adequate nutrition and be instructed to discontinue any weight control diets during the course of treatment.

If improvements in a patient's nutritional status is one of your management objectives, mark the checklist. You should then decide which aspects of nutritional deficiencies are to be treated and describe how this is to be done.

☐ ☐ Improve nutritional deficiencies
    ☐ Improve caloric and protein intake. How? _____ ☐ ☐
    ☐ Improve fluid intake. How? _____ ☐ ☐
    ☐ Improve vitamin/mineral intake. How? _____ ☐ ☐

Treatment Options to Improve Nutritional Deficiencies

The following treatment methods can be used to improve each of the categories of nutritional deficiencies:

☐ **Improve Caloric and Protein Intake**

- **Instruct patient to eat well-balanced meals** with at least 170 grams (6 oz.) of protein and a total caloric content of about 3,000 calories per day. This can only be advised for patients who **do not** have difficulties swallowing.
- **Liquid diets** with high protein and high caloric values.
- **Admit patient to the hospital** where nutritional intake can be closely controlled and supplemented with I.V. feeding when necessary.

☐ **Improve Fluid Intake**

Dehydration and salt imbalances are common in patients who have had a serious infection for several days prior to seeking treatment, or can become a serious problem during treatment. Fluid intake should be at least 3 liters per day including water intake and water content of foods.
- **Advise patient to drink 8-10 glasses of fluid per day.**
- **Admit patient to hospital** and place on I.V. fluids.

☐ **Improve Vitamin and Mineral Intake**

Vitamin and mineral deficiencies can be present in older patients who have not eaten well, in patients suffering from alcoholism, drug addiction, or in otherwise healthy patients who have a debilitating infection. Since many vitamins are precursors to essential metabolic co-enzymes, they are essential factors for improving body defense systems.
- **Advise patient to take over-the-counter vitamins.**
- **Prescribe vitamins and minerals.**
- **Place patient in hospital if severe** vitamin and dietary deficiencies exist.

☐ ☐ **Manage Alcohol Consumption**

Alcohol can produce serious drug interaction problems when consumed with pain control agents or antibiotics.

Treatment Options to Control Use of Alcohol

- Advise patients to **discontinue alcohol consumption immediately** and not resume consumption of alcohol until infection has resolved and all medications have been discontinued.
- Patient **should be hospitalized** if high consumption of alcohol is expected during treatment. **Any patient with a potential for D.T.s if alcohol is withdrawn must be hospitalized.**

☐ ☐ **Manage Drug Abuse Problems**

Drug abusers, especially narcotic addicts, can present major problems to you during treatment of a painful infection. They may overstate their pain and demand more potent analgesics and then sell these drugs to others rather than taking them as prescribed. Often these patients will see multiple dentists for the same infection to obtain narcotic prescriptions. In addition, these patients may not be responsible enough to obtain (and take) antibiotic prescriptions.

Treatment Options

- **Verify patient's story with his/her drug counselor**, if on methadone program.
- **Substitute non-narcotic analgesics** (aspirin, Ibuprofen, acetaminophen) for mild to moderate pain control (since most non-narcotic analgesics are peripheral acting they may not provide effective pain relief).
- **Prescribe combinations of aspirin** (or acetaminophen) and codeine.
- **Refer** patient with drug addiction problem to oral surgeon or hospital for management.

These patients can be a difficult management problem for anyone treating them.

☐ ☐ **Improve Psychological Factors**

A patient's psychological status can have significant effect on his/her ability to follow your instructions. Such conditions as **extreme anxiety, hysteria, senile dementia, schizophrenia, marked depression,** or **mental retardation** can be of major significance. If you cannot rely upon your patient to carry out your instructions or to make return visits to your office for monitoring results, your patient should be referred or hospitalized.

Treatment Options for Managing Psychological Factors

- **Discuss problem** with patient and/or family.
- Refer patient for **outpatient counseling.**
- **Hospitalize** patient if problem is acute.

☐ ☐ **Improve Family and Social Factors**

Improvements in your patient's surrounding environment are often necessary. Persons living alone may require assistance and persons with heavy family responsibilities may require temporary removal from this environment. Hospitalization may be your only way to improve family and/or social factors.

Treatment Options to Improve Family and Social Factors

- **Obtain responsible care** for persons living alone including relative, friend, or even public health nurse.
- **Hospitalize patients** to place them into a controlled environment free from family and social distractions.

☐ ☐ Promote Localization

If allowed to pursue their natural course, non-localized bacterial infections will usually localize (become fluctuant), develop pus, form an abscess, and establish intraoral or extraoral drainage. This sequence of events assumes that the infection does not involve vital structures, produce septicemia or systemic toxicity. Many clinicians believe the application of heat will promote pus formation (localization) and cause the abscess to "point" in the direction of the heat source. Heat may be applied **intraorally** or **extraorally. The key to the use of heat is to localize an infection or encourage drainage without promoting the extension of the infection to adjacent areas or causing the infection to "point" to an area where facial scarring will result.** If you plan to apply heat to promote localization you should follow the guidelines below:

Guidelines for Heat Application

1. Heat applied to non-suppurative infections appears to hasten the onset of suppuration. Heat will hasten movement of suppuration to the surface along natural pathways, but transcending of anatomical barriers is unclear.

2. Heat applied to a cellulitis without also using antibiotics (or other treatment) is likely to cause the infection to spread.

3. Once antibiotic is shown to be effective in treating a cellulitis, heat may be applied to speed resolution, but antibiotic must be continued.

4. Heat applied after pus has formed may increase presure in the abscess and cause extension of the infection if drainage is not first established.

5. If lymph nodes are involved, continue antibiotic and heat application. This will either resolve the lymph node involvement **or** lead to suppuration and drainage of the involved lymph nodes.

6. Once drainage has been established extraoral (and intraoral) heat application will encourage drainage.

Treatment Options to Promote Localization

- **Intraoral heat** can be applied using warm water or saline. Generally one teaspoon of table salt (NaCl) is dissolved in an 8-10 oz. glass of warm water. The water temperature should be just hot enough to be tolerated by oral tissues, but not too hot to cause tissue damage. Your patient should hold the warm saline in his/her mouth as long as it remains warm, then discard the solution and repeat with another mouthful. Advise patients not to swallow the saline solution. Patients should repeat this procedure about **once per hour** during waking hours for 1-2 days.

- **Extraoral heat** can be applied by the use of a heating pad, hot water bottle, hot towel or washcloth heated with hot tap water. Extraoral heat may be used once adequate drainage has been established.

  Application of extraoral heat is rarely used in the treatment of non-localized dental infections because extraoral drainage of fascial space infections can result in permanent facial scarring. If extraoral drainage is indicated, you should refer your patient to a specialist.

You should never apply heat to a non-localized infection WITHOUT ANTIBIOTIC COVERAGE. Application of heat to a diffuse swelling can cause accelerated spread to adjacent areas before localization and fluctuance have developed.

☐ ☐ **Controlling Pain**

Pain accompanying an infection may require analgesic therapy to alleviate suffering and provide enough comfort for your patient to eat and rest. Pain from infection can vary with the severity of the infection as well as with the individual. Pain from infections can be very severe and often requires central-acting analgesics. Once pressure from an abscess is released the degree of pain usually diminishes and a peripherally acting analgesic will be effective. A combination of central-acting and peripheral-acting analgesics is often indicated.

Medication Options for Controlling Pain

- Advise patient to take aspirin, 650 mg or Acetaminophen, 600-1,000 mg. This can be **given for mild pain** and has additional antipyretic effects. (q4h)
- For **moderate pain** prescribe a combination of aspirin (or acetaminophen) plus a narcotic such as codeine (or narcotic derivative such as oxycodone).
- **Hospitalize patient** for administration of analgesic such as I.M. meperidine 75 mg every 3 hours. This may be necessary in cases of severe cellulitis.

   Pain from odontogenic infections is real and significant. Constant pain can prevent rest and may prolong your patient's recovery time.

STUDY EXERCISES

Treatment options for **obtaining adequate rest** *include:*
- limit strenuous activity
- stay home
- admit to hospital if unable to comply

Treatment options to improve a **patient's nutritional status** *include:*

Caloric & Protein	**Fluids**	**Vitamins & Minerals**
balanced diet	8-10 glass fluid/day	OTC vitamin
liquid diet	hospital if unable to comply	Rx vitamins
hospital if unable to comply		hospital

Treatment options to **control alcohol** *consumption and possible D.T.s include:*
- hospital
- withdraw from its consumption

Treatment options to **manage drug abuse** *problems include:*
- hospital
- drug consulting consult
- substitute non narcotic drugs
- Rx combination aspirin & codeine

Treatment options to improve **psychological factors** *include:*
- hospitalize
- discuss w/ family
- outpatient counseling

Treatment options to improve **family and social factors** *include:*
- Obtain care of responsible person
- hospitalize

Treatment methods to **promote localization** *of an infection include:*
- intraoral heat
- extraoral heat

Treatment methods to help **control pain** *include:*
- Mild pain   aspirin
- Moderate pain   aspirin + codeine
- Severe pain   hospitalize + demerol

STUDY QUESTIONS

*For each of the following cases, complete the checklist for **improving body resistance**.*

Case #1. *You have just diagnosed a 65-year-old patient to have a fluctuant submandibular space infection which has developed 4 days after you extracted his non-vital, periapically abscessed, left mandibular first molar. The patient is single and retired and lives alone in a hotel without bath and toilet facilities in his room. He smokes two packs (40) of cigarettes and consumes one pint (325 ml) of whiskey per day. He lacks cooking facilities and normally obtains one meal per day at a local mission consisting of a bowl of soup and piece of bread. Currently he complains of moderate to severe pain in the area of swelling which has kept him awake for the past two nights. His past medical history taken at the time of surgery (four days ago) indicated severe edema of the ankles and shortness of breath when climbing the one flight of stairs to your office. His blood pressure is currently 180/95, Pulse = 82, Temp = 38.2°C and R.R. = 18.*

Improving body resistance

Yes No
- ☒ ☐ Manage systemic medical problems. How? __CHF__
- ☒ ☐ Manage possible drug interaction problems. How? __Alcohol__
- ☒ ☐ Obtain adequate rest .... ☐ Limit activities ☐ Home or bed rest _____
- ☒ ☐ Improve nutritional deficiencies
  - ☐ Improve caloric and protein intake. How? __hospital__
  - ☐ Improve fluid intake.   How? __"__
  - ☐ Improve vitamin/mineral intake. How? __"__
- ☒ ☐ Control alcohol consumption   How? _____
- ☐ ☐ Manage drug addiction problem   How? _____
- ☐ ☐ Improve psychological factors   How? _____
- ☐ ☐ Improve family & social factors   How? _____
- ☒ ☐ Promote localization — Heat ☐ Intraoral ☐ Extraoral How _____
- ☒ ☐ Control pain   ☐ Analgesic_____ Dose_____ Route __IV__
  - ☐ Sedative dressing_____

Case #2. *A 45-year-old female with a 20-year history of diabetes mellitus and rheumatic heart disease returns to your office with a non-fluctuant submental spce infection two days after you began endodontic treatment of her mandibular left central incisor. Prior to initiating endodontic treatment you reviewed her medical history and found her taking the following medications: **insulin** (40 units I.M. in the morning); **Digoxin; Hydrochlorthiazide** (diuretic); and the **codeine** (30 mg) with aspirin (320 mg) which you prescribed following her endodontic treatment. Prior to beginning endodontic treatment you believed her diabetes to be under control and she was premedicated with phenoxymethyl penicillin 1.0 gm one hour before treatment and continuing to today. She lives at home with her husband and 18-year-old daughter. She does not consume alcohol (on advice of her physician) and she has no significant psychological or family problems. **Clinical** examination revealed a moderately firm, reddish swelling confined to the anterior portion of the submental space. Temp = 38.0°C, B.P. = 160/80; Pulse = 83; Resp. Rate = 17.*

Improving body resistance

Yes No
- ☒ ☐ Manage systemic medical problems. How? __diabetes & RHD__
- ☒ ☐ Manage possible drug interaction problems. How? _____
- ☒ ☐ Obtain adequate rest .... ☐ Limit activities ☐ Home or bed rest _____
- ☐ ☐ Improve nutritional deficiencies
  - ☐ Improve caloric and protein intake. How? _____
  - ☐ Improve fluid intake.   How? _____
  - ☐ Improve vitamin/mineral intake. How? _____
- ☐ ☒ Control alcohol consumption   How? _____
- ☐ ☒ Manage drug addiction problem   How? _____
- ☐ ☐ Improve psychological factors   How? _____
- ☐ ☐ Improve family & social factors   How? _____
- ☒ ☐ Promote localization — Heat ☐ Intraoral ☐ Extraoral How _____
- ☒ ☐ Control pain   ☒ Analgesic __Asp + Codn__ Dose_____ Route __ORAL__
  - ☐ Sedative dressing_____

STUDY EXERCISES

*Case #3. A healthy 18-year-old male patient of yours comes to your office complaining of pain in the back of his mouth and some soreness when he opens his mouth. The problem began 3 days ago and is getting worse. A review of his **medical history** indicates he is in excellent health and is not currently taking any medications. He has adequate nutritional intake at this time. He is an aerobic dance instructor and spends 6 hours per day exercising with his classes. For the last two nights he has only been able to sleep for 2-3 hours because of the pain. Your **clinical examination** revealed no serious conditions; Temp = 38°C, Pulse 60, BP 120/50, Resp. rate = 15. You observe a localized, non-fluctuant reddish area distal to a partially erupted mandibular right third molar with minor swelling of the anterior pillar area. While pain is elicited, no restriction of mouth opening is seen. Local pre-disposing signs are negative. Radiographs are negative. **Diagnosis** was moderate pericoronitis around mandibular right third molar extending into the pterygomandibular space with no modifying factors which would increase patient risk.*

Improving body resistance

Yes No
- [ ] [x] Manage systemic medical problems. How? _____ [ ] [ ]
- [ ] [x] Manage possible drug interaction problems. How? _____ [ ] [ ]
- [x] [ ] Obtain adequate rest .... [x] Limit activities [x] Home or bed rest _____ [ ] [ ]
- [ ] [x] Improve nutritional deficiencies [ ] [ ]
  - [ ] Improve caloric and protein intake. How? _____ [ ] [ ]
  - [ ] Improve fluid intake. How? _____ [ ] [ ]
  - [ ] Improve vitamin/mineral intake. How? _____ [ ] [ ]
- [ ] [x] Control alcohol consumption How? _____ [ ] [ ]
- [ ] [x] Manage drug addiction problem How? _____ [ ] [ ]
- [ ] [x] Improve psychological factors How? _____ [ ] [ ]
- [ ] [x] Improve family & social factors How? _____ [ ] [ ]
- [ ] [x] Promote localization — Heat [ ] Intraoral [ ] Extraoral How _____ [ ] [ ]
- [x] [ ] Control pain [x] Analgesic *Asp, Codien* Dose_____ Route *Oral* [ ] [ ]
  - [ ] Sedative dressing _____

Discussion of Cases

Case #1 Discussion.

Improving body resistance

Yes No
- [x] [ ] Manage systemic medical problems. How? *Possible Undiagnosed Heart Disease* [x] [x]
- [ ] [x] Manage possible drug interaction problems. How? _____ [ ] [ ]
- [ ] [ ] Obtain adequate rest .... [ ] Limit activities [ ] Home or bed rest _____ [ ] [ ]
- [x] [ ] Improve nutritional deficiencies
  - [ ] Improve caloric and protein intake. How? *Past history of very Poor Nutrition* [ ] [x]
  - [ ] Improve fluid intake. How? *Hospital referral needed* [ ] [x]
  - [ ] Improve vitamin/mineral intake. How? _____ [ ] [x]
- [x] [ ] Control alcohol consumption How? *Hospitalize* [ ] [x]
- [ ] [ ] Manage drug addiction problem How? _____ [ ] [ ]
- [ ] [ ] Improve psychological factors How? _____ [ ] [x]
- [x] [ ] Improve family & social factors How? *Hospitalize* [ ] [x]
- [x] [ ] Promote localization — Heat [ ] Intraoral [ ] Extraoral How _____ [x] [x]
- [x] [ ] Control pain [x] Analgesic_____ Dose_____ Route *I.V.* [ ] [ ]
  - [ ] Sedative dressing _____

In management of this patient you should first consider management of possible undiagnosed heart disease (swollen ankles and shortness of breath). His family and social factors (living conditions) contribute significantly to his nutritional deficiencies, alcohol consumption, and lack of an adequate living environment for suportive care. In addition, pain may be preventing adequate rest. All of these factors indicate that the patient would best be treated in a hospital environment.

In retrospect, a more thorough patient evaluation should have been performed prior to tooth extraction and the patient referred to a specialist for the initial tooth extraction. Control of his compromising conditions prior to tooth extraction may have reduced the probability for this current infection.

Case #2 Discussion.

Improving body resistance

Yes No

☑ ☐ Manage systemic medical problems. How? *Significant Diabetes & Rheumatic Heart Dis.* ☐ ☑

☑ ☐ Manage possible drug interaction problems. How? *may need close medical management* ☐ ☑

☐ ☑ Obtain adequate rest . . . . ☐ Limit activities ☐ Home or bed rest _____ ☐ ☐

☐ ☑ Improve nutritional deficiencies

    ☐ Improve caloric and protein intake. How? _____ ☐ ☐

    ☐ Improve fluid intake. How? _____ ☐ ☐

    ☐ Improve vitamin/mineral intake. How? _____ ☐ ☐

☐ ☑ Control alcohol consumption How? _____ ☐ ☐

☐ ☑ Manage drug addiction problem How? _____ ☐ ☐

☐ ☑ Improve psychological factors How? _____ ☐ ☐

☐ ☑ Improve family & social factors How? _____ ☐ ☐

☑ ☐ Promote localization – Heat ☑ Intraoral ☐ Extraoral How *Intraoral Rinses hourly* ☐ ☐

☑ ☐ Control pain ☑ Analgesic *Codeine + Asprin* Dose *C·30 mg/A·325 Q3H* Route *orally* ☐ ☐

    ☐ Sedative dressing _____ ☐ ☐

Significant medical problems exist with this patient. Infections can be more difficult to control in diabetic patients because phagocytotic activity can be decreased. Other drug interaction problems must be monitored for possible drug interaction problems. This patient should be referred for specialized care and hospitalization may be justified. Continuation of pain control and localization of the infection are also important management objectives for improving body resistance. Other difficulties may also be involved in **eliminating the microorganism(s)** *and* **controlling anatomical factors.**

Case #3 Discussion.

Improving body resistance

Yes No

☐ ☑ Manage systemic medical problems. How? _____ ☐ ☐

☐ ☑ Manage possible drug interaction problems. How? _____ ☐ ☐

☑ ☐ Obtain adequate rest . . . . ☑ Limit activities ☑ Home or bed rest _____ ☐ ☐

☐ ☑ Improve nutritional deficiencies

    ☐ Improve caloric and protein intake. How? _____ ☐ ☐

    ☐ Improve fluid intake. How? _____ ☐ ☐

    ☐ Improve vitamin/mineral intake. How? _____ ☐ ☐

☐ ☑ Control alcohol consumption How? _____ ☐ ☐

☐ ☑ Manage drug addiction problem How? _____ ☐ ☐

☐ ☑ Improve psychological factors How? _____ ☐ ☐

☐ ☑ Improve family & social factors How? _____ ☐ ☐

☐ ☑ Promote localization – Heat ☑ Intraoral ☐ Extraoral How *Intraoral rinses hourly* ☐ ☐

☑ ☐ Control pain ☐ Analgesic *Codeine + Asprin* Dose *C·30 mg/A·325 Q3H* Route *orally* ☐ ☐

    ☐ Sedative dressing _____ ☐ ☐

In the area of improving patient resistance, no medical, drug, nutritional deficiency, alcohol, psychological or family and social problems require management. However, his strenuous work and pain (which is causing lack of sleep) may be slowly reducing his natural body resistance. These factors need management. The patient should stay home from work, and taking codeine (30 mg) and aspirin (325 mg) should control these factors. Application of hot rinses may pomote localization of the infection. Management of anatomical factors and methods for eliminating the causative microorganism(s) will be discussed later.

Eliminating the Causative Microorganism(s)

Fundamental to the treatment of any infection is the elimination of the causative microorganism(s). While the body defense mechanisms have capacities to eliminate microorganisms, intervention by health care specialists is frequently required to reduce the numbers of microorganism(s) present in an abscess to a level that can be managed by the patient's normal defense mechanisms. Page 4 of the checklist summarizes treatment options directed toward minimizing the numbers of microorganisms with the overall treatment objectives of:

- Controlling the spread of microorganisms
- Reducing swelling, pressure and pain
- Shortening the resolution time
- Minimizing any long- or short-term deformities that could result from prolonged infection

If infection is non-fluctuant, efforts to obtain drainage may be unsuccessful until fluctuance develops. You should attempt needle aspiration of the swelling prior to incision and drainage. If pus is obtained, send it to the lab for culturing. If no pus, delay I & D until fluctuance develops.

The treatment methods directed toward elimination of microorganisms from body tissues are described below. You should check the appropriate box on the checklist if drainage is indicated and check the treatment method you have selected. Describe where and how drainage is to be accomplished in the space to the right side.

Elimination of causative microorganisms

☐ ☐ Drainage
   ☐ Irrigation with water or saline _____
   ☐ Curettage around the following teeth _____
   ☐ Endodontic treatment of the following teeth _____
   ☐ Extraction of the following teeth _____
☐ ☐ Incise and Drain . . . . . Location _____
   ☑ Intraoral . . . . Where? _____
   ☑ Extraoral . . . . Where? _____
☐ ☐ Remove sequestrum . . Where? _____
☐ ☐ Antibiotic therapy _____ Dose _____ Duration _____

☐ ☐ Obtaining Local Drainage (Without Incision)

Many infections which are localized to the alveolar ridges can be managed by drainage methods that do not involve incision of tissues. While these methods should be considered first, you should not hesitate to perform intraoral incision and drainage for soft tissue infections that cannot be controlled by local drainage methods.

☐ Irrigation with Water or Saline

Irrigation with tap water or a saline solution can be helpful especially when treating mild forms of pericoronitis or for certain periodontal abscesses. Patients may be given 25 ml plastic syringes fitted with a curved plastic tip and/or rubber bulb with a curved tip) and instructed to squirt water under the tissue flap (operculum) overlying the partially erupted tooth or into the gingival sulcus or furcation area. Frequently this irrigation will induce drainage of local infection and partial or complete resolution will occur. The partially erupted mandibular third molar should be removed following resolution of any pericoronitis.

If this treatment method fails to decrease the problem in 1-2 days, more aggressive treatment is needed.

This treatment should always be used in conjunction with more aggressive methods if moderate or serious pericoronitis or periodontal abscess has spread to any of the fascial spaces.

☐ **Curettage of Periodontal Pockets**

Localized periodontal abscesses may frequently be drained through curettage of the gingival sulcus and removal of subgingival and supragingival calculus which often blocks the natural drainage of the sulcus. Patients may be instructed to keep the sulcus open by using a toothpick, small dental instrument, or other small device. Following resolution of the infection, surgical correction of the deep periodontal pocket may be required to prevent recurrence of the problem. You should refer your patient to a periodontist for consultation.

This treatment method may be inadequate if used alone in the treatment of a moderate to severe periodontal abscess with the spread of infection to fascial spaces or buccal vestibule.

☐ **Endodontic Treatment**

Drainage of periapical abscesses may be accomplished by opening the tooth and enlarging the root canals to allow pus to drain intraorally. Your training in the field of endodontics will generally explain this procedure.

Often insufficient drainage is obtained by this method alone. This is especially true if the infection has progressed into the fascial spaces of the head and neck.

☐ **Extraction of the Involved Tooth**

Extraction of an abscessed tooth (or teeth) with forceps and/or elevators has long been the method of choice for treating dental infections. Extraction of the involved tooth can remove the cause of the infection and allow drainage through the tooth socket. However, the use of modern endodontic techniques followed by tooth restoration, make this treatment option less desirable. Non-restorable decayed teeth or root fragments, non-correctable periodontally involved teeth, partially erupted impacted teeth, vertically fractured teeth, or teeth in the line of jaw fracture should be extracted.

If the infection has spread to facial spaces, additional treatment methods should also be used because drainage through the extraction socket may be insufficient.

Performing surgical extractions involving flap surgery can result in the spread of infection to surrounding fascial spaces or areas. You should attempt to resolve the infection then later extract the first tooth. If this approach is not possible, then close patient follow-up is essential.

STUDY EXERCISES

Summarize the following methods for obtaining drainage of alveolar ridge infections:
Irrigation with water or saline: _25ml plastic syringe, irrigate under operculum_
Curettage of periodontal pockets: _toothpick or small device to keep sulcus open_
Endodontic treatment: _allow drainage through tooth_
Extraction of involved tooth: _allow drainage through socket_

☐   ◻ Incision and Drainage

Incision and drainage is a treatment method which involves placing an incision through soft tissue extending into an area of localized abscess and allowing suppuration (pus) to drain from the abscess. **A drain is then placed to allow continued drainage.**

Incision and drainage procedures can contribute to the resolution of **acute localized infections** in the following ways:

- It is the most effective method for rapidly removing large numbers of microorganisms from a fluctuant abscess.
- It can reduce pain, trismus, or other loss of function associated with soft tissue swelling by reducing the pressure within the abscess.
- It can improve local blood circulation by reducing pressure in the area.
- It will reduce the probability of the infection spreading to adjacent fascial spaces or anatomical areas due to the increased pressure within the abscess.
- It will allow the removal of pus from the tissue, thus promoting more rapid soft tissue repair.
- It often alters the oxidation-reduction potential in the tissue, thereby preventing growth of facultative or anaerobic microbes.
- **Incision and drainage is GENERALLY INEFFECTIVE in the management of NON-FLUCTUANT infectious swellings such as acute cellulitis, actinomycosis and fungal infections.**

If incision and drainage is one of your treatment objectives you should check the "yes" column on the checklist and select the appropriate site. If the best site is extraoral or is a difficult intraoral site, refer your patient to an oral and maxillofacial surgeon.

Site Selection for Incision and Drainage

The incision should be placed **into healthy tissue adjacent to the most fluctuant area of the abscess.** Placement of incisions into inflamed and/or infected skin or mucosa can cause unnecessary scarring. The relative degree of difficulty associated with incision placement relates to the following:

- Ease of surgical access
- Potential damage to nerves, arteries, or salivary glands and/or ducts
- Potential for permanent scarring

Incision and drainage may be accomplished by either **intraoral** or **extraoral routes. Figure VIII-3** summarizes the range of difficulties associated with incision and drainage of various anatomical areas.

SITE SELECTION FOR INCISION AND DRAINAGE

INTRAORAL		EXTRAORAL	
LESS DIFFICULT	**MORE DIFFICULT**	**LESS DIFFICULT**	**MORE DIFFICULT**
• Maxillary buccal vestibule	• Sublingual space	• Mentalis space	• Submandibular space
• Maxillary labial vestibule	• Lateral pharyngeal		• Submental
• Hard palate	• Retropharyngeal		• Lateral pharyngeal
• Mentalis space	• Peritonsillar		• Submasseteric space
• Buccal space	• Pterygomandibular		• Infraorbital
• Mandibular facial vestibule except in area of mental nerve and facial artery	• Area of mental nerve		• Temporal spaces
	• Area of facial artery		• Cervical spaces
	• Infratemporal space		• Parotid space
• Infraorbital area	• Infraorbital area		

Figure VIII-3. Summary of the relative difficulties associated with intraoral and extraoral incision and drainage sites.

☑ Intraoral Incision and Drainage

Once you have determined the need for intraoral incision and drainage and have made the decision to perform this procedure yourself (rather than referring your patient), the following steps should be performed:

Site Selection

- **Identify** the area of fluctuance visually and by palpation.
- Select a site for incision which is **directly over** the fluctuant area (when possible) but **avoid important underlying anatomical structures** (nerves, arteries, salivary glands and ducts).

Particular care should be used in evaluating site selection. This process can be made more difficult if the area of swelling distorts the normal soft tissue landmarks.

Pain Control

During an intraoral incision and drainage procedure, the **majority of discomfort is associated with incision of the mucosal tissue.** Less pain is associated with procedures involving the abscess cavity and most deeper structures (procedures involving periosteum may also produce significant discomfort without adequate anesthesia). The following anesthetic techniques can minimize (or eliminate) much of the discomfort associated with intraoral incision and drainage:
- **Topical anesthetic** applied to mucosal surface in the surgical area.
- **Superficial infiltration** of local anesthetic solution.
- Regional block anesthesia.

Usually, the area of inflammation is hypersensitive to pain. You should avoid injecting anesthetic solutions into the abscessed or inflamed areas because:
- The products of inflammation can deactivate the anesthetic agents.
- Microorganisms may be carried into deeper tissues along the needle track.
- Additional fluid pressure produced by additional anesthetic solutions may force the infection into previously uninvolved areas.

Infection Involves	Problem	Solution
• Medial retromolar or anterior pillar areas	Infection spread to pterygomandibular space with "low block" technique for inferior alveolar nerve anesthesia	Use modified block technique — "high block"
• Maxillary buccal vestibule in 2nd and 3rd molar area	Infection spread to infratemporal space and pterygoid plexus possible with posterior superior alveolar nerve anesthesia	Use infraorbital block technique

NOTE: General anesthesia may be required to obtain adequate pain control for incision and drainage of deep fascial spaces, or may be necessary for extremely apprehensive patients and/or children.

Figure VIII-4. Problems associated with obtaining nerve block anesthesia when infection involves the needle path normally used for anesthesia.

NOTE: **Adequate pain control is essential to obtaining patient cooperation during an incision and drainage process. Inadequate pain control can lead to an inadequate attempt at incision and drainage and necessitate a repeat procedure and/or delays in resolution of the infection.**

Surface Decontamination

When possible (and if not performed at the time of specimen collection), surface decontamination of the oral mucosa should be performed prior to making the incision. Introducing oral flora into deeper tissue spaces may initiate a new and different infection or may add new organisms to the infection and influence future culture results.

Placing the Incision and Blunt Dissection

The **incision** should be made superficially through the mucosa and submucosa into the abscess cavity (site selection for the incision was previously discussed) and avoid important anatomical structures. It should be only large enough to allow placement of a quarter- or half-inch drain.

Following placement of the incision, a **blunt dissection** of the underlying tissue is performed with a straight or curved hemostat. In the blunt dissection technique, the tips of the **closed (but not locked) hemostat** are first inserted into the incision. Opening the hemostat then separates the underlying tissue. Blunt dissection should proceed until the abscess cavity is reached and suppuration (pus) exudes from the incision. If multiple spaces or areas are involved (e.g. maxillary buccal vestibule and infraorbital area), intraoral blunt dissection should be extended into the additional spaces or areas as well.

Drain Placement

The purpose of drain placement is to **keep the incision open** until the abscess cavity has completely drained. Without the aid of a drain the incision could close prematurely.

After exposing the abscess cavity with blunt dissection, an appropriate sterile rubber drain (¼″ Penrose drain) of adequate length is selected. By clipping the hemostat to the leading edge of the drain, the drain can be inserted through the incision to the depth of the abscess cavity. The hemostat is then opened and, with care, is withdrawn without inadvertently removing the drain. A suture is placed through the drain and mucosal tissue to stabilize the position of the drain and prevent premature removal. The suture should be placed in healthy tissue. Placement in highly inflamed mucosa may result in loss of the suture by tearing of the tissue and subsequent premature loss of the drain.

Intraoral drains should remain in place until drainage of the tissue space(s) has been completed and resolution of the infection is underway. Usually, intraoral drains are left in place for 2-7 days. Drains are to be removed by cutting the suture and removing the entire drain. When used for draining deep spaces, **progressive withdrawal** of the drain will promote healing of deeper tissues first.

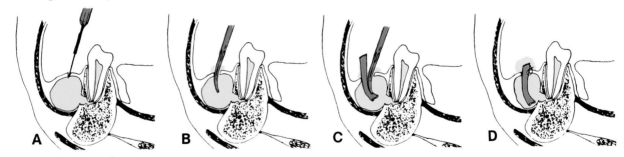

Figure VIII-5. Summary of the steps involved in intraoral incision and drainage. A. Incision is placed through decontaminated mucosal tissue. B. Blunt dissection of tissue is performed with a hemostat. C. Drain is inserted into abscess cavity with the aid of a hemostat. D. Drain position is secured by the placement of a suture.

On the **treatment summary checklist**, we have color coded the **degree of difficulty** for intraoral incision and drainage as both **blue** and **red** to reflect the wide range of difficulty associated with surgical access and avoidance of important underlying anatomical structures. If intraoral incision and drainage is indicated, you should **analyze** these variables and decide whether to perform this procedure **yourself** or **refer** this surgery to a specialist and/or hospital.

☑ Extraoral Incision and Drainage

A greater level of training and clinical experience is generally required to perform **extraoral** incision and drainage procedures. Detailed knowledge of the anatomical structures underlying the skin is essential to prevent damage to nerves, major blood vessels, salivary glands and ducts, especially if deeper spaces are involved. Sites for extraoral incisions must be chosen with care to minimize unsightly facial scarring. With the possible exception of infections involving the **mentalis, submental,** and **some submandibular** spaces, infections requiring extraoral incision and drainage are best referred to a dental specialist experienced in extraoral surgery. For these reasons, the need for extraoral incision and drainage has been color coded **yellow/red** indicating this technique should usually be referred to a specialist and/or hospital. We will, however, briefly review the procedure for extraoral incision and drainage to highlight the similarities and differences between extraoral and intraoral techniques.

Site Selection

The incision site for extraoral incision and drainage should be the **most dependent location** (a dependent location is the lowest point of the abscess cavity when the head is in an upright position) to allow suppuration to drain from the inferior aspect of the abscess cavity. The skin incision should be placed in an **inconspicuous location** on the head (usually below the inferior border of the mandible, along the hair line, or in or paralleling natural skin folds).

The incision should **avoid damaging important anatomical structures** such as the **facial** and **trigeminal nerves, major arteries** and **saliary glands** and **ducts.**

As you can see, selecting the optimal site for an extraoral incision is more involved than for intraoral site selection. Extraoral incision requires both detailed knowledge of facial anatomy and specialized clinical training.

Surface Decontamination

Prior to placing the incision through skin, the surgical site should be decontaminated with Betadine® or Phisohex® surgical scrub to remove as much normal skin flora as possible and a sterile surgical drape is often positioned. The exclusion of skin flora from the surgical site is fundamental to any surgical procedure.

Pain Control

The skin is the most sensitive tissue encountered when performing an extraoral incision and drainage. However, unlike oral mucosa, the skin is impermeable to topical application of anesthetics. Therefore, pain control can only be accomplished by **local infiltration of anesthetic.**

Regional intraoral nerve blocks (e.g. mandibular nerve, posterior superior alveolar nerve, etc.) may help to reduce pain from deeper soft tissues and periosteum. **General anesthetics** are frequently used when deeper fascial spaces are approached from extraoral routes. **The use of a general anesthetic during the treatment of Ludwig's angina or a severe neck infection with associated respiratory difficulty can be dangerous.** (See Ludwig's angina, page 194.)

Incision and Blunt Dissection

Once the incision site has been carefully selected and prepared, an **incision** is placed **only through the skin and subcutaneous** tissue and should be only **large enough to accommodate the drain size selected** (¼", ½", or 1"). Blunt dissection using a hemostat is used to separate deeper tissues and is slowly advanced into the abscess cavity. It is important to **determine whether more than one abscess cavity is present** and to **establish adequate drainage of all involved areas. Multilocular** abscess cavities often occur and **require careful blunt dissection** to expose each area.

Drain Placement and Removal

While there are many types of drains and considerable variation in the number of drains used for extraoral incision and drainage, the principles of drainage remain the same. Sterile rubber drains are used to maintain an opening between the abscess cavity and the skin surface to prevent closure of the incision and allow drainage to continue.

The drain is first grasped by a hemostat near its **leading edge** and carried into the abscess cavity by insertion of the hemostat through the skin incision. The drain is then **released** and the **hemostat is carefully withdrawn, leaving the drain in place.**

Frequently long drains are placed **through** an abscess cavity, entering through a skin incision on one side and exiting through a skin incision on the other side. These **"through-and-through"** drains are believed to better facilitate drainage and may allow irrigation procedures if indicated.

The drain must then be secured to prevent accidental displacement or removal. As with intraoral drains, a suture (usually a 3-0 or 4-0 nylon monofilament) is placed through the drain and the skin. Through-and-through drains are often not sutured, but both ends are joined by a "safety pin."

A **sterile dressing** is then placed over the drain to **reduce environmental contamination of the wound area** and **collect suppuration.**

Since a drain is a foreign body irritant and potential source of new infection, it should be removed as soon as suppuration has ceased to flow. Gram stains and culturing attempts which show absence of microorganisms can also be used as a guide for determining the appropriate time for drain removal. Clinical experience with extraoral drains will enable you to distinguish between suppurative drainage and drainage resulting from the drain itself and normal tissue weepage. Usually, extraoral drains remain in place for 2-7 days. Drains placed in deep spaces are usually removed progressively over a period of days to allow the abscess cavity to close and heal from the deepest area first.

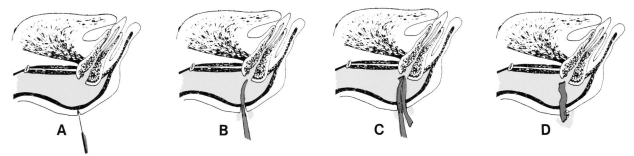

Figure VIII-6. Summary of the steps involved in extraoral incision and drainage of a submental space abscess. A. Incision is placed through decontaminated skin. B. Blunt dissection of tissue is performed with a hemostat. C. Drain is inserted into the abscess cavity with the aid of a hemostat. D. Drain position is secured with a suture.

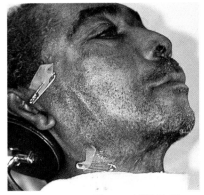
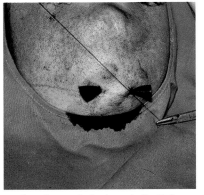
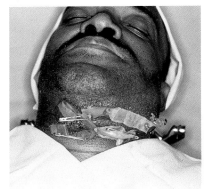

Figure VIII-7. Examples of extraoral drains: left, "Through-and-through" drain; center, "Bow-tie" drain; right, multiple drains as used in the treatment of Ludwig's angina

□ □ Remove Sequestrum (Debridement)

The term **sequestrectomy** is used to describe the removal of sequestra of necrotic bone. **Debridement** refers to the removal of devitalized soft tissue from a wound surface. Just as the key to successful root canal fillings depends upon the removal of necrotic pulp tissue, removal of necrotic bone and/or soft tissue may be the key to successful management of oral and/or maxillofacial infections. **The presence of necrotic tissue, with** or **without viable microorganisms, can stimulate the inflammatory process leading to further tissue breakdown and/or delay the healing process.**

Drainage (and/or incision and drainage) of oral and/or maxillofacial **soft tissue** infections is generally effective and **rarely** requires removal of necrotic proliferative granulation tissue. On the other hand, infections of **bone** (osteomyelitis and osteoradionecrosis) result in sequestra formation and resolution of bone infections will be delayed **until these sequestra are either resorbed or removed.** While small pieces of **uncontaminated avascular bone** (often resulting from surgical procedures) can be resorbed by the body, the resorption of **necrotic bone resulting from microbial infections** may take weeks, months or even years. The surgical removal of infected sequestra can **assist** the healing process and **reduce** healing time.

Surgical procedures used to remove necrotic bone can range from relatively **simple procedures** for removing small alveolar bone spicules (which have been retained under a surgical flap following tooth extraction) to **major surgical procedures** involving removal of entire sections of the mandible requiring reconstruction of surgical deformities with bone grafts, etc.

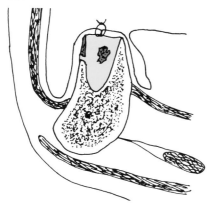

Figure VIII-8. Post-operative infections from surgical debris or inflammation from retained bone spicules can usually be managed by flap reflection and removal of the irritant. Sharp, avascular bone spicules are trimmed with a rongeurs.

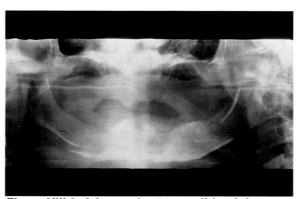

Figure VIII-9. Advanced osteomyelitis of the mandible requiring major sequestrectomy and reconstructive surgery.

If removal of sequestra is indicated, you should **assess** the amount of bone removal necessary. If it involves extensive areas of the maxilla or mandible, you should **refer** your patient to an oral and maxillofacial surgeon for management.

□ □ Antibiotic Therapy

The goal of this section is to present a **clinically useful approach** to the use of antibiotic therapy in the management of oral and/or maxillofacial infections.

Indications for the Use of Antibiotics

Antibiotics **can be** a valuable tool in the management of infections. On the other hand, indiscriminant and/or inappropriate use of these agents can actually be detrimental to both individual patients with infections and to the continued value of antibiotics in the treatment of all infections. The misuse of antibiotics in the treatment of infected patients **is of little therapeutic value** (but adds significant and/or unnecessary cost to patients) and can **complicate the clinical picture**, thus **seriously compromising subsequent treatment**. Widespread misuse of antibiotics can also **increase the numbers of resistant species** and **increase the number of allergic patients**, thus **diminishing** the long-term clinical value of these agents.

ANTIBIOTICS: INDICATIONS AND CONTRAINDICATIONS

ANTIBIOTICS ARE INDICATED	ANTIBIOTICS ARE NOT INDICATED
• For treatment of any acute diagnosed infection	• In minor chronic, well-localized oral infections (i.e. chronic periodontal abscess)
• When host defenses are seriously compromised by medical conditions and/or medications	• To promote wound healing
	• As prophylactic coverage for minor surgical or dental procedures
• For prophylactic coverage in patients with RHD, heart murmur, prosthetic heart appliances or other prosthetic devices	• To sterilize root canals
• When it is established that an infection has systemic involvement	• For treatment of chronic pericoronitis or gingivitis
• When facial or cervical cellulitis is present	• For treatment of localized osteitis, acute osteitis, or acute alveolar osteitis (dry socket)
• For acute pericoronitis	
• For osteomyelitis	• For prophylactic treatment of minor oro-antral perforations resulting from maxillary tooth extraction
• For fungal infection	• As post-surgical therapy for surgery involving the oral mucosa
• For acute periapical and periodontal abscesses if adequate endodontic and/or surgical drainage cannot be obtained	

Figure VIII-9. General indications and contraindications for the use of antibiotics.

NOTE: ANTIBIOTICS WILL NOT REMOVE PUS. Incision and drainage of suppurative material is the cornerstone of infection management. Antibiotics will help control and confine non-localized (non-fluctuant) infections until drainage can be obtained.

General Guidelines

When, in the management of oral and maxillofacial infections, the need for antibiotics **has been established**, the following **general guidelines** should be considered:
1. **Collect a specimen** from infected area **before** beginning antibiotic therapy when possible.
2. Ideally, obtain culture and susceptibility data **before selecting** an antibiotic.
3. If antibiotics are needed **prior** to receiving culture and susceptibility data, attempt to **obtain Gram stain data as a basis** for antibiotic selection.
4. If antibiotics are needed and **neither** culture and susceptibility nor Gram stain data are available, choose the antibiotic which is **"most likely"** to be effective against the presumed microorganism(s) based on the historical data and clinical data.
5. If two antibiotics are believed to be equally effective, choose the one with the **least side effects** and/or **lowest toxicity, and is the most cost effective for the patient.**

6. **Use larger doses of antibiotics for shorter periods of time** rather than lower doses for longer periods of time.

7. Parenterally administered (I.V. and I.M.) antibiotics attain more rapid and more reliable blood levels. **Anaphylactic reactions** are more likely to occur with parenterally administered antibiotics. Parenteral administration of antibiotics is usually performed by specialists with or without hospital support.

8. In severe, life-threatening infections requiring immediate antibiotic treatment (and where no C & S data is available), I.V. administration of high doses of multiple antibiotics under hospital conditions may be required. The antibiotics used are selected to kill a broad spectrum of microorganisms including both Gram (+) and Gram (−) forms. With some infections, even this approach will be unsuccessful.

When antibiotics are indicated in the treatment of an infection, your ability to choose the "ideal antibiotic" is greatly influenced by the following factors:

• The **degree of urgency** of the infection. The degree of urgency can range from:

  Not urgent, as seen often with chronic, low-grade infections (actinomycosis or fungal infections) which do not produce significant systemic effects and cannot be removed by drainage techniques.

  Urgent, as seen with a spreading cellulitis, especially if it is producing early signs of systemic involvement.

  Acute emergency, as seen with infections which have progressed to systemic toxicity, respiratory compromise, CNS involvement, etc.

• The **amount of information available** as to the identity, characteristics, and antibiotic susceptibilities of the microorganism(s) involved. Available information can range from **none** to definitive species identification and antibiotic susceptibilities.

Figure VIII-10 below summarizes the relationship between the above factors and your ability to select the "ideal antibiotic."

GUIDELINES FOR ANTIBIOTIC SELECTION BASED ON CLINICAL URGENCY

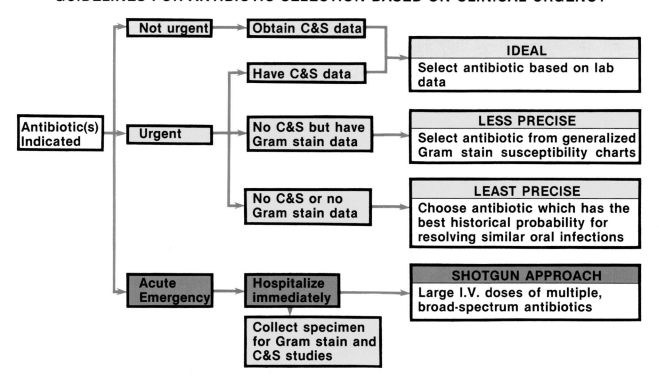

Figure VIII-10. Flow chart for selecting antibiotics based on clinical urgency.

Choosing the Appropriate Antibiotic

When choosing an appropriate antibiotic for the treatment of an oral and/or maxillofacial infection, a **careful evaluation of all relevant information is essential**. The following areas should be reviewed:

- **The overall health of the patient** (see the historical data checklist).
- **The specific clinical signs and symptoms** of the infection (see the clinical data checklists for signs and symptoms, anatomical location and radiographic data).
- **The results of any laboratory studies** (see the laboratory data checklists)
- **The evaluation of modifying factors.**
- **The clinical results of previous initial treatment.**

NOTE: Any uncontrolled oral and/or maxillofacial infection which requires the use of antibiotics should be monitored on a daily basis. If your initial antibiotic is not effective, immediately consult with a specialist and/or refer your patient.

If You Have Culture and Susceptibility (C&S) Data (Urgent and Not Urgent, see page 263)
If C&S data are available, you can prescribe an antibiotic which is very likely to control the infection (in conjunction with other treatment). If C&S data show **multiple drug susceptibilities**, you should **consult appropriate reference sources** and **select the drug of first choice** or an alternative drug if the first drug is unacceptable (e.g. allergy, recent antibiotic use, etc.). While the correlation between laboratory results and clinical effectiveness is **usually** quite high, you **should not always assume** this to be the case. Occasionally the lab data may indicate susceptibility to an antibiotic, but clinically the antibiotic may not be effective. The converse of this also may occur. **Regardless of laboratory data**, an antibiotic which **appears clinically effective should be continued.**

The chart in **Figure VIII-11** was developed to **assist physicians** in antibiotic selection for body infections. It is extremely useful as a quick reference for choosing an appropriate antibiotic once identification of the microorganism is established. (Unfortunately this chart does not include many of the oral flora involved in oral infections and the results may not apply to mixed infections from oral flora.)

If You Have Gram Stain Data But No C&S Data (Urgent but not an Acute Emergency)
In the absence of C&S data, the Gram stain results can often provide information useful in selecting an antibiotic. Gram stain results can be rapidly obtained (within about 20 minutes) and can:

- Establish presence of Gram (+) and/or Gram (−) microbes, identify morphology (cocci, rods and filamentous forms), describe growth characteristics (chains, clumps, large, small).
- Identify apparent single species or mixed infections and determine relative abundance of various Gram stain groups in a mixed infection (e.g. 4(+) Gram (+) cocci in clumps with 2(+) Gram (−) rods).

Gram stain results can be of great assistance but:

- **May not detect** small Gram (−) rods (often anaerobes) or microbes present in small numbers.
- **May not** be able to distinguish between species within the major Gram stain categories or **cannot** distinguish between aerobes and anaerobes.

When selecting an antibiotic with **only Gram stain** data:

- First, **if Gram stain provides sufficient data**, use the chart shown in **Figure VIII-11** (e.g., the presence of Gram (+) cocci in clumps often indicates presence of *staphylococci* and thus the drug of choice would be cloxacillin or dicloxacillin).
- If Gram stain data **is not this specific**, then refer to **Figure VIII-12** and select an antibiotic which is effective for the **most abundant organism** shown in the Gram stain specimen. See additional references (e.g. **Accepted Dental Therapeutics** or **Management of Infections of the Oral and Maxillofacial Regions** by Topazian and Goldberg).

Figure VIII-11 (Gram Negative Bacilli):

GRAM NEG. BACILLI	PENICILLIN	METHICILLIN-CLOXACILLIN	AMPICILLIN	CARBENICILLIN	CEPHALOSPORINS	ERYTHROMYCIN	TETRACYCLINE	CHLORAMPHENICOL	STREPTOMYCIN	KANAMYCIN	GENTAMICIN OR TOBRAMYCIN	POLYMYXIN	CLINDAMYCIN	SULFONAMIDES	AMIKACIN	TMP-SMX
Acinetobacter			R	3	R		R	R		1	1	2				S
Bacteroides fragilis	R			S	R⁴	R	2	1		R	R		1²			R
Bacteroides (other)	1		S	S	S	2	S	S	S	R	R		S			R
Bordetella pertussis						1	2									
Brucella							1	2	2	2	2					
Campylobacter						S			S	S						
Cholera							1	2								
E. coli			1	S	2	R	S	S		S	2				S	S
E. coli (urine)			S	S	S	R	S	S	S	S				S	S	S
Enterobacter			R	2	R⁴	R		S			1			1		1
Haemophilus influenzae			1	S	2³	R	S	S						3		S
Klebsiella			R	R	1¹	R		3	3	S	2¹					S¹
Pasteurella multocida	1		S				2	2								
Proteus (indole pos)			R	2	R⁴	R	R	S			2	1				S
Proteus mirabilis			1	S	2	R	R	S		S	S					S
Pseudomonas			R	1¹	R	R	R	R	R		1¹					S¹
Salmonella			2	S	S	R	S	1		S	S				S	S
Serratia			R	2	R⁴	R		2		1	1	R				S
Shigella			1	S	S	R	S	2		S	S					S
Yersinia pestis (Plague)									1		1					

1 = First Choice
2 = Second Choice
3 = Third Choice
R = Resistant
S = Sensitive

Superscripts
¹ May be used in combination for synergism
² Given IV
³ Cephalosporins ineffective for Haemophilus influenzae meningitis. Chloramphenicol alternative drug of choice in this situation. (Also true for meningococcal and pneumococcal meningitis.)
⁴ May be sensitive to expanded spectrum cephalosporins (cefoxitin, cefamandole).

Figure VIII-11 (Gram Positive Cocci, etc.):

	PENICILLIN	METHICILLIN-CLOXACILLIN	AMPICILLIN	CARBENICILLIN	CEPHALOSPORINS	ERYTHROMYCIN	TETRACYCLINE	CHLORAMPHENICOL	STREPTOMYCIN	KANAMYCIN	GENTAMICIN	VANCOMYCIN	CLINDAMYCIN	SPECTINOMYCIN	RIFAMPIN	SULFONAMIDES	TMP-SMX
GRAM POS. COCCI																	
Microaerophilic strep	1		2														
Pneumococci	1		2		2	S							3				
Staph (Coag neg.)	2	1	2										3				
Staph (Coag. pos.)		1	2		3									S	S⁸	2	
Strep Group A	1		2		2												
Strep fecalis (Enterococcus)	2⁶	1	3								2⁶	S					
Strep viridans	1⁵		2		2												
GRAM NEG. COCCI																	
Neis. gonorrheae	1		2		3	2	2							2			
Neis. meningitidis	1		3		3	1⁷	S								1⁷		
Clostridium perfringens	1				2	2	2	3					3				
Coryne. diphtheriae	2				1								3	3			
Listeria monocytogenes		1			2												
SPIROCHETES																	
Borrelia	2				1		1										
Leptospira	1				2		2										
Trep. pallidum	1				3	2	3										
ACTINOMYCETES																	
Actinomyces	1			2	2								S				
Nocardia					2	2⁵										1	S
MISCELLANEOUS																	
Chlamydia						S	S									S	S S
Mycoplasma						1	2										
Psittacosis							1	2									
Rickettsia							1	2									

Superscripts
⁵ Doxycycline, minocycline only.
⁶ Combined therapy of gentamicin plus penicillin or cephalosporin.
⁷ For carriers only; tetracycline prophylaxis refers to minocycline.
⁸ First choice if resistant to methicillin for serious infections.

Figure VIII-11. Selection of antibiotics based upon species identification and Gram stain reaction (from *Antimicrobial Therapy and Infectious Diseases*, Eisenberg, Furukawa, Ray, W.B. Saunders Co. 1980, with permission. **NOTE:** Publisher's errata sheet indicates strep. viridans reaction to penicillin should be 1⁶, not 1⁵.

If You Have NO Gram Stain or C&S Data (Urgent but not an Acute Emergency)

If **no lab data are available**, first, **obtain a specimen.** See **Figure VIII-12.** Then **choose** the antibiotic with the **best historical probability** for controlling oral infections. Usually **penicillin** (1.0g initial dose followed by 500 mg q6h for up to 7 days) will be effective. Monitor daily. If no improvement is seen **within two days**, consult with a specialist or refer.

NOTE: *Bacteroides fragilis* is generally resistant to penicillin. It can become the dominant organism in the presence of penicillin and rapidly cause a life-threatening infection.

Acute Emergency (No data)

Refer patient to hospital. Specialists will **first** obtain a specimen for lab studies, then administer **multiple I.V.** antibiotics in hope that "something" will work fast enough to save the patient's life.

%	Microorganisms	1st Choice	2nd Choice
	GRAM (+) COCCI		
60	Streptococci	Penicillin	Erythromycin Cephalosporin
8	Streptococcus fecalis	Ampicillin	Penicillin (+ gentamicin)
5	Staphylococcus	Penicillinase-resistant penicillin	Cephalosporin Clindamycin
18	Peptococcus } Peptostreptococcus }	Penicillin	Clindamycin
	GRAM (+) RODS		
7	Lactobacillus	Penicillin	
2	Bifidobacterium	Penicillin	
2	Eubacterium	Penicillin	
5	Actinomyces	Penicillin	Erythromycin Tetracycline

%	Microorganisms	1st Choice	2nd Choice
	GRAM (−) COCCI		
10	Neisseria	Penicillin	Amoxicillin Spectinomycin
20	Veillonella paruvla	Penicillin	
	GRAM (−) RODS		
15	Klebsiella-Enterobacter	Aminoglycoside	Cephalosporin TMP
15	Escherichia coli	Aminoglycoside	
20	Bacteroides species	Penicillin	Metronidazole Clindamycin
1	Bacteroides fragilis	Clindamycin	
5	Fusobacterium	Penicillin	
9	Eikenella Corrodens	Penicillin	Ampicillin Tetracycline

Figure VIII-12. Approximate percent occurrence of microorganisms involved in oral infections and the antibiotic(s) that can be used to control these organisms. You will notice that the total percentages exceed 100%, indicating mixed infections are common. See additional references for additional data.

Improving Anatomical Factors

Development of inflammation and/or accumulation of pus can produce signs and symptoms unique to the anatomical location of the infection. You should always evaluate the need to manage problems relating to the anatomical location of the infection.

NOTE: Drainage and/or incision and drainage of suppurative material (pus) is the cornerstone of infection management. Drainage can both remove large numbers of microorganisms and reduce problems associated with the anatomical location of the infection.

While incision and drainage will promote resolution of most problems associated with the anatomical location of an infection, it is generally ineffective if performed before the infection has localized (developed fluctuance). The management of the following signs and symptoms related to the anatomical location will be discussed in this section.

Improving Anatomical Factors
☐ ◼ Relieve trismus ...... How? _____ ☐ ☐
☐ ◼ Preserving airway .... How? _____ ☐ ☐
☐ ◼ Space decompression How? _____ ☐ ☐

☐ ◼ **Relieve Trismus**

Trismus is the painful condition which impairs the extension of the muscles associated with mastication. Trismus results from **inflammation** and/or **accumulation of toxins** in **muscle** fibers of this muscle group.

The **resolution** of trismus resulting from infection involves the **removal** of inflammatory exudates and/or toxins from the muscle fibers by blood and lymphatic circulation. The treatment of trismus, therefore, depends upon the **removal of the cause of inflammation** and **increasing the circulation** to the involved area. Assuming the cause of inflammation is being managed, the following treatment options can be used. However, these management techniques are mostly palliative.

Treatment Options to Relieve Trismus

- **Increase fluid intake 8-10 glasses of fluid/day.** This will promote circulation in the involved area and result in removal and excretion of inflammatory and microbial toxins.
- **Application of heat.** Heat application will increase local circulation and thus promote both localization of an infection and a reduction in trismus.
    Intraoral heat — Hot saline rinses (see page 249)
    Extraoral heat (see methods, page 249)

    NOTE: Never apply heat to non-localized infections without antibiotic coverage.

☐ ◼ **Preserving Airway**

Any patient who is having airway problems associated with an infection must be immediately referred to a specialist and/or hospital. The following discussion is mostly provided for your information and is **not** intended to suggest endorsement of these techniques for use by practitioners of general dentistry.

If a patient is having airway problems, **sedative agents** (strong narcotics) or **muscle relaxants** (diazepam) **should be avoided.** These patients may be relying upon the accessory muscles of respiration or body posturing to maintain respiration, and the use of these drugs may relax the patient sufficiently **to cause respiratory collapse.**

Preservation of the airway is **essential** in patients with infections involving posterior mandibular, pharyngeal, or cervical areas. The **accumulation of pus** can produce enough swelling to close off the upper airway, and **edema of the glottis and epiglottis** can obstruct the opening into the trachea. Two approaches can be used to maintain a compromised airway:

- **Intubation.** This technique involves placement of a tube (airway) from the upper respiration area into the trachea. The tube will prevent collapse of the soft tissue airway. Blind intubation, however, can puncture pharyngeal abscesses, causing suppuration to drain into the lungs or cause irritation of the epiglottis, producing edema and closure of the airway before the tube can be inserted. The use of a fiberoptic bronchoscope has, however, made this technique easier to perform and has also reduced the risks. Intubation is frequently performed prior to tracheostomy.

- **Establish new airway below the area of involvement.** This approach may be accomplished by coniotomy, tracheostomy or cricothyrotomy. A tracheostomy with local anesthesia is usually performed if general anesthesia is required for incision and drainage of the involved area.

☐ ☐ **Space Decompression**

In certain areas of the head and neck, acute swelling from inflammation and/or pus can compress vital structures and impair function. **Space decompression** may be necessary to **reduce the pressure** in a space **generated by the presence of inflammation and/or suppuration.** Methods for space decompression may be used both **prior to** or **after localization (fluctuance) has developed.**

- **Prior to localization.** A massive cellulitis of the neck may produce swelling which exceeds the elasticity of the skin and further swelling can then only proceed inward at the expense of the upper airway. **Incising the skin** of the throat area will permit external expansion and relieve internal pressure to the airway. This technique can be extremely valuable even if no drainage is obtained. The photo to the right illustrates an example of this technique. **Generally oral surgeons prefer to use horizontal incisions** rather than vertical incisions to minimize post-surgical scarring.

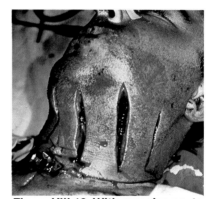

Figure VIII-13. With massive acute cellulitis of the neck region (Ludwig's angina), incising the skin of the throat may permit space decompression and relieve internal pressure on the airway. Multiple horizontal incisions are currently preferred.

- **After localization.** Usually, **incision and drainage** will relieve pressure within the abscess cavity once localization has occurred. **Aspiration** with a needle and syringe may also be used to remove small localized collections of pus. While the cause of the infection is being treated, **aspiration** of **small areas** of pus may remove the products of inflammation, eliminating the need for extraoral incision and drainage. Some **subperiosteal, palatal, mentalis, anterior submental** and **submasseteric space abscesses** can be managed by aspiration.

NOTE: Repeated aspirations may be necessary and the patient should be closely followed. This technique is likely to be ineffective if the source of the infection is not controlled or viable microorganisms remain in the abscess cavity.

268 Odontogenic Infections

DEFINITIVE TREATMENT

Definitive treatment can be initiated after a **definitive diagnosis** is obtained. As previously discussed, a **definitive diagnosis is developed from**:
- Laboratory data
- Additional radiographic data
- Additional clinical data
- Evaluation of the progress of initial treatment

Laboratory identification of an infectious microorganism and **determination** of the **antibiotic susceptibility** usually requires two to six days and occasionally longer if special stains, biopsy or other techniques are involved. During this time period many infections will be controlled through appropriate selection of initial treatment methods, thus a definitive diagnosis in these instances may be more precisely termed a **confirming diagnosis** since the problem may have resolved before the additional data becomes available.

However, if the problem **is not under control** by the time you receive these additional data, then a definitive diagnosis allows you to **assess** your **initial diagnosis, initial management objectives**, and **initial treatment methods** to determine the need for alternative treatment methods tailored to the **specific microorganism(s)** or new **problems**. Typically you may find that the microorganism(s) are not sensitive to the initial antibiotic and a different antibiotic is needed. You may **also** discover that other changes in your management objectives are necessary because **the patient's health may have deteriorated** (or improved) or additional (or fewer) anatomical areas are involved.

Thus, **definitive management objectives** are established and specific **definitive treatment methods** are selected from the treatment options described in the initial treatment section. A **definitive treatment checklist** has been designed to assist you in identifying the need to alter treatment based upon your definitive diagnosis.

DEFINITIVE TREATMENT
- ☐ No change from initial therapy required
- ☐ Changes from initial therapy required (describe) _____ ☐ ☐
    - ☐ ☐ Manage critical systemic conditions _____ ☐ ☐
    - ☐ ☐ Improving body resistance _____ ☐ ☐
        - ☐ Change pain medication _____ ☐ ☐
        - ☐ Other _____ ☐ ☐
    - ☐ ☐ Elimination of microorganism(s) _____ ☐ ☐
        - ☐ Change antibiotic(s) to _____ dose _____ duration _____ ☐ ☐
            - _____ dose _____ duration _____ ☐ ☐
        - ☐ Other _____ ☐ ☐
    - ☐ ☐ Manage anatomical factors _____ ☐ ☐
        - ☐ Obtain additional drainage _____ ☐ ☐
        - ☐ Other _____ ☐ ☐
- Comments_____

If your definitive management must involve significant changes, you should select another management checklist, cross out "initial treatment" and re-label it as "definitive treatment," date it, and identify your current **definitive management objectives** and describe your new treatment methods.

NOTE: If an infection is progressing rapidly in spite of your initial treatment methods you would be well advised to immediately refer your patient to a specialist without waiting to receive the laboratory data. This information should be forwarded to the specialist as soon as it is available.

STUDY EXERCISES

For the following clinical situation, describe the need for changes in initial treatment methods based upon initial treatment results and receipt of additional data.

Case Description: *Four days ago you performed endodontic drainage of a cariously involved, non-vital, mandibular left second premolar for a diet-controlled diabetic 24-year-old male. At the time of endodontic treatment only a small drop of suppuration was obtained, even with enlargement of the apical foramen. At that time a small, fluctuant, red swelling was also present in the lingual vestibule and you aspirated a specimen of pus and sent it to your clinical microbiology lab for analysis. Your initial diagnosis was "small sublingual space abscess secondary to an endodontic abscess of the mandibular left second premolar." Treatment consisted of endodontic access, medication of the pulp chamber with CMCP, closure of the orifice with temporary cement. Based upon STAT Gram stain report of 4 + Gram (+) cocci occurring in short chains, and 2 + Gram (+) cocci occurring in clumps, you wrote him a prescription for 10 days of oral penicillin (500 mg q6h) and advised him to take aspirin (650 mg) prn. The patient then left town for three days.*

The patient has now returned to your office. The sublingual swelling is larger and he complains of dull pain on swallowing which was not controlled by aspirin. His enlarged and tender left submandibular lymph node and the area under his chin appear swollen. Earlier that morning you received the lab report which indicated 4(+) **peptostreptococcus** *susceptible to penicillin, oxacillin, and erythromycin; 2(+) penicillinase-producing* **staphylococcus aureus** *susceptible to oxacillin, methicillin and dicloxacillin.*

Would the current clinical and laboratory data alter your initial diagnoses and treatment of this infection? ____yes____ If so, complete the checklist below.

DEFINITIVE TREATMENT

- ☐ No change from initial therapy required
- ☑ Changes from initial therapy required (describe) _____ ☐ ☐
  - ☐ ☐ Manage critical systemic conditions _____ ☐ ☐
  - ☐ ☐ Improving body resistance _____ ☐ ☐
    - ☐ Change pain medication _____ ☐ ☐
    - ☐ Other _____ ☐ ☐
  - ☐ ☐ Elimination of microorganism(s) _____ ☐ ☐
    - ☑ Change antibiotic(s) to _oxacillin_ dose _____ duration _____ ☐ ☐
      - _____ dose _____ duration _____ ☐ ☐
    - ☐ Other _____ ☐ ☐
  - ☑ ☐ Manage anatomical factors _____ ☐ ☐
    - ☑ Obtain additional drainage _____ ☐ ☐
    - ☐ Other _____ ☐ ☐
- Comments _____

Analysis: *A* **change** *from initial therapy is* **definitely required** *based on the* **clinical course of this infection** *and the* **laboratory data**. *The initial management of the infection was well done with the possible exception of the prescription for penicillin V instead of methicillin since the STAT Gram stain showed possible penicillinase-producing staphylococci (in lesser numbers, however, than the dominant streptococcal microorganisms). It was unfortunate that the patient left town for 3 days and was not available for daily recall and evaluation.*

Your **definitive diagnosis** *differs from your initial diagnosis only in regards to the presumed antibiotic susceptibility of the involved microorganisms. Currently additional anatomical areas are involved and your* **definitive course of action** *could be to either* **refer** *this patient to a specialist (not an unwise decision because of the potential complication of diabetes) or continue treatment in your office but monitor the results on a daily basis. Treatment should now consist of:*

Improving Body Resistance: *Restrict strenuous activities, maintain adequate nutrition through diet, and pain control (30 mg codeine prn)*

Elimination of Causative Microorganisms: *Open, drain and re-medicate the root canal (possibly instrumenting through the apex to induce additional drainage); incise and drain the sublingual abscess intraorally, and place a drain (this may be a difficult surgical procedure because of the anatomical area involved); continue penicillin and prescribe oxacillin (500 mg q6h) for 7-10 days. Usually, the surgical drain will be removed in 2-7 days and continued monitoring of drain site healing is advised.*

Improving Anatomical Factors: *May prescribe intraoral warm rinses and extraoral hot packs.*

NOTE: If you do not manage moderate infections regularly in your office, you should promptly refer this patient to a specialist. You should also transmit a description of what was done to date and a copy of the lab report.

NOTE: If patient's condition does not improve dramatically within 48 hours, referral to a specialist is essential.

MONITORING TREATMENT RESULTS

Any patient undergoing treatment for an oral and/or maxillofacial infection should be closely monitored to observe the results of treatment. There will be times when your **initial treatment methods** will **fail to control** a patient's problem. In addition, your patient **may not (or cannot) follow your instructions** and your planned treatment will not be carried out. Regardless of the reasons for ineffective treatment, you must **keep informed** of the results in time to either modify treatment or refer your patient.

NOTE: **Close monitoring of oral and/or maxillofacial infections will minimize the risk for serious complications. The frequency of monitoring must be determined according to the overall severity of the infection.**

General Guidelines

Selection of a monitoring schedule is based upon the **degree of severity** of the infection. The **severity** of oral infections can range from **low risk** (chronically draining fistula confined to the alveolar process) to **high risk** (massive, acute cellulitis or acute abcess involving critical fascial spaces). In addition, your **patient's health** may range from excellent to severely compromised and the **microorganism(s)** can be **slow growers** or **highly invasive**. Therefore, options for monitoring patients with oral infections can include:
- **Continuous monitoring in a hospital**
- **Daily** return visits to the dental office
- **Weekly** return visits
- **Monthly** or multiple month return visits

When monitoring the results of treatment, your **first concern** is to **establish that acute** (or potentially acute) **problems are controlled** and next that your treatment is effectively restoring the **overall health** of your patient. While this process may involve consultation with or referral to specialists, a general dentist will usually be responsible for long-term follow-up and definitive dental treatment.

> **EXAMPLE:** A patient presented to a general practitioner (general dentist) complaining of dental pain and soreness below his lower jaw. The presence of a submandibular space abscess with cellulitis secondary to pulpal necrosis of his mandibular left second molar was correctly diagnosed. Endodontic drainage and penicillin (500 q6h) therapy were immediately begun. However, this treatment **did not** resolve the problem and the infection spread to additionally involve the sublingual and submental spaces. The sequence of events was as follows:
> 1. Patient saw dentist who initially diagnosed the problem and instituted root canal access, prescribed penicillin and sent an aspirate specimen to the microbiology lab.
>   a. Patient was seen **the next day** and showed no improvement.
>   b. Patient seen on the following day, at which time swelling had crossed the midline and also involved sublingual and submental spaces. Culture results showed penicillin-resistant Gram (−) rods consistent with *Bacteriodes fragilis.*
> 2. Patient was **immediately** taken to hospital where an oral surgeon administered appropriate I.V. antibiotics and performed extraoral space decompression after tracheostomy.
>   a. Patient received continuous monitoring in the hospital for the next 10 days.
>   b. Patient then returned regularly to the oral surgeon's office for management of the incision and drainage site.
> 3. Patient later returned to the general dentist's office for **completion of root canal therapy**, for **long-term follow-up** of the root canal therapy and placement of a gold crown on the involved tooth.

The above scenario had a happy ending because the general dentist initially monitored the problem on a daily bais. If early detection of Ludwig's had not been made and appropriate referral not been made at that time, the outcome may have resembled that of the unfortunate case presented at the beginning of this book.

GUIDELINES FOR MONITORING TREATMENT RESULTS

MONITORING OPTIONS	WHEN USED
• Continuous monitoring in a hospital	• Life threatening infections • Debilitated or medically compromised patients • Infections from unusual microorganisms
• Daily office visits	• Any infection involving fascial spaces • Non-localized cellulitis • When an antibiotic was selected without C & S or Gram stain data and effectiveness is not established
• 2-3 day office visits	• Minor alveolar ridge infections • Infections that are resolving with appropriate treatment • Observation of I & D sites
• Weekly office visits	• Controlled infections requiring some follow up to monitor resolution • Treatment of chronic infections of known etiology (e.g. actinomycotic infections)
• Long-term follow up (monthly)	• Long-term follow up to determine success of treatment, frequently combined with 6-month or yearly dental check-ups

Figure VIII-14. Summary of monitoring options for evaluation of treatment results.

NOTE: Telephone communication should not be substituted for direct patient examination when an infection is active. However, telephone communication can be a valuable tool for detecting the presence of complicating factors and arranging direct patient examination.

Monitoring Schedule Checklist

The following monitoring schedule is provided on the management checklist to guide treatment follow up. You should date **Day 0** as the time when you were first contacted by the patient and instituted initial treatment. You should then plan the appropriate monitoring schedule, **date** these times and **reappoint** the patient for follow up. When the **patient returns**, you should check this box in the column headed "seen" (often patients fail to keep follow-up appointments or delay returning to your office until the problem has become more serious). During **each visit** you should briefly review the data collection and diagnosis portions of the checklist and **note** any changes in your patient's condition. At each visit you should determine whether the patient's condition is **getting worse, unchanged, improving** but not resolved, **resolved**, or at what stage your patient should be **referred**.

MONITORING TREATMENT RESULTS

	Patient Appt.	Patient Seen	Worse	Same	Better	Resolved	Referred Specialist	Referred Hospital	Comments
Day 0		☒					☐	☐	
Day 1	☐	☐	☐	☐	☐	☐	☐	☐	_____
Day 2	☐	☐	☐	☐	☐	☐	☐	☐	_____
Day 3	☐	☐	☐	☐	☐	☐	☐	☐	_____
Day 4	☐	☐	☐	☐	☐	☐	☐	☐	_____
Day 5	☐	☐	☐	☐	☐	☐	☐	☐	_____
Day 6	☐	☐	☐	☐	☐	☐	☐	☐	_____
Day 7	☐	☐	☐	☐	☐	☐	☐	☐	_____
Day 10	☐	☐	☐	☐	☐	☐	☐	☐	_____
Day 14	☐	☐	☐	☐	☐	☐	☐	☐	_____
Long term	☐	☐	☐	☐	☐	☐	☐	☐	_____

NOTE: Use of this monitoring format can help you keep informed of the results of treatment and permit early changes in treatment or timely referral. You must, however, determine the appropriate monitoring schedule for each individual patient.

POST-TEST — UNIT VIII

- *Answer each of the following questions.*
- *Check your answers with the correct answers beginning on page 277.*
- *If all questions are answered correctly, review Unit IX on page 280 to see how all of the checklists fit together to form a comprehensive system for managing oral and/or maxillofacial infections. Then, give yourself a* **gold star for persistence** *and take your spouse and/or your friend to dinner at a fine restaurant to celebrate your successful completion of this formidable text (unfortunately, Stoma Press is* **unable** *to pay the bill).*
- *If you are not able to answer all of the questions correctly, re-read and re-study the contents of this unit, re-do the post-test, then proceed as above.*

Questions:

1. *Assuming no critical conditions are present, the* **first step** *in planning the treatment of an oral and/or maxillofacial infection is to define a list of (a) _management_ objectives to identify the need for managing signs and symptoms associated with improving your (b) _patient's_ _health_, eliminating the (c) _problems (microbes)_(s) involved, and decreasing problems associated with the (d) _anatomical_ _cause_ _location_ of the problem. You can then select specific (e) _treatment_ _tx_ or determine the need for referral to a (f) _specialist_ or (g) _hospital_ if an appropriate treatment option requires skills, actions or facilities beyond your control. Once you have observed the results of initial treatment and have received additional data (e.g. micro lab reports), a (h) _definitive_ diagnosis can be made and (i) _definite_ treatment can be instituted. The progress of treatment should be closely (j) _monitored_ on a regular basis to assess the clinical progress of the infection and permit modification of treatment methods.*

2. *Which of the following signs and symptoms* **indicate** *the presence of a* **critical condition requiring immediate referral** *to a specialist and/or hospital?*

    a. *Patient complains of pain in the mandibular right posterior area, a stiffness in his neck, and has a temperature of 103°F.*

    b. *Patient developed a cellulitis involving the infraorbital and periorbital areas 4 days ago and now says he is tired, irritated by bright lights, and his eyes won't focus clearly.*

    c. *Patient complains of increased pain and swelling of the submandibular area 3 days after you surgically removed a partially erupted mandibular third molar. He also complains of difficulties in swallowing and a slight difficulty in breathing.*

    d. *Two days after you began endodontic treatment of a mandibular left canine, your patient's wife telephones your office stating her husband has developed fever, chills, and a rapid, thready pulse, and complains of pain in his lower left jaw.*

    e. *Six days after extraction of a maxillary right first molar, your patient's mother phones your office to cancel her son's appointment. You ask her about his condition and she says he has an intense headache and has been vomiting since yesterday.*

3. Given the following clinical situations, **choose the number** of the **appropriate** treatment option for **managing systemic medical problems** as shown in **bold** to the right:

a. _2_ Patient with diet-controlled diabetes has a palatal abscess secondary to a periapical abscess of a maxillary left lateral incisor.

b. _3_ A chronic alcoholic patient has an acute cellulitis involving the buccal space and infraorbital abscess of his maxillary right second premolar.

c. _2_ A patient with mild asthma requiring antihistamines has a fluctuant mentalis space abscess secondary to a chronic periapical abscess of his mandibular right central incisor.

1. **Will not influence your treatment of infection.**
2. **Proceed with treatment, but follow closely for complications.**
3. **Refer to specialist.**
4. **Refer to hospital.**

4. Given the following clinical situations, choose the **number of the appropriate** treatment option for **improving nutritional deficiencies** as shown in **bold** to the right.

a. _1_ Patient has been on a quick weight loss program and has a submandibular space abscess secondary to an abscessed mandibular left second molar.

b. _3_ 75-year-old patient with an acute cellulitis of the infraorbital area lives alone and eats one meal per day at the local mission.

c. _3_ 38-year-old female has been sick with a submandibular space infection for 3 days, during which time she has not been able to swallow food or water.

1. **Instruct patient to eat balanced meals totaling over 3,000 calories/day and drink 8-10 glasses of water per day.**
2. **Prescribe liquid diet with 8-10 glasses of water per day.**
3. **Patient needs hospitalization.**

5. For each of the following clinical situations, choose the **number** (or numbers) **of the appropriate** treatment option shown in **bold** to the right.

a. _1 2_ A 42-year-old male attorney is a
   _3 4_ heavy "social drinker" and requires both antibotics and a narcotic analgesic in the treatment of a moderately serious oral infection.

b. _3_ A 28-year-old male with current puncture wounds from a heroin habit says he needs a strong analgesic like Percodan® to control pain from a minor dental infection. He says he is on a methadone program, and codeine and/or aspirin is not effective.

c. _1 2_ A 36-year-old female who consumes one pint (375 ml) of vodka per day needs a moderate to strong analgesic to control pain from an acute infraorbital cellulitis.

1. **Advise patient to discontinue use of alcohol while taking their prescribed medications.**
2. **Patient should be referred and hospitalized during management of the infection.**
3. **Verify patient's story with his drug counselor.**
4. **Prescribe non-narcotic pain medication.**

6. Given the following data and assuming the need for antibiotic therapy, choose the appropriate antibiotic (you may use the reference charts on page 265).

a. _pen_ Patient has an acute (rapid onset) cellulitis of the infraorbital area. You have no lab data.

b. _pen_ Patient has a submental space infection which shows: 4+ Gram (+) cocci in clusters, 1+ Gram (−) rods.

c. _erythro_ Lab reports 4+ small Gram (−) cocci and 3+ Gram (+) rods on STAT Gram stain.

d. _clinda_ Penicillin, your initial antibiotic, has failed to improve an infection after 48 hours. Lab studies indicate probable **Bacteroides fragilis**, but they do not have sensitivity results yet.

7. For each of the following clinical situations, choose the **number** (or numbers) **of the appropriate** treatment option shown in **bold** to the right.

   a. _3_ A 25-year-old Down's syndrome patient requires an antibiotic for treatment of a submental cellulitis of dental origin. He is employed at a local hospital, lives alone and has no close friends or family nearby.

   b. _X_ A 62-year-old retired salesman requires an antibiotic for treatment of an acute pericoronitis. He has extreme anxiety over this problem and is afraid of taking drugs of any kind.

   c. _1_ A 26-year-old, low-income, graduate student who lives alone requires an antibiotic to control a staphylococcus infection of dental origin. You wish to prescribe oxacillin for seven days, but when informed of the cost by the pharmacist, the patient refused the prescription.

   1. **Discuss problem with patient and/or family.**
   2. **Refer patient for counseling.**
   3. **Obtain responsible care from friends, relatives, or public health nurse.**
   4. **Hospitalize patient.**

8. For each of the following clinical situations, choose the **number** (or numbers) **of the appropriate** treatment option shown in **bold** to the right.

   a. _1,2_ Patient has an acute infraorbital cellulitis. No pus was obtained by an endodontic route. You will prescribe penicillin as initial treatment.

   b. _X_ Patient had a submandibular space abscess which is draining intraorally by incision and drainage.

   c. _X_ Patient has a buccal space cellulitis which you plan to drain intraorally once it becomes fluctuant. Penicillin is to be prescribed.

   d. _4_ Patient has a fluctuant anterior sublingual space abscess which is not draining from the involved endodontically "opened" tooth.

   1. **Intraoral heat.**
   2. **Extraoral heat.**
   3. **Do not apply heat of any kind at this time.**
   4. **Refer to a specialist for management.**

9. For each of the following clinical situations, choose the **number** (or numbers) **of the appropriate** treatment option shown in **bold** to the right.

   a. _1,2_ Patient has mild pain from a low-grade, chronic pericoronal abscess.

   b. _1,2_ Patient has acute inflammation around a partially erupted mandibular third molar with trismus.

   c. _4_ Patient has a carious, unrestorable tooth and advanced periodontal disease. At this time she has a vestibular periodontal abscess (fluctuant) from this tooth.

   d. _4_ Patient has a fistula on the maxillary buccal alveolar ridge from a chronic abscess of his maxillary second premolar. Patient declines endodontic therapy.

   1. **Irrigate with water or saline.**
   2. **Local curettage.**
   3. **Endodontic treatment.**
   4. **Extract involved tooth at this time.**

10. Describe what can be done to **relieve trismus.** _I & D, antibiotics_

11. When might **space decompression** be necessary and what benefit can be derived? _parapharyngeal & neck involvement_

12. Describe the important factors to consider in each of the steps involved in performing an **intraoral** I&D procedure.

    a. Site selection _know anatomy of area._
    b. Pain control _Infiltrate, Topical_
    c. Surface decontamination _decontaminate w/ Betadine_
    d. Placing the incision _not on inflamed turn_
    e. Blunt dissection _w/ close hemostat work into & open_
    f. Drain placement _place w/ hemostat_
    g. Drain removal _once suppuration is about complete_

13. Describe the important factors to consider in each of the steps involved in performing an **extraoral** I&D procedure.
    a. Site selection _____ *know anatomy*
    b. Pain control _____ *infiltrate*
    c. Surface decontamination _____ *Betadine*
    d. Placing the incision _____
    e. Blunt dissection _____
    f. Drain placement _____
    g. Drain removal _____

14. For each of the following clinical situations, choose the **number** (or numbers) **of the appropriate** treatment option shown in **bold** to the right.
    a. __5__ Patient has a chronic (slowly growing) submandibular swelling. You performed an intraoral tissue biopsy in the mandibular posterior buccal sulcus which, with Gram stain, demonstrated presence of filamentous microorganisms.
    b. __4__ Patient has a fluctuant swelling in the maxillary buccal vestibule and infraorbital area.
    c. ____ Patient has an acute cellulitis involving the right lateral pharyngeal space secondary to an acute pericoronitis.
    d. __1__ Patient has a large fluctuant swelling of the left lateral palate secondary to a non-vital maxillary left lateral incisor.
    e. __4__ Patient has a fluctuant swelling in the left temporal region and submasseteric space (above the zygomatic arch) believed to be secondary to a chronic pericoronal abscess around the mandibular left third molar.

    1. **Intraoral I&D indicated.**
    2. **Extraoral I&D.**
    3. **No I&D indicated at this time.**
    4. **Refer to a specialist for I&D.**
    5. **Refer to a specialist for management.**

15. Describe the treatment for an infection resulting from the post-surgical entrapment of a non-vital piece of bone under your surgical flap. _____ *open & irrigate* _____

16. Describe the differences between initial and definitive management objectives and what additional data is needed to plan definitive treatment. *Initial: w/o lab data - immediate. Definitive - know what / found*

17. For each of the following clinical situations, choose the **number** (or numbers) **of the appropriate** treatment option shown in **bold** to the right.
    a. __2__ Patient requires antibiotic therapy for an acute cellulitis of the base of the upper lip. Endodontic treatment produced no drainage.
    b. __1__ Patient has an acute right lateral pharyngeal swelling, fever, is lethargic, and has trouble swallowing.
    c. ____ Patient has had an intraoral surgical drain placed in the mandibular buccal vestibule which is successfully draining a large buccal space abscess.
    d. ____ Patient was given penicillin for treatment of a post-surgical infection which resulted after an impacted mandibular third molar was removed. No lab data is available.

    1. **Continuous hospital monitoring.**
    2. **Daily office visits.**
    3. **2-3 day office visits.**
    4. **Weekly office visits.**

18. Why should you indicate the date of the initial appointment and the date of the next follow-up appointment on the checklist for diagnosing and managing oral infections? _____ *record progress* _____

19. Assuming that **you will treat** the following patient, **complete the treatment summary checklist** (on the next page) for **initial management objectives** and **outline** the **specific treatment methods** that should be used **at this time**, including planning of the **appropriate monitoring schedule.**

> **Case Description:** A 16-year-old male, who lives at home with his parents (mother not employed outside of the home), presents to your office in pain and with facial swelling involving the submandibular and buccal spaces which is secondary to a non-vital, cariously destroyed mandibular left first molar. The pain began in the area of this tooth two days ago, subsided a little, then the facial swelling began yesterday. Currently these spaces are mildly swollen, firm and indurated to palpation, red, warm, and non-fluctuant. A moderate amount of trismus is present, but the patient has only a minor problem with swallowing and no problems with breathing. The patient has had a loss of appetite since yesterday, consuming a small quantity of soft food and three glasses of fluid (diet beverage) in the last 24 hours. A **review of past medical history** is non-contributory for conditions which would compromise body defenses (except possibly the 250 mg of tetracycline he takes per day to control acne). Current **vital signs** are as follows: Temp. 102.4°F; Pulse 78; Resp. Rate 17; B.P. 120/75. A left submandibular lymph node was enlarged and tender. A **periapical radiograph** of the involved tooth showed extensive caries extending into the roots (such that the tooth cannot be restored) and 2x2 mm radiolucent lesions at the apices of both the mesial and distal roots. Due to the potential seriousness of this case, you attempted aspiration of the buccal space adjacent to the first molar. No aspirate was recovered, so you injected 0.5 ml of sterile saline and withdrew this in the syringe. The specimen was sealed in the syringe with tape and a sterile rubber stopper was used to plug the needle. A blood specimen was collected and both specimens were submitted to your clinical laboratory (lab does both hematology and microbiology studies). **STAT WBC** showed WBC = 12,000 with increase in polys and shift to left (stabs or immature neutrophils). **STAT Gram** stain showed presence of mixed infection (4 + Gram (+) cocci, 2+ Gram (−) rods, plus occasional other forms) and the lab reported it as "normal oral flora." You instruct the lab to do both anaerobic and aerobic mixed culture susceptibility and also begin definitive C&S studies.

Complete the checklist on page 277 based on this initial data and determine your **initial treatment.** Then proceed with the case data below.

> **The Next Day (24 hours later):** This patient appropriately returns to your office the next day. He is in less pain and is now taking fluids as prescribed. Food intake has improved. The buccal and submandibular space swellings are now fluctuant. **Vital signs** are: Temp 99.6°F; Pulse 64; B.P. 110/70; Resp. Rate 16. Micro lab reports positive aerobic and anaerobic mixed culture susceptibility to oxacillin, clindomycin, but not to penicillin.

Based upon the **first day** results, determine which treatment methods are now appropriate. Re-evaluate your initial treatment and add any **new treatment** to the checklist **using a different** colored marker.

> **The Second Day (48 hours later):** On the second day after beginning initial treatment, the area of swelling continues to decrease and the drains are removed 48 hours later. Temperature is 98.6°F; patient feels much better and has only mild discomfort in the drainage site.

Based upon the 48-hour results, complete the monitoring schedule on the checklist, assuming the infection continues to improve.

MANAGEMENT SUMMARY

MANAGEMENT OF CRITICAL CONDITIONS

Yes	No	Condition Present	Describe Condition	Refer	Hospitalize
☑	☐	Abnormally high fever	102.4 _____	☐	☐
☐	☑	Respiratory problems..................	_____	☐	☐
☐	☑	CNS involvement	_____	☐	☐
☐	☑	Systemic toxicity	_____	☐	☐
☐	☑	Dehydration (moderate to severe)	_____	☐	☐
☐	☑	Inadequate nutrition (moderate to severe) ..	_____	☐	☐
☑	☐	Spread to critical areas	_____	☐	☐
☐	☑	Medically compromised patient	_____	☐	☐
☐	☑	High potential for alcohol or drug withdrawal	_____	☐	☐

INITIAL TREATMENT (based on initial diagnosis)

Improving body resistance

Yes	No		Refer	Hospitalize
☐	☑	Manage systemic medical problems. How? _____	☐	☐
☐	☑	Manage possible drug interaction problems. How? _____	☐	☐
☑	☐	Obtain adequate rest .... ☑ Limit activities ☑ Home or bed rest _____	☐	☐
☑	☐	Improve nutritional deficiencies		
		☑ Improve caloric and protein intake. How? _____	☐	☐
		☑ Improve fluid intake. How? _____	☐	☐
		☐ Improve vitamin/mineral intake. How? _____	☐	☐
☐	☑	Control alcohol consumption How? _____	☐	☐
☐	☑	Manage drug addiction problem How? _____	☐	☐
☐	☑	Improve psychological factors How? _____	☐	☐
☐	☑	Improve family & social factors How? _____	☐	☐
☑	☐	Promote localization — Heat ☑ Intraoral ☐ Extraoral How _____	☐	☐
☑	☐	Control pain ☐ Analgesic _____ Dose _____ Route _____	☐	☐
		☐ Sedative dressing _____	☐	☐

Elimination of causative microorganisms

			Refer	Hospitalize
☐	☑	Drainage		
		☐ Irrigation with water or saline _____		
		☐ Curettage around the following teeth _____		
		☐ Endodontic treatment of the following teeth _____	☐	
		☐ Extraction of the following teeth _____	☐	☐
☐	☑	Incise and Drain ..... Location _____	☐	☐
		☑ Intraoral .... Where? _____	☐	☐
		☑ Extraoral .... Where? _____	☐	☐
☐	☑	Remove sequestrum... Where? _____	☐	☐
☑	☐	Antibiotic therapy _Pen_ _____ Dose _____ Duration _____	☐	☐

Improving Anatomical Factors

			Refer	Hospitalize
☐	☑	Relieve trismus ...... How? _____	☐	☐
☐	☑	Preserving airway .... How? _____	☐	☐
☐	☑	Space decompression How? _____	☐	☐

DEFINITIVE TREATMENT

☐ No change from initial therapy required
☑ Changes from initial therapy required (describe) _____

			Refer	Hospitalize
☐	☑	Manage critical systemic conditions _____	☐	☐
☑	☐	Improving body resistance _____	☐	☐
		☑ Change pain medication	☐	☐
		☐ Other	☐	☐
☑	☐	Elimination of microorganism(s) _____	☐	☐
		☐ Change antibiotic(s) to _oxacillin_ dose _____ duration _____	☐	☐
		_____ dose _____ duration _____	☐	☐
		☐ Other _____	☐	☐
☑	☐	Manage anatomical factors _____	☐	☐
		☑ Obtain additional drainage _____	☐	☐
		☐ Other _____	☐	☐

Comments _____

MONITORING TREATMENT RESULTS

	Patient Appt.	Seen	Clinical Course of Infection Worse	Same	Better	Resolved	Referred Specialist	Hospital	Comments
Day 0		☒	☐	☐		☐	☐	☐	_____
Day 1	☐	☐	☐	☐	☑	☐	☐	☐	_____
Day 2	☐	☐	☐	☐	☐	☐	☐	☐	_____
Day 3	☐	☐	☐	☐	☐	☐	☐	☐	_____
Day 4	☐	☐	☐	☐	☐	☐	☐	☐	_____
Day 5	☐	☐	☐	☐	☐	☐	☐	☐	_____
Day 6	☐	☐	☐	☐	☐	☐	☐	☐	_____
Day 7	☐	☐	☐	☐	☐	☐	☐	☐	_____
Day 10	☐	☐	☐	☐	☐	☐	☐	☐	_____
Day 14	☐	☐	☐	☐	☐	☐	☐	☐	_____
Long term	☐	☒	☐	☐	☐	☐	☐	☐	_____

POST-TEST ANSWERS

1. a. management; b. patient's health; c. microorganism(s); d. anatomical location; e. initial; f. specialist; g. hospital; h. definitive; i. definitive; j. monitored

2. All of these situations require immediate referral to a specialist and/or hospital.

3. a = 2; b = 3; c = 2

4. a = 1; b = 3; c = 3

5. a = 1 (or 2 if 1 is unsuccessful)
   b = 3, or 4, or 2
   c = 1 (or 2 if 1 is unsuccessful)

6. a = penicillin
   b = penicillin
   c = penicillin
   d = clindamycin

7. a = 3 (or 4)
   b = 1 (or 4 if 1 is unsuccessful)
   c = 1 (hopefully prescribe dicloxicillin if this is acceptable. If not, then 4)

8. a = 2 (4); b = 1 and/or 2; c = 1; d = 3

9. a = 1, 2 (4 is OK); b = 1, 2 (not 4); c = 4 (1); d = 4

10. see page 266

11. see page 267

12. see pages 257-258

13. see pages 258-260

14. a = 3, 5; b = 1 (5); c = 3, 5; d = 1; e = 2, 4 (5)

15. see page 261

16. see page 268

17. a = 2; b = 1; c = 3; d = 2

18. see page 271

19. **Discussion of Case:** *The complete initial management summary is given on the next page. The* **initial management** *(day 0) is* **shown in red**. *Treatment instituted the following day (day 1 results) is* **shown in blue**. *The results of* **subsequent follow-up** *are shown in black. The overall strategy for management includes:*

Initial Management Strategy (Day 0):
   1. Controlling the fascial space cellulitis.
   2. Discontinuing previous antibiotic (tetracycline)
   3. Instituting immediate antibiotics (penicillin V, 1.0 gm to build blood level, then 500 mg qid). Penicillin is the best choice for mixed infections when you have no specific data.
   4. Improving nutritional deficiencies.
   5. Promoting localization: saline holds (intraoral heat application) should be prescribed. Extraoral heat is generally not recommended until drainage is established.
   6. Establishing a potential path of drainage (endo). **Note: Surgical extraction would be unwise in the presence of fascial space cellulitis.**
   7. Pain control.

After 24-Hour Recall (Day 1 revision in treatment):
   1. Since cellulitis is now controlled (fluctuant abscesses present), **removal** of the cause (unrestorable tooth) **and drainage** of pus is essential. Endodontic drainage alone cannot guarantee effective drainage. Tooth extraction will definitely help, but intraoral I&D is the most effective treatment. Extraoral heat application at this time will help promote drainage.
   2. Even though the lab data indicated penicillin may not be effective, the infection has localized and no new antibiotic is indicated. Continue penicillin for the 7-day duration of the prescription.

After 48-Hour Recall (Day 2 plan strategy for follow-up):
   Monitor results and follow treatment closely the 3rd day. If the patient continues to improve, extend the re-call period to 2-3 day intervals and then longer until both the infection and surgical sites have resolved.

MANAGEMENT SUMMARY

MANAGEMENT OF CRITICAL CONDITIONS

Yes	No	Condition Present	Describe Condition	Refer	Hospitalize
☐	☐	Abnormally high fever	Day 0 - No critical conditions	☐	☐
☐	☐	Respiratory problems....................	Day 1 - No critical conditions	☐	☐
☐	☐	CNS involvement	Day 2 - No critical conditions	☐	☐
☐	☐	Systemic toxicity	Day 3 - No critical conditions	☐	☐
☐	☐	Dehydration (moderate to severe)	Day 5 - No critical conditions	☐	☐
☐	☐	Inadequate nutrition (moderate to severe) ..		☐	☐
☐	☐	Spread to critical areas		☐	☐
☐	☐	Medically compromised patient		☐	☐
☐	☐	High potential for alcohol or drug withdrawal		☐	☐

INITIAL TREATMENT (based on initial diagnosis)

Improving body resistance

Yes No

- ☐ ☑ Manage systemic medical problems. How? _____
- ✓ ☐ Manage possible drug interaction problems. How? _stop tetracycline_
- ✓ ☐ Obtain adequate rest .... ☐ Limit activities ✓☐ Home or bed rest _____
- ✓ ☐ Improve nutritional deficiencies
  - ✓☐ Improve caloric and protein intake. How? _____
  - ✓☐ Improve fluid intake. How? _____
  - ☐ Improve vitamin/mineral intake. How? _____
- ☐ ✓☐ Control alcohol consumption How? _____
- ☐ ✓☐ Manage drug addiction problem How? _____
- ☐ ✓☐ Improve psychological factors How? _____
- ☐ ✓☐ Improve family & social factors How? _____
- ✓ ☐ Promote localization — Heat ✓☐ Intraoral ✓☐ Extraoral How _Saline holds moist heat_
- ✓ ☐ Control pain ✓☐ Analgesic _Codeine + Aspirin_ Dose _30 mg/650 mg_ Route _oral_
  - ☐ Sedative dressing _____

Elimination of causative microorganisms

- ✓☐ ☐ Drainage
  - ☐ Irrigation with water or saline _____
  - ☐ Curettage around the following teeth _____
  - ✓☐ Endodontic treatment of the following teeth _open mand left first molar to drain_
  - ✓☐ Extraction of the following teeth _mandibular left first molar_
- ✓☐ ☐ Incise and Drain ..... Location
  - ✓☐ Intraoral .... Where? _left buccal space_
  - ✓☐ Extraoral .... Where? _____
- ☐ ☐ Remove sequestrum.. Where? _____
- ✓☐ ☐ Antibiotic therapy _Penicillin-V_ Dose _1.0 Gm stat 500 mg qid_ Duration _____

Improving Anatomical Factors

- ☐ ✓☐ Relieve trismus ...... How? _____
- ☐ ✓☐ Preserving airway .... How? _____
- ☐ ✓☐ Space decompression How? _____

DEFINITIVE TREATMENT

- ☑ No change from initial therapy required — _initial therapy is working_
- ☐ Changes from initial therapy required (describe) _____
  - ☐ ☐ Manage critical systemic conditions _____
  - ☐ ☐ Improving body resistance _____
    - ☐ Change pain medication _____
    - ☐ Other _____
  - ☐ ☐ Elimination of microorganism(s) _____
    - ☐ Change antibiotic(s) to _____ dose _____ duration _____
      - _____ dose _____ duration _____
    - ☐ Other _____
  - ☐ ☐ Manage anatomical factors _____
    - ☐ Obtain additional drainage _____
    - ☐ Other _____

Comments _infection is resolving with initial treatment_ _Infection resolving - stop lab analysis_

MONITORING TREATMENT RESULTS

	Patient Appt.	Patient Seen	Worse	Same	Better	Resolved	Referred Specialist	Hospital	Comments
Day 0	☐	☒	☐	☐	☐	☐	☐	☐	Control cellulitis
Day 1	☑	☑	☐	☐	☑	☐	☐	☐	localized: I+D, extraction
Day 2	☑	☑	☐	☐	☑	☐	☐	☐	swelling↓ patient improving
Day 3	☑	☑	☐	☐	☑	☐	☐	☐	remove drain temp. normal
Day 4	☐	☐	☐	☐	☐	☐	☐	☐	
Day 5	☑	☑	☐	☐	☑	☐	☐	☐	trismus↓, minimal swelling
Day 6	☐	☐	☐	☐	☐	☐	☐	☐	
Day 7	☐	☐	☐	☐	☐	☐	☐	☐	
Day 10	☐	☐	☐	☐	☐	☐	☐	☐	
Day 14	☑	☑	☐	☐	☐	☑	☐	☐	infection resolved, I+D closed,
Long term	☐	☐	☐	☐	☐	☐	☐	☐	extraction site healing normally

Unit IX
CHECKLIST FOR DIAGNOSING AND MANAGING
ORAL AND/OR MAXILLOFACIAL SWELLINGS

OVERVIEW AND OBJECTIVES

The purpose of this unit is to assemble all of the individual checklists presented in the data collection, diagnostic decisions, and management sections of this book into a clinical guide for diagnosing and managing oral and/or maxillofacial swellings. Ideally, we would have several complete cases for you to work through using this 4-page checklist; however, you've probably had enough practice using the components of this checklist and can integrate the components yourself if given the opportunity. Therefore, the objective for this unit is:

1. Given a patient presenting with an oral and/or maxillofacial swelling: collect all relevant data, develop an initial diagnosis, develop a definitive diagnosis if necessary, define your initial management objectives and the treatment methods necessary, determine the necessary monitoring schedule and evaluation of treatment progress and, finally, identify all areas of this procedure for which referral to a specialist or hospital are indicated.

Unit IX
CHECKLIST FOR DIAGNOSING AND MANAGING
ORAL AND/OR MAXILLOFACIAL SWELLINGS

The complete checklist is presented on pages 281-284. As you can see, this checklist stresses the **systematic collection of data** (historical, clinical, radiographic and laboratory data) as a basis for **diagnostic** and **management decisions.** We have **color coded** this checklist to signify the relative degree of seriousness for many categories of information to help you avoid the many potential pitfalls involved in the management of oral and/or maxillofacial infections. **You may find this checklist to be extremely helpful in your practice for planning management and documentation of moderate infections.**

ADDITIONAL COPIES OF THIS CHECKLIST
MAY BE OBTAINED FROM THE PUBLISHER.

We sincerely hope you have found this material helpful as a **beginning tool** in understanding the potential complexities involved in managing oral infections. We encourage your continued professional growth in this area through additional reading and continuing education courses. Proper management of oral swellings, be they of non-microbial or microbial origins, can be of the greatest importance to you and your patients. Always keep in mind that early referral to specialists and/or a hospital may avert acute emergencies and avoid the scenario described at the beginning of this book.

CHECKLIST FOR DIAGNOSING AND MANAGING ORAL AND/OR MAXILLOFACIAL SWELLINGS©

HISTORICAL DATA

Patient Name _____ (Ref. #_____) Date of Data Collection _____

CHIEF COMPLAINT (present problem)_____

HISTORY OF PRESENT PROBLEM

☐ Onset of Illness _____

☐ Duration of Illness_____

☐ Episodic Nature _____

☐ Patient Symptoms

   a) Pain _____

   b) Swelling _____

   c) Dysfunction_____

   d) Other _____

   _____

   _____

☐ Previous Treatment _____

   _____

☐ Factors Improving Condition_____

_____

☐ Factors Exacerbating Condition _____

_____

☐ Local Trauma

   a) Injury_____

   b) Post surgical _____

☐ Associated Oral Disease

   a) Caries _____

   b) Periodontal disease _____

   c) Nonvital teeth_____

   d) Other _____

PAST MEDICAL FACTORS THAT WOULD COMPROMISE HOST DEFENSES

Specific Medical Factors

Yes No

☐ ☐ Disease process(es) _____ Effect _____

☐ ☐ Medication(s) _____ Effect _____

☐ ☐ Allergies _____

☐ ☐ Recent antibiotic therapy. Drug _____ Dosage _____ How long ago _____

☐ ☐ Radiation therapy_____

General Factors Predisposing to Infections

☐ ☐ Age ____ years .... ☐ Age related factors present_____

☐ ☐ Nutritional status ... ☐ Adequate ☐ Inadequate: ☐ Protein & Caloric ☐ Fluids ☐ Vitamins & minerals

☐ ☐ Alcohol consumption ☐ Non-user ☐ Low withdrawal potential ☐ High withdrawal potential

☐ ☐ Drug abuse .... Drug(s) _____ Dosage _____ Duration _____ ☐ Low Risk ☐ High Risk

☐ ☐ Psychological status . ☐ Favorable· ☐ Unfavorable: Why? _____

☐ ☐ Family & social status ☐ Favorable ☐ Unfavorable: Why? _____

CLINICAL DATA

SERIOUS GENERAL SIGNS

Degree of Severity & Course of Action

Yes No

☐ ☐ **Toxic Appearance** ..... _____

☐ ☐ **Respiratory Difficulty** .. _____

☐ ☐ **CNS Changes** .... _____

☐ ☐ **Dehydration**.......... _____

☐ ☐ **Inadequate Diet** .... _____

VITAL SIGNS

Temp _____°F _____°C B.P. ___/___/___ mm Hg Describe Abnormality(ies)_____

Pulse Rate _____ beats/min Resp. Rate _____ cycles/min

_____

SIGNS OF INFLAMMATION

Yes No

☐ ☐ **Swelling** (see details in Anatomic Areas involved)   Additional characteristics

   ☐ Intraoral size _____ ☐ Generalized ☐ Non-fluctuant _____

   ☐ Extraoral size _____ ☐ Localized ☐ Fluctuant _____

☐ ☐ **Increased Temperature of Involved Area** _____

☐ ☐ **Pain & Tenderness** .... ☐ Generalized ☐ Localized Where?_____

☐ ☐ **Redness** .... ☐ Intraoral ☐ Extraoral

   ☐ Red ☐ Reddish purple ☐ Purple _____

☐ ☐ **Loss of Function**

   ☐ Trismus .... ☐ Slight ☐ Moderate ☐ Severe _____

   ☐ Dysphagia .... ☐ Slight ☐ Moderate ☐ Severe _____

   ☐ Respiratory Difficulty . ☐ Slight ☐ Moderate ☐ Severe _____

LOCAL PREDISPOSING SIGNS

☐ ☐ Recent Local Trauma .... ☐ Accidental injury ☐ Surgical trauma ☐ Other _____

☐ ☐ Associated Oral Diseases ☐ Caries ☐ Periodontal disease ☐ Non-vital teeth_____

☐ ☐ Altered vascularity .... ☐ Reduced vascularity ☐ Increased vascularity ☐ Radiation therapy

HEAD AND NECK EXAMINATION

General Comments _____

_____

LYMPH NODE INVOLVEMENT:

	R	L			R	L	
	☐	☐	1. Posterior auricular		☐	☐	7. Infraorbital
	☐	☐	2. Occipital		☐	☐	8. Buccal
	☐	☐	3. Superficial cervical		☐	☐	9. Mental
	☐	☐	4. Posterior cervical		☐	☐	10. Submental
	☐	☐	5. Inferior deep cervical		☐	☐	11. Submandibular
	☐	☐	6. Anterior auricular		☐	☐	12. Jugulo omo-hyoid

Yes No
☐   ☐   Abnormal node(s). Which group(s)? _____
☐   ☐   Tender node(s). Which group(s)?_____
☐   ☐   Enlarged node(s). Which group(s)?_____
☐   ☐   Indurated node(s). Which group(s)? _____

ANATOMICAL LOCATION OF SWELLING

RIGHT VIEW   **FRONT VIEW**   **LEFT VIEW**   **SAGITTAL**

FRONTAL   **CORONAL**   **FRONTAL**

MAXILLA, MANDIBLE, TEETH   **PRIMARY TEETH**   **INTRA-ORAL**

SUMMARY OF INVOLVED ANATOMICAL AREAS

Involves dento-alveolar ridges
☐ Maxillary ridge. Where? _____
☐ Mandibular ridge. Where? _____

Mandible & Below
☐ 1 Facial vestibule of mandible
☐ 2 Body of mandible
☐ 3 Mentalis space
☐ 4 Submental space
☐ 5 Sublingual space
☐ 6 Submandibular space

Cheek & Lateral Face
☐ 7 Buccal vestibule of maxilla
☐ 8 Buccal space
☐ 9 Submasseteric space
☐ 10 Deep Temporal space
☐ 10 Superficial Temporal
☐ 11 Infratemporal
☐ 12 Parotid space

Pharyngeal Spaces
☐ 13 Pterygomandibular
☐ 14 Parapharyngeal
    — Lateral pharyngeal
    — Retropharyngeal
☐ 15 Peritonsillar

☐ 16 Cervical Spaces

Mid-face Region
☐ 17 Palatal
☑ 18 Infraorbital
☐ 19 Periorbital
☑ 20 Base of upper lip
☐ 21 Maxillary sinus

RADIOGRAPHIC DATA

Views taken
- ☐ Panoramic
- ☐ Periapical
- ☐ Occlusal
- ☐ Other

Findings (record any abnormalities)
_____
_____
_____
_____

Additional Radiographic Views Needed
_____

Results _____
_____
_____

LABORATORY DATA

Yes No
- ☐ ☐ Culture material available at this time
- ☐ ☐ STAT Gram stain indicated
- ☐ ☐ Specimen collected for micro lab
- ☐ ☐ Specimen collected for histopathologic exam
- ☐ ☐ Hematology studies needed. Which? _____

STAT Gram Stain Results
- ☐ Single specie ☐ Mixed ☐ No microbes present
- ☐ Gram (+) cocci _____ ☐ Gram (−) cocci _____
- ☐ Gram (+) rods _____ ☐ Gram (−) rods _____
- ☐ Other _____

DIAGNOSTIC DECISIONS

SUMMARY OF PATIENT'S PROBLEMS

1. _____
2. _____
3. _____
4. _____
5. _____
6. _____
7. _____
8. _____
9. _____
10. _____
11. _____
12. _____
13. _____
14. _____
15. _____

PROCESS FOR INITIAL DIAGNOSIS

Problem is . . . . ☐ Microbial ☐ Non-Microbial ☐ Unknown_____

Source of Infection is . . ☐ Odontogenic ☐ Non-odontogenic ☐ From Dental Tx ☐ Unknown _____

Soft Tissue (dentally related)
- ☐ Periodontal Abscess
- ☐ Pericoronal Abscess
- ☐ Dento-Alveolar Abscess
- ☐ Post-surgical Infection
- ☐ Post-injection Infection
- ☐ Maxillary Sinusitis
- ☐ Other _____
  _____

Periosteum
- ☐ Subperiosteal abscess
- ☐ Post-Injection
- ☐ Periostitis

Hard Tissue
- ☐ Acute alveolar osteitis (dry socket)
- ☐ Osteitis
- ☐ Osteomyelitis
- ☐ Osteoradionecrosis

Special sigificance
- ☐ Acute cellulitis
- ☐ Ludwig's angina
- ☐ Osteo-radionecrosis
- ☐ Cavernous sinus thrombosis

Soft tissue (non-dental)
- ☐ Maxillary sinusitis
- ☐ Peritonsillar abscess
- ☐ Salivary gland infection
- ☐ Ear infection
- ☐ Superficial skin infection
- ☐ Superficial mucosal infection
- ☐ Other _____

Progress of Infection is . ☐ Chronic (slow) ☐ Acute (rapid) ☐ Dangerously Acute (fulminating) _____

EVALUATION OF MODIFYING FACTORS

Patient's Health
- ☐ Serious medical risk
- ☐ Moderate medical risk
- ☐ Low medical risk
- ☐ No medical risk
Why? _____
_____

Anatomical Factors
- ☐ High risk space(s)
- ☐ Multiple spaces (bi)
- ☐ Involves adjacent areas but controllable
- ☐ Confined to alveolar ridge
Where? _____
_____

Microbial Factors
- ☐ Acute cellulitis
- ☐ Systemic toxicity
- ☐ Extreme swelling
- ☑ Fever
- ☐ Chronic infection
- ☐ Recent antibiotic
- ☐ Poor O.H./perio disease

- ☐ Culture indicated but not taken
- ☐ No Gram stain
- ☐ Culture taken
- ☐ Gram stain obtained
- ☐ Culture not indicated
Other _____

INITIAL DIAGNOSIS
_____
_____
_____

INITIAL COURSE OF ACTION
- ☐ Treat in office ☐ Refer to a specialist ☐ Hospitalize. Who/Where? _____
- ☐ Need additional data. What data? _____

PROCESS FOR DEFINITIVE DIAGNOSIS

Summary of Laboratory Data

MICROBIOLOGY LAB
- ☐ Single species ☐ Mixed ☐ None
Predominant species: _____
_____
- ☐ Aerobic ☐ Anaerobic
Antibiotic Sensitivity:
  1st choice _____
  2nd choice _____
  3rd choice _____

HEMATOLOGY LAB
- ☐ WBC count _____
- ☐ WBC Differential:
  Polys _____% Eosinophils _____%
  Lymphocytes _____% Basophils _____%
  Monocytes _____% Immature? _____
  ESR _____mm/hr
  Blood Culture _____
  _____

HISTOPATHOLOGY LAB
Tissue specimen analysis _____
_____
_____
_____
_____
_____
_____

DEFINITIVE DIAGNOSIS
- ☐ Agrees/Consistent with initial diagnosis
- ☐ Differs from initial diagnosis _____
_____

DEFINITIVE COURSE OF ACTION
- ☐ Treat in office ☐ Refer to a specialist ☐ Hospitalize. Who/Where? _____
- ☐ Need additional data. What data? _____
_____

MANAGEMENT SUMMARY

MANAGEMENT OF CRITICAL CONDITIONS

Yes	No	Condition Present	Describe Condition	Refer	Hospitalize
☐	☐	Abnormally high fever	_____	☐	☐
☐	☐	Respiratory problems..................	_____	☐	☐
☐	☐	CNS involvement	_____	☐	☐
☐	☐	Systemic toxicity	_____	☐	☐
☐	☐	Dehydration (moderate to severe)	_____	☐	☐
☐	☐	Inadequate nutrition (moderate to severe) ..	_____	☐	☐
☐	☐	Spread to critical areas	_____	☐	☐
☐	☐	Medically compromised patient	_____	☐	☐
☐	☐	High potential for alcohol or drug withdrawal	_____	☐	☐

INITIAL TREATMENT (based on initial diagnosis)

Improving body resistance

Yes No

☐ ☐ Manage systemic medical problems. How? _____ ☐ ☐
☐ ☐ Manage possible drug interaction problems. How? _____ ☐ ☐
☐ ☐ Obtain adequate rest .... ☐ Limit activities ☐ Home or bed rest _____ ☐ ☐
☐ ☐ Improve nutritional deficiencies
    ☐ Improve caloric and protein intake. How? _____ ☐ ☐
    ☐ Improve fluid intake. How? _____
    ☐ Improve vitamin/mineral intake. How? _____
☐ ☐ Control alcohol consumption How? _____ ☐ ☐
☐ ☐ Manage drug addiction problem How? _____ ☐ ☐
☐ ☐ Improve psychological factors How? _____ ☐ ☐
☐ ☐ Improve family & social factors How? _____ ☐ ☐
☐ ☐ Promote localization — Heat ☐ Intraoral ☐ Extraoral How _____ ☐ ☐
☐ ☐ Control pain ☐ Analgesic_____ Dose_____ Route_____ ☐ ☐
    ☐ Sedative dressing _____ ☐ ☐

Elimination of causative microorganisms

☐ ☐ Drainage
    ☐ Irrigation with water or saline _____
    ☐ Curettage around the following teeth _____
    ☐ Endodontic treatment of the following teeth _____ ☐
    ☐ Extraction of the following teeth _____ ☐ ☐
☐ ☐ Incise and Drain ..... Location _____ ☐ ☐
    ☑ Intraoral .... Where? _____ ☐ ☐
    ☑ Extraoral .... Where? _____ ☐ ☐
☐ ☐ Remove sequestrum.. Where? _____ ☐ ☐
☐ ☐ Antibiotic therapy_____ Dose_____ Duration_____ ☐ ☐

Improving Anatomical Factors

☐ ☐ Relieve trismus ...... How? _____ ☐ ☐
☐ ☐ Preserving airway .... How? _____ ☐ ☐
☐ ☐ Space decompression How? _____ ☐ ☐

DEFINITIVE TREATMENT

☐ No change from initial therapy required
☐ Changes from initial therapy required (describe) _____ ☐ ☐
  ☐ ☐ Manage critical systemic conditions _____
  ☐ ☐ Improving body resistance _____ ☐ ☐
    ☐ Change pain medication_____ ☐ ☐
    ☐ Other _____
  ☐ ☐ Elimination of microorganism(s) _____ ☐ ☐
    ☐ Change antibiotic(s) to _____ dose _____ duration _____ ☐ ☐
    _____ dose _____ duration _____ ☐ ☐
    ☐ Other _____
  ☐ ☐ Manage anatomical factors _____ ☐ ☐
    ☐ Obtain additional drainage _____ ☐ ☐
    ☐ Other _____ ☐ ☐

Comments_____

MONITORING TREATMENT RESULTS

	Patient		Clinical Course of Infection				Referred		Comments
	Appt.	Seen	Worse	Same	Better	Resolved	Specialist	Hospital	
Day 0		☒					☐	☐	_____
Day 1	☐	☐	☐	☐	☐	☐	☐	☐	_____
Day 2 ..	☐	☐	☐	☐	☐	☐	☐	☐	_____
Day 3	☐	☐	☐	☐	☐	☐	☐	☐	_____
Day 4	☐	☐	☐	☐	☐	☐	☐	☐	_____
Day 5	☐	☐	☐	☐	☐	☐	☐	☐	_____
Day 6 ..	☐	☐	☐	☐	☐	☐	☐	☐	_____
Day 7	☐	☐	☐	☐	☐	☐	☐	☐	_____
Day 10 ..	☐	☐	☐	☐	☐	☐	☐	☐	_____
Day 14	☐	☐	☐	☐	☐	☐	☐	☐	_____
Long term ..	☐	☐	☐	☐	☐	☐	☐	☐	_____

REFERENCES
and
ADDITIONAL SOURCES OF INFORMATION

The following additional sources of information are provided for your benefit if you are interested in expanding your knowledge in the area of diagnosing and treating patients with oral and/or maxillofacial infections.

TEXTBOOKS

American Dental Association, Council on Dental Therapeutics. **Accepted Dental Therapeutics.** Chicago, Illinois (new edition published annually).

Archer, W.H. **Oral and Maxillofacial Surgery**, ed 5. Philadelphia, W.B. Saunders Co., 1975, pp. 513-514.

Eisenberg, M.S., Furukawa, C., Ray, C.G. **Manual of Antimicrobial Therapy and Infectious Diseases.** W.B. Saunders Company, 1980.

Goldberg, M.H.: **Infections of the Maxillofacial Regions** in Hayward, J.R.: **Oral Surgery.** Springfield, Illinois, Charles C Thomas, 1976.

Hollingshead, W.H. **Anatomy for Surgeons**, vol. 1. The head and neck, ed 2. New York, Hoeber-Harper, 1968.

Killey, H.C., Seward, G.R., Kay, L.W. **An Outline of Oral Surgery, Part I.** The maxillary sinus and its dental implications, H.C. Killey & L.W. Kay, John Wright & Sons, Ltd., Bristol, U.K., 1975.

Killey, H.C., Seward, G.R., Kay, L.W. **An Outline of Oral Surgery, Part II.** The maxillary sinus and its dental implications, H.C. Killey & L.W. Kay, John Wright & Sons, Ltd., Bristol, U.K., 1975.

Kruger, G.O., Ed. **Textbook of Oral and Maxillofacial Surgery**, Ed. 5, St. Louis, C.V. Mosby Co. 1979.

Thoma, K.H. **Oral Surgery**, 5th ed., vol. 11. St. Louis, C.V. Mosby Co., 1969.

Topazian, R.G. and Goldberg, M.H. **Management of Infections of the Oral and Maxillofacial Regions**, W.B. Saunders Company, 1981.
> As of our publication date, this text is the most complete summary of this topic in print and should become an essential component of a dental practitioner's library. This text amplifies on many of the areas which are beyond the scope of this book.

United States Pharmacopeial Convention, **United States Pharmacopeia Dispensing Information**, Rockville, Maryland, 1980 (revised annually).

Williams, P., and Warwick, R. **Gray's Anatomy**, ed. 36. Philadelphia, W.B. Saunders Co., 1980.

NEWSLETTER

Thomas J. Pallasch, Editor, **Dental Drug Service Newsletter**, P.O. Box 1912, Glendale, CA 91209. **Principles of Antibiotic Therapy** beginning Volume 2, No. 10 (Oct. 1981).
> This newsletter provides current information of extreme value, is well written, and summarizes a wide range of relevant topics.

JOURNAL ARTICLES

Beck, A.L.: **Deep neck infection.** Ann. Otol. 51:592, 1942.

Beck, A.L.: **The influence of the chemotherapeutic and antibiotic drugs on the incidence and course of deep neck infections.** Ann. Otol. Rhinol. Laryngol., 61:515, 1952.

Fielding, A.F., Cross, S., Matise, J.L., Mohnac, A.M. **Cavernous sinus thrombosis: report of case.** JADA Vol. 106, No. 3 (March) 1983, pp. 342-344.

Grodinsky, M., and Holyoke, E.A.: **Fasciae and fascial spaces of head, neck and adjacent regions.** Am. J. Anat., 63:367, 1938.

Haymaker, W. **Fatal infections of the central nervous system and meninges after tooth extraction, with an analysis of twenty-eight cases.** Am. J. Orthod. 31:117-188, 1945.

Laskin, D.M.: **Anatomic considerations in diagnosis and treatment of odontogenic infections.** JADA, 69:308, 1964.

Shapiro, H.H., Sleeper, E.L. and Guralnick, W.C.: **Spread of infection of dental origin — anatomical and surgical considerations.** Oral Surg., 3:1407, 1950.

Spilka, C.J.: **Pathways of dental infections.** J. Oral Surg., 24:111, 1966.

Williams, A.C., and Guralnick, W.C.: **The diagnosis and treatment of Ludwig's angina.** New Engl. J. Med., 228:443, 1943.

INDEX